DIET AND NUTRITION
SOURCEBOOK

SIXTH EDITION

Health Reference Series

DIET AND NUTRITION
SOURCEBOOK

SIXTH EDITION

Provides Basic Consumer Health Information about Federal Dietary Guidelines and Food Guidance System, Portion Sizes, Healthy Dietary Supplements, and Elements of Good Nutrition and Its Requirement through Lifespan, the Medical Concerns, and Healthy Food Choices

Along with the Importance of Nutrition in Weight Management, a Glossary of Related Terms, and a Directory of Nutrition Support Organizations and Programs

OMNIGRAPHICS

615 Griswold St., Ste. 520, Detroit, MI 48226

Bibliographic Note

Because this page cannot legibly accommodate all the copyright notices, the Bibliographic Note portion of the Preface constitutes an extension of the copyright notice.

* * *

OMNIGRAPHICS
Kevin Hayes, *Managing Editor*

* * *

ISBN 978-0-7808-1711-1
E-ISBN 978-0-7808-1712-8

Library of Congress Cataloging-in-Publication Data

Names: Hayes, Kevin (Editor of health information), editor. | Omnigraphics, Inc., issuing body.

Title: Diet and nutrition sourcebook / edited by Kevin Hayes.

Description: Sixth edition. | Detroit, MI : Omnigraphics, Inc., 2021. | Series: Health reference series | Includes index. | Summary: " Provides basic consumer health information about nutrition through the lifespan including facts about dietary guidelines and healthy eating, weight management, and other medical concerns. Includes index, glossary of related terms, and other resources"-- Provided by publisher.

Identifiers: LCCN 2019021352 (print) | LCCN 2019021861 (ebook) | ISBN 9780780817111 (library binding) | ISBN 9780780817128 (ebook)

Subjects: LCSH: Nutrition--Popular works. | Diet--Popular works. | Health--Popular works. | Consumer education.

Classification: RA784 .D534 2019 (print) | RA784 (ebook)

LC record available at https://lccn.loc.gov/2019021352
LC ebook record available at https://lccn.loc.gov/2019021861

Printed in the United States

Table of Contents

Part 2. The Elements of Good Nutrition

Part 3. Nutrition through the Life Span

Part 6. Importance of Nutrition in Weight Management

Part 7. The Role of Nutrition in People with Other Medical Concerns

Part 8. Additional Help and Information

Preface

ABOUT THIS BOOK

Nutrition and diet play a crucial role in maintaining health, well-being, quality of life, and longevity. Nutrition is not just important for the present generations but also helps in keeping future generations healthy across their lifespan. According to the *Dietary Guidelines for Americans 2020-2025*, Americans have fallen far short of meeting their diet recommendations and diet-related chronic disease is continuing to be the major public-health concern. The statistics provided by the Centers for Disease Control and Prevention (CDC) in 2015 states that only 12 percent and 9 percent of adults consumed the recommended fruits and vegetables, respectively. The consumption of fruits and vegetables can help prevent various chronic diseases that include diabetes, heart disease, cancer, and obesity.

Diet and Nutrition Sourcebook, Sixth Edition, provides information on nutrition and health, including information from the recently updated *Dietary Guidelines for Americans.* It details the importance of good nutrition and its major role in every part of life right from the toddler to older ages. This book also describes the importance of nutrition in weight management such as childhood obesity, healthy weight loss, diets and supplements, and the other medical concerns associated with it. The book concludes with a glossary of related terms and a directory of related nutrition programs and organizations.

HOW TO USE THIS BOOK

This book is divided into parts and chapters. Parts focus on broad areas of interest. Chapters are devoted to single topics within a part.

Part 1: Guidelines for Healthy Eating provides basic information about the *Dietary Guidelines* based on the *2020–2025 Dietary Guidelines for Americans.* The importance of portion sizes, Nutrition Facts label, and the safe and healthy use of dietary supplements are also explained.

Part 2: The Elements of Good Nutrition details down the structure of food and explains the nutritional values and good effects of different food on our body. The role of carbohydrates, proteins, vitamins, minerals, fats, along with the key takeaways from nutrition, are also discussed.

Part 3: Nutrition through the Life Span describes the nutrition levels that are required at different age groups of life. It covers age groups such as infants and toddlers, kids and children, teens and adolescents, women, adults, and older adults.

Part 4: Lifestyle and Nutrition gives tips on healthy shopping, vegetarian diet, healthy cooking, and food and alcohol consumption at home and outside. It helps people to understand the value of a healthy and necessary diet to maintain a balanced lifestyle.

Part 5: Nutrition-Related Health and Safety Concerns gives information about health and safety concerns relating to food and diet. It explains about natural sugars, artificial sugars, additives, food coloring, sodium, commercial beverages, and the health consequences of nutrition misinformation.

Part 6: Importance of Nutrition in Weight Management discusses the risks of overweight and obesity in adults and children. Tips for healthy weight loss, the pros and cons of dietary supplements for weight loss, and popular fad diets are explained.

Part 7: The Role of Nutrition in People with Other Medical Concerns explains the health conditions such as diabetes, cholesterol, food allergies, lactose intolerance, along with other diseases such as cancer and celiac disease.

Part 8: Additional Help and Information consists of a glossary of related terms and a directory of organizations that support nutritional programs.

BIBLIOGRAPHIC NOTE

This volume contains documents and excerpts from publications issued by the following U.S. government agencies: Centers for Disease Control and Prevention (CDC); *Dietary Guidelines for Americans* (DGA); Economic Research Service (ERS); *Eunice Kennedy Shriver* National Institute of Child Health and Human Development (NICHD); Federal Trade Commission (FTC); Food and Nutrition Service (FNS); National Cancer Institute (NCI); National Center for Complementary and Integrative Health (NCCIH); National Center on Birth Defects and Developmental Disabilities (NCBDDD); National Diabetes Information Clearinghouse (NDIC);

National Digestive Diseases Information Clearinghouse (NDDIC); National Heart, Lung, and Blood Institute (NHLBI); National Institute of Diabetes and Digestive and Kidney Diseases (NIDDK); National Institute on Aging (NIA); National Institutes of Health (NIH); *NIH News in Health*; Office of Dietary Supplements (ODS); Office of Disease Prevention and Health Promotion (ODPHP); Office on Women's Health (OWH); U.S. Department of Agriculture (USDA); U.S. Department of Health and Human Services (HHS); U.S. Department of Homeland Security (DHS); U.S. Department of Veterans Affairs (VA); and U.S. Food and Drug Administration (FDA).

It also contains original material produced by Omnigraphics and reviewed by medical consultants.

ABOUT THE *HEALTH REFERENCE SERIES*

The *Health Reference Series* is designed to provide basic medical information for patients, families, caregivers, and the general public. Each volume provides comprehensive coverage on a particular topic. This is especially important for people who may be dealing with a newly diagnosed disease or a chronic disorder in themselves or in a family member. People looking for preventive guidance, information about disease warning signs, medical statistics, and risk factors for health problems will also find answers to their questions in the *Health Reference Series*. The *Series*, however, is not intended to serve as a tool for diagnosing illness, in prescribing treatments, or as a substitute for the physician–patient relationship. All people concerned about medical symptoms or the possibility of disease are encouraged to seek professional care from an appropriate healthcare provider.

A NOTE ABOUT SPELLING AND STYLE

Health Reference Series editors use *Stedman's Medical Dictionary* as an authority for questions related to the spelling of medical terms and *The Chicago Manual of Style* for questions related to grammatical structures, punctuation, and other editorial concerns. Consistent adherence is not always possible, however, because the individual volumes within the *Series* include many documents from a wide variety of different producers, and the editor's primary goal is to present material from each source as accurately as is possible. This sometimes means that information in different chapters or sections may follow other guidelines and alternate spelling authorities. For example, occasionally a copyright holder may require that eponymous terms be shown in possessive forms (Crohn's disease vs. Crohn disease) or that British spelling norms be retained (leukaemia vs. leukemia).

MEDICAL REVIEW

Omnigraphics contracts with a team of qualified, senior medical professionals who serve as medical consultants for the *Health Reference Series*. As necessary, medical consultants review reprinted and originally written material for currency and accuracy. Citations including the phrase "Reviewed (month, year)" indicate material reviewed by this team. Medical consultation services are provided to the *Health Reference Series* editors by:

Dr. Vijayalakshmi, MBBS, DGO, MD
Dr. Senthil Selvan, MBBS, DCH, MD
Dr. K. Sivanandham, MBBS, DCH, MS (Research), PhD

HEALTH REFERENCE SERIES UPDATE POLICY

The inaugural book in the *Health Reference Series* was the first edition of *Cancer Sourcebook* published in 1989. Since then, the *Series* has been enthusiastically received by librarians and in the medical community. In order to maintain the standard of providing high-quality health information for the layperson the editorial staff at Omnigraphics felt it was necessary to implement a policy of updating volumes when warranted.

Medical researchers have been making tremendous strides, and it is the purpose of the *Health Reference Series* to stay current with the most recent advances. Each decision to update a volume is made on an individual basis. Some of the considerations include how much new information is available and the feedback we receive from people who use the books. If there is a topic you would like to see added to the update list, or an area of medical concern you feel has not been adequately addressed, please write to:

Managing Editor
Health Reference Series
Omnigraphics
615 Griswold St., Ste. 520
Detroit, MI 48226

Part 1 | **Guidelines for Healthy Eating**

Chapter 1 | **Federal Dietary Guidelines and Food Guidance System**

Chapter Contents

Section 1.1 | **Introduction to the Dietary Guidelines for Americans**

This section includes text excerpted from "*Dietary Guidelines for Americans, 2020-2025,*" *Dietary Guidelines for Americans* (DGA), U.S. Department of Agriculture (USDA), December 2020.

The foods and beverages that people consume have a profound impact on their health. The scientific connection between food and health has been well documented for many decades, with substantial and increasingly robust evidence showing that a healthy lifestyle – including following a healthy dietary pattern – can help people achieve and maintain good health and reduce the risk of chronic diseases throughout all stages of the lifespan: infancy and toddlerhood, childhood and adolescence, adulthood, pregnancy and lactation, and older adulthood. The core elements of a healthy dietary pattern are remarkably consistent across the lifespan and across health outcomes.

The federal *Dietary Guidelines* is designed for policymakers and nutrition and health professionals to help all individuals and their families consume a healthy, nutritionally adequate diet. The information in the *Dietary Guidelines* is used to develop, implement, and evaluate federal food, nutrition, and health policies and programs. It also is the basis for federal nutrition education materials designed for the public and for the nutrition education components of USDA and HHS nutrition programs. state and local governments, schools, the food industry, other businesses, community groups, and media also use *Dietary Guidelines* information to develop programs, policies, and communication for the general public.

The aim of the *Dietary Guidelines* is to promote health and prevent disease. Because of this public-health orientation, the *Dietary Guidelines* is not intended to contain clinical guidelines for treating chronic diseases. Chronic diseases result from a complex mix of genetic, biological, behavioral, socioeconomic, and environmental factors, and people with these conditions have unique healthcare requirements that require careful oversight by a health professional. The body of scientific evidence on diet and health reviewed to inform the *Dietary Guidelines* is representative of the United States population – it includes people who are healthy, people at risk for diet-related chronic conditions and diseases, such as cardiovascular disease, type 2 diabetes, and obesity, and some people who are living with one or more of these diet-related chronic illnesses. At the same time, it is essential that federal agencies, medical organizations, and health professionals adopt the *Dietary Guidelines* to meet the specific needs of their patients as part of an individual, multifaceted treatment plan for the specific chronic disease.

IMPORTANCE OF DIETARY GUIDELINES

The *Dietary Guidelines* translates the current science on diet and health into guidance to help people choose foods and beverages that comprise a healthy and enjoyable dietary pattern – the "what" and "how much" of foods and beverages to consume to achieve good health, reduce risk of diet-related chronic diseases, and meet nutrient needs. The *Dietary Guidelines* is just one piece of the nutrition guidance landscape, however. Other guidance is designed to address requirements for the specific nutrients contained in foods and beverages or to address treatments for individuals who have a chronic disease.

DIETARY GUIDELINES FOR AMERICANS: WHAT IT IS, WHAT IT IS NOT

Quantitative Guidance on Foods, Not Nutrient Requirements

Nutrient requirements are established and updated by the National Academies of Sciences, Engineering, and Medicine (NASEM). At the request of the United States and Canadian federal governments, the academies set the quantitative requirements or limits – known as "Dietary Reference Intakes" (DRI) – on nutrients, which include macronutrients (i.e., protein, carbohydrates, and fats), vitamins and minerals (e.g., vitamin C, iron, and sodium), and food components (e.g., dietary fiber). Because foods provide an array of nutrients and other components that have benefits for health, nutritional needs should be met primarily through foods. Thus, the *Dietary Guidelines* translates the academies' nutrient requirements into food and beverage recommendations. The *Dietary Guidelines* recognize, though, that in some cases, fortified foods and dietary supplements are useful when it is not possible otherwise to meet needs for one or more nutrients (e.g., during specific life stages such as pregnancy).

Health Promotion, Not Disease Treatment

At its core, the *Dietary Guidelines* have a public-health mission – that is, health promotion and disease prevention. Medical and nutrition professionals may use or adapt the *Dietary Guidelines* to encourage their patients or clients to follow a healthy dietary pattern.

Because of this public-health orientation, the *Dietary Guidelines* are not intended to be a clinical guideline for treating chronic diseases. However, the *Dietary Guidelines* often have served as a reference for federal, medical, voluntary, and patient care organizations as they develop clinical nutrition guidance tailored for people living with a specific medical condition.

IMPLEMENTING THE DIETARY GUIDELINES

The United States government uses the *Dietary Guidelines* as the basis of its food assistance and meal programs, nutrition education efforts, and decisions about national health objectives. For example, the National School Lunch Program (NSLP) and the Older Americans Act (OAA) Nutrition Program incorporate the *Dietary Guidelines* in menu planning; the Special Supplemental Nutrition Program for Women, Infants, and Children (WIC) applies the *Dietary Guidelines* in its program and educational materials; and the Healthy People objectives for the nation include objectives based on the *Dietary Guidelines.*

The *Dietary Guidelines* also provide a critical structure for state and local public-health promotion and disease prevention initiatives. In addition, it provides foundational, evidence-based nutrition guidance for use by individuals and those who serve them in public and private settings, including health professionals, public health and social service agencies, healthcare and educational institutions, researchers, agricultural producers, food and beverage manufacturers, and more.

Section 1.2 | **Major Food Groups and MyPlate Food Guidance System**

This section includes text excerpted from "*Dietary Guidelines for Americans, 2020-2025*," *Dietary Guidelines for Americans* (DGA), U.S. Department of Agriculture (USDA), December 2020.

Eating an appropriate mix of foods from the food groups and subgroups – within an appropriate calorie level – is important to promote health at each life stage. Each of the food groups and their subgroups provides an array of nutrients, and the amounts recommended reflect eating patterns that have been associated with positive health outcomes. Foods from all of the food groups should be eaten in nutrient-dense forms.

FOOD GROUP TYPES

Vegetables

Healthy dietary patterns include a variety of vegetables from all five vegetable subgroups – dark green; red and orange; beans, peas, and lentils; starchy; and others. These include all fresh, frozen, canned, and dried options in cooked or raw forms, including 100 percent vegetable juices. Vegetables in their nutrient-dense forms have limited additions such as salt, butter, or creamy sauces.

VEGETABLE SUBGROUPS

- **Dark green vegetables.** All fresh, frozen, and canned dark green leafy vegetables and broccoli, cooked or raw: for example, amaranth leaves, bok choy, broccoli, chamnamul, chard, collards, kale, mustard greens, poke greens, romaine lettuce, spinach, taro leaves, turnip greens, and watercress.
- **Red and orange vegetables.** All fresh, frozen, and canned red and orange vegetables or juice, cooked or raw: for example, calabaza, carrots, red or orange bell peppers, sweet potatoes, tomatoes, 100 percent tomato juice, and winter squash.

- **Beans, peas, lentils.** All cooked from dry or canned beans, peas, chickpeas, and lentils: for example, black beans, black-eyed peas, bayo beans, chickpeas (garbanzo beans), edamame, kidney beans, lentils, lima beans, mung beans, pigeon peas, pinto beans, and split peas. Does not include green beans or green peas.
- **Starchy vegetables.** All fresh, frozen, and canned starchy vegetables: for example, breadfruit, burdock root, cassava, corn, jicama, lotus root, lima beans, plantains, white potatoes, salsify, taro root (dasheen or yautia), water chestnuts, yam, and yucca.
- **Other vegetables.** All other fresh, frozen, and canned vegetables, cooked or raw: for example, asparagus, avocado, bamboo shoots, beets, bitter melon, Brussels sprouts, cabbage (green, red, napa, savoy), cactus pads (nopales), cauliflower, celery, chayote (mirliton), cucumber, eggplant, green beans, kohlrabi, luffa, mushrooms, okra, onions, radish, rutabaga, seaweed, snow peas, summer squash, tomatillos, and turnips.

HEALTH BENEFITS OF VEGETABLES*

- As part of an overall healthy diet, eating foods such as vegetables that are lower in calories per cup instead of some other higher-calorie food may be useful in helping to lower calorie intake.
- Eating a diet rich in vegetables as part of an overall healthy diet may reduce the risk for heart disease, including heart attack and stroke.
- Eating a diet rich in some vegetables as part of an overall healthy diet may protect against certain types of cancers.
- Adding vegetables can help increase the intake of fiber and potassium, which are important nutrients that many Americans do not get enough of in their diet.

**Text excerpted from "Vegetables," MyPlate, U.S. Department of Agriculture (USDA), December 30, 2020.*

Fruits

All fresh, frozen, canned, and dried fruits and 100 percent fruit juices: for example, apples, Asian pears, bananas, berries (e.g., blackberries, blueberries, currants, huckleberries, kiwifruit, mulberries, raspberries, and strawberries); citrus fruit (e.g., calamondin, grapefruit, lemons, limes, oranges, and pomelos); cherries, dates, figs, grapes, guava, jackfruit, lychee, mangoes, melons (e.g., cantaloupe, casaba, honeydew, and watermelon); nectarines, papaya, peaches, pears, persimmons, pineapple, plums, pomegranates, raisins, rhubarb, sapote, and soursop.

HEALTH BENEFITS OF FRUITS†

- As part of an overall healthy diet, eating foods such as fruits that are lower in calories per cup instead of some other higher-calorie food may be useful in helping to lower calorie intake.
- Eating a diet rich in fruits as part of an overall healthy diet may reduce the risk for heart disease, including heart attack and stroke.
- Eating a diet rich in some fruits as part of an overall healthy diet may protect against certain types of cancers.
- Adding fruit can help increase the intake of fiber and potassium which are important nutrients that many Americans do not get enough of in their diet.

†*Text excerpted from "Fruits," MyPlate, U.S. Department of Agriculture (USDA), December 30, 2020.*

Grains

- **Whole grains.** All whole-grain products and whole grains used as ingredients: for example, amaranth, barley (not pearled), brown rice, buckwheat, bulgur, millet, oats, popcorn, quinoa, dark rye, whole-grain cornmeal, whole-wheat bread, whole-wheat chapati, whole-grain cereals and crackers, and wild rice.
- **Refined grains.** All refined-grain products and refined grains used as ingredients: for example, white breads,

refined-grain cereals and crackers, corn grits, cream of rice, cream of wheat, barley (pearled), masa, pasta, and white rice. Refined grain choices should be enriched.

HEALTH BENEFITS OF GRAINS‡

- Consuming whole grains as part of a healthy diet may reduce the risk of heart disease.
- Consuming whole-grain foods that contain fiber, as part of an overall healthy diet, can support healthy digestion.
- Eating whole grains, as part of an overall healthy diet, may help with weight management.
- Eating grain products fortified with folate helps prevent neural tube defects (NTDs) when consumed as part of an overall healthy diet before and during pregnancy.

‡*Text excerpted from "Grains," MyPlate, U.S. Department of Agriculture (USDA), December 29, 2020.*

Dairy and Fortified Soy Alternatives

All fluid, dry, or evaporated milk, including lactose-free and lactose-reduced products and fortified soy beverages (soy milk), buttermilk, yogurt, kefir, frozen yogurt, dairy desserts, and cheeses. Most choices should be fat-free or low fat. Cream, sour cream, and cream cheese are not included due to their low-calcium content.

HEALTH BENEFITS OF DAIRY AND FORTIFIED SOY ALTERNATIVES§

Calcium and vitamin D are important nutrients at any age. Intake of dairy products that contain these nutrients help to:

- Improve bone health especially in children and adolescents, when bone mass is being built.
- Promote bone health and prevent the onset of osteoporosis in adults, most of whom do not get enough of these nutrients.

§*Text excerpted from "Dairy," MyPlate, U.S. Department of Agriculture (USDA), December 29, 2020.*

Protein Foods

- **Meats, poultry, eggs.** Meats include beef, goat, lamb, pork, and game meat (e.g., bison, moose, elk, deer). Poultry includes chicken, Cornish hens, duck, game birds (e.g., ostrich, pheasant, and quail), goose, and turkey. Organ meats include chitterlings, giblets, gizzard, liver, sweet breads, tongue, and tripe. Eggs include chicken eggs and other birds' eggs. Meats and poultry should be lean or low fat.
- **Seafood.** Examples of seafood that are lower in methylmercury include anchovy, black sea bass, catfish, clams, cod, crab, crawfish, flounder, haddock, hake, herring, lobster, mullet, oyster, perch, pollock, salmon, sardine, scallop, shrimp, sole, squid, tilapia, freshwater trout, light tuna, and whiting.
- **Nuts, seeds, soy products.** Nuts and seeds include all nuts (tree nuts and peanuts), nut butter, seeds (e.g., chia, flax, pumpkin, sesame, and sunflower), and seed butter (e.g., sesame or tahini and sunflower). Soy includes tofu, tempeh, and products made from soy flour, soy protein isolate, and soy concentrate. Nuts should be unsalted.

HEALTH BENEFITS OF PROTEIN FOODS[#]

- Proteins function as building blocks for bones, muscles, cartilage, skin, and blood. They are also building blocks for enzymes, hormones, and vitamins. Proteins are one of three nutrients that provide calories (the others are fat and carbohydrates).
- Nutrients provided by various protein foods can differ. Varying your protein food choices can provide your body with a range of nutrients designed to keep your body functioning well. Vitamin B help build tissue and aid in forming red blood cells. Iron can prevent anemia. Magnesium helps build bones and supports muscle function. Zinc can support your immune systems.

- EPA and DHA are omega-3 fatty acids found in varying amounts in seafood. Eating 8 ounces per week of seafood may help reduce the risk for heart disease.

#Text excerpted from "Protein Foods," MyPlate, U.S. Department of Agriculture (USDA), December 30, 2020.)

OTHER DIETARY COMPONENTS

Oils

Oils are important to consider as part of a healthy dietary pattern as they provide essential fatty acids. Commonly consumed oils include canola, corn, olive, peanut, safflower, soybean, and sunflower oils. Oils also are naturally present in nuts, seeds, seafood, olives, and avocados. The fat in some tropical plants, such as coconut oil, palm kernel oil, and palm oil, are not included in the oils category because they contain a higher percentage of saturated fat than do other oils.

Beverages

When choosing beverages in a healthy dietary pattern, both the calories and nutrients that they provide are important considerations. Beverages that are calorie-free – especially water – or that contribute beneficial nutrients, such as fat-free and low-fat milk and 100 percent juice, should be the primary beverages consumed. Coffee, tea, and flavored waters also are options, but the most nutrient-dense options for these beverages include little if any, sweeteners or cream.

Caffeine

Caffeine is a dietary component that functions in the body as a stimulant. Most intake of caffeine in the United States comes from coffee, tea, and soda. Caffeine is a substance that is generally recognized as safe (GRAS) in cola-type beverages by the U.S. Food and Drug Administration (FDA). For healthy adults, the FDA has cited 400 milligrams per day of caffeine as an amount not generally associated with dangerous, negative effects.

Section 1.3 | The Science behind Healthy Eating Patterns

This section includes text excerpted from documents published by two public domain sources. Text under the headings marked 1 are excerpted from "*Dietary Guidelines for Americans, 2020-2025*," *Dietary Guidelines for Americans (DGA)*, U.S. Department of Agriculture (USDA), December 2020; Text under the heading marked 2 is excerpted from "USDA Food Patterns," National Institute on Aging (NIA), National Institutes of Health (NIH), April 29, 2019.

THE FUNDAMENTALS OF HEALTHY DIETARY PATTERN[1]

A fundamental premise of the *Dietary Guidelines* is that almost everyone, no matter an individual's age, race, or ethnicity, or health status, can benefit from shifting food and beverage choices to better support healthy dietary patterns.

FOLLOWING A HEALTHY DIETARY PATTERN AT EVERY LIFE STAGE[1]

Healthy eating starts at birth with the exclusive consumption of human milk, if possible, for about the first 6 months. If human milk is unavailable, infants should be fed an iron-fortified commercial infant formula (i.e., labeled "with iron") regulated by the U.S. Food and Drug Administration (FDA), which are based on standards that ensure nutrient content and safety. Healthy eating continues with the introduction of complementary foods and beverages at about 6 months of age. By 12 months, infants should maintain their healthy eating as they transition to developmentally appropriate foods and beverages. Healthy eating continues in each life stage thereafter. Even though nutrient needs vary across life stages, the foods and beverages that individuals should eat over the lifespan are remarkably consistent.

WHAT IS A DIETARY PATTERN?[1]

Over the course of any given day, week, or year, individuals consume foods and beverages in combination – a dietary pattern. A dietary pattern represents the totality of what individuals habitually eat and drink, and the parts of the pattern act synergistically to affect health. As a result, the dietary pattern may better predict overall health status and disease risk than individual foods or nutrients.

A healthy dietary pattern consists of nutrient-dense forms of foods and beverages across all food groups, in recommended amounts, and within calorie limits. Achieving a healthy dietary pattern at each life stage not only supports health at that point in time, but also supports health in the next life stage and possibly for future generations. If healthy dietary patterns can be established early in life and sustained thereafter, the impact on health could be significant. Establishing and maintaining a healthy dietary pattern can help minimize diet-related chronic disease risk. Conversely, consuming foods and beverages that are not nutrient-dense may lead to disease expression in later years. High intakes of such foods (i.e., an unhealthy dietary pattern) throughout the lifespan can increase the risk of developing chronic diseases.

The good news is that at any stage of life, individuals can make efforts to adopt a healthy dietary pattern and improve their health. The Healthy U.S.-Style Dietary Pattern, the USDA's primary Dietary Pattern, provides a framework for healthy eating that all Americans can follow. It is based on the types and proportions of foods Americans of all ages, genders, races, and ethnicities typically consume, but in nutrient-dense forms and appropriate amounts.

The healthy Mediterranean-Style Dietary Pattern and the healthy vegetarian dietary pattern are variations of the Healthy U.S.-Style Dietary Pattern that have the same core elements. The USDA Dietary Patterns are meant to be tailored to meet cultural and personal preferences and used as guides to plan and serve meals for individuals, households, and in a variety of institutions and other settings. The dietary approaches to stop hypertension (DASH) dietary pattern is an example of a healthy dietary pattern and has many of the same characteristics as the Healthy U.S.-Style Dietary Pattern.

For most individuals, no matter their age or health status, achieving a healthy dietary pattern will require changes in food and beverage choices. Some of these changes can be accomplished by making simple substitutions, while others will require greater effort to accomplish. Although individuals ultimately decide what and how much to consume, their personal relationships; the settings in which they live, learn, work, play, and gather; and other contextual factors – including their ability to consistently access healthy and affordable food – strongly influence their choices. Health professionals, communities, businesses and industries, organizations, government, and other segments of society all have a role to play in supporting individuals and families in making choices that align with the *Dietary Guidelines* and ensuring that all people have access to a healthy and affordable food supply. Resources, including federal programs that support households, regardless of size and make-up, in choosing a healthy diet and improving access to healthy food, are highlighted throughout this edition of the *Dietary Guidelines for Americans.*

HEALTHY UNITED STATES-STYLE DIETARY PATTERN[1]

Table 1.1. Healthy U.S.-Style Dietary Pattern at the 2,000-Calorie Level, with Daily or Weekly Amounts from Food Groups, Subgroups, and Components

Food Group or Subgroup	Daily Amount[a] of Food From Each Group (Vegetable and protein foods subgroup amounts are per week.)
Vegetables (cup eq/day)	**2 ½**
	Vegetable Subgroups in Weekly Amounts
Dark Green Vegetables (cup eq/wk)	1 ½
Red and Orange Vegetables (cup eq/wk)	5 ½
Beans, Peas, Lentils (cup eq/wk)	1 ½
Starchy Vegetables (cup eq/wk)	5
Other Vegetables (cup eq/wk)	4
Fruits (cup eq/day)	**2**
Grains (ounce eq/day)	**6**
Whole Grains (ounce eq/day)	≥ 3
Refined Grains (ounce eq/day)	< 3
Dairy (cup eq/day)	**3**
Protein Foods (ounce eq/day)	**5 ½**

Table 1.1. Continued

Food Group or Subgroup	**Daily Amount[a] of Food From Each Group (Vegetable and protein foods subgroup amounts are per week.)**
	Protein Foods Subgroups in Weekly Amounts
Meats, Poultry, Eggs (ounce eq/wk)	26
Seafood (ounce eq/wk)	8
Nuts, Seeds, Soy Products (ounce eq/wk)	5
Oils (grams/day)	**27**
Limit on Calories for Other Uses (kcal/day)[b]	**240**
Limit on Calories for Other Uses (%/day)	12%

[a]Food group amounts shown in cup or ounce equivalents (eq). Oils are shown in grams. Amounts will vary for those who need <2,000 or >2,000 calories per day.

[b]Foods are assumed to be in nutrient-dense forms, lean or low fat, and prepared with minimal added sugars, refined starches, saturated fat, or sodium. If all food choices to meet food group recommendations are in nutrient-dense forms, a small number of calories remain within the overall limit of the pattern (i.e., a limit on calories for other uses). The amount of calories depends on the total calorie level of the pattern and the amounts of food from each food group required to meet nutritional goals. Calories up to the specified limit can be used for added sugars, saturated fat, and/or alcohol, or to eat more than the recommended amount of food in a food group.

OTHER HEALTHY DIET PATTERNS[2]

Healthy Mediterranean-Style eating pattern. This eating pattern contains more fruits and seafood and less dairy than the Healthy U.S.-Style Eating Pattern. There is also less calcium and vitamin D because it includes fewer dairy foods.

Healthy Vegetarian eating Pattern. This eating pattern contains no meat, poultry, or seafood. Compared with the Healthy U.S.-Style Eating Pattern, it contains more soy products, eggs, beans and peas, nuts and seeds, and whole grains.

THE HEALTH BENEFITS OF A HEALTHY DIETARY PATTERN[1]

Science is the foundation of the *Dietary Guidelines* recommendations on what Americans should eat and drink to promote health, reduce risk of chronic disease, and meet nutrient needs. The science shows that following a healthy dietary pattern, meeting food group and nutrient needs with nutrient-dense foods and beverages, and limiting the intake of foods and beverages that are not nutrient dense are related to many health benefits. Science also supports the idea that every life stage provides an opportunity to make food choices that promote health and well-being, achieve and maintain appropriate weight status, and reduce the risk of diet-related chronic disease.

Evidence on the association between dietary patterns and reduced risk of diet-related chronic diseases has expanded in recent years and supports the use of dietary patterns as a foundation for the recommendations in the *Dietary Guidelines for Americans, 2020-2025*. Consistent evidence demonstrates that a healthy dietary pattern is associated with beneficial outcomes for all-cause mortality, cardiovascular disease, overweight and obesity, type 2 diabetes, bone health, and certain types of cancer (breast and colorectal).

Common characteristics of dietary patterns associated with positive health outcomes include a relatively higher intake of vegetables, fruits, legumes, whole grains, low- or nonfat dairy, lean meats and poultry, seafood, nuts, and unsaturated vegetable oils, and relatively lower consumption of red and processed meats, sugar-sweetened foods and beverages, and refined grains. The evidence examined showed broad representation across a number of populations and demographic groups. This suggests a consistent association no matter the region or cultural context in which a healthy dietary pattern is consumed. In addition, dietary patterns characterized by higher intake of red and processed meats, sugar-sweetened foods and beverages, and refined grains are, in and of themselves, associated with detrimental health outcomes.

A HEALTHY DIETARY PATTERN SUPPORTS APPROPRIATE CALORIE LEVELS[1]

The total number of calories a person needs each day varies depending on a number of factors, namely the person's age, sex, height, weight, level of physical activity, and pregnancy or lactation status.

Due to reductions in basal metabolic rate that occur with aging, calorie needs generally decrease for adults as they age. In addition, a need to lose, maintain, or gain weight affects how many calories should be consumed. Estimated amounts of calories needed are based on age, sex, and level of physical activity. These estimates are based on the Estimated Energy Requirement (EER) equations established by the National Academies of Sciences, Engineering, and Medicine (NASEM) or National Academies using reference heights (average) and reference weights (healthy) for each age-sex group. These amounts are estimates. The best way to evaluate calorie intake, in comparison to calorie needs, is by measuring body weight status.

CUSTOMIZE AND ENJOY FOOD AND BEVERAGE CHOICES TO REFLECT PERSONAL PREFERENCES, CULTURAL TRADITIONS, AND BUDGETARY CONSIDERATIONS[1]

Eating should be enjoyed, and a healthy dietary pattern can be enjoyable, from early life to older adulthood. The science reviewed to inform the *Dietary Guidelines* represents the diversity of Americans, including all ages and life stages, different racial and ethnic backgrounds, and a range of socioeconomic statuses. A healthy dietary pattern can benefit all individuals regardless of age, race or ethnicity, or current health status.

The *Dietary Guidelines* provide a framework intended to be customized to fit individual, household, and federal program participants' preferences, as well as the foodways of the diverse cultures in the United States. The United States population is diverse in myriad ways. The *Dietary Guidelines* framework purposely provides recommendations by food groups and subgroups – not specific foods and beverages – to avoid being prescriptive. This framework approach ensures that people can "make it their own" by selecting healthy foods, beverages, meals, and snacks specific to their needs and preferences. The food groups include a broad variety of nutrient-dense food and beverage choices. In every setting, across all cultures, and at any age or budget, there are foods and beverages that can fit within the *Dietary Guidelines* framework.

Start with Personal Preferences

Exposure to different types of food is important early in life to better develop a child's interest and willingness to eat and enjoy a variety of foods. Through each life stage that follows, a key starting point for establishing and maintaining a healthy dietary pattern is to ensure that individual and/or family preferences – in nutrient-dense forms – are built into day-to-day choices.

Incorporate Cultural Traditions

Cultural background can have a significant influence on food and beverage choices. Customizing the *Dietary Guidelines* framework to reflect specific cultures and traditions is an important strategy to help communities across the country eat and enjoy a healthy dietary pattern. Nutrient dense culturally relevant foods and beverages are part of all of the food groups. Spices and herbs can help flavor foods when reducing added sugars, saturated fat, and sodium, and they also can add to the enjoyment of nutrient-dense foods, dishes, and meals that reflect specific cultures. Relying on the expertise of professionals in nutrition and in specific cultural foodways can help people prepare foods healthfully while retaining heritage.

Consider Budget

Despite a common perception that eating healthfully is expensive, a healthy dietary pattern can be affordable and fit within budgetary constraints. There are a range of strategies that can be used to help individuals and families follow a healthy dietary pattern including advanced planning; considering regional and seasonal food availability; and incorporating a variety of fresh, frozen, dried, and canned options. The USDA food plans – thrifty, low-cost, moderate-cost, and liberal-cost food plans – each represent a nutritious diet at a different cost level. These plans are scheduled to be revised, with an updated Thrifty Food Plan (TFP) published by the end of 2022 to reflect updated food availability and food cost data.

Chapter 2 | **Portion Sizes and Servings**

Chapter Contents

Section 2.1 | Just Enough for You: About Food Portions

This section includes text excerpted from "Just Enough for You: About Food Portions," National Institute of Diabetes and Digestive and Kidney Diseases (NIDDK), December 2016. Reviewed May 2021.

To reach or stay at a healthy weight, how much you eat is just as important as what you eat. Do you know how much food is enough for you? Do you understand the difference between a portion and a serving? The information below explains portions and servings and provides tips to help you eat just enough for you.

WHAT IS THE DIFFERENCE BETWEEN A PORTION AND A SERVING?

A portion is how much food you choose to eat at one time, whether in a restaurant, from a package, or at home. A serving, or serving size, is the amount of food listed on a product's Nutrition Facts, or food label (see Figure 2.1).

Different products have different serving sizes, which could be measured in cups, ounces, grams, pieces, slices, or numbers - such as three crackers. A serving size on a food label may be more or less than the amount you should eat, depending on your age, weight, whether you are male or female, and how active you are. Depending on how much you choose to eat, your portion size may or may not match the serving size.

As a result of updates to the Nutrition Facts label in May 2016, some serving sizes on food labels may be larger or smaller than they had been before. For instance, a serving size of ice cream is now 2/3 cup, instead of 1/2 cup. The serving size of yogurt is six ounces rather than eight ounces. The U.S. Food and Drug Administration (FDA) changed some food and beverage serving sizes so that labels more closely match how much people actually eat and drink.

Serving Size and Servings per Container

Go back to the updated food label in Figure 2.1. To see how many servings a container has, you would check "servings per container" listed at the top of the label above "Serving size." The serving size is 2/3 cup, but the container has eight servings. If you eat two

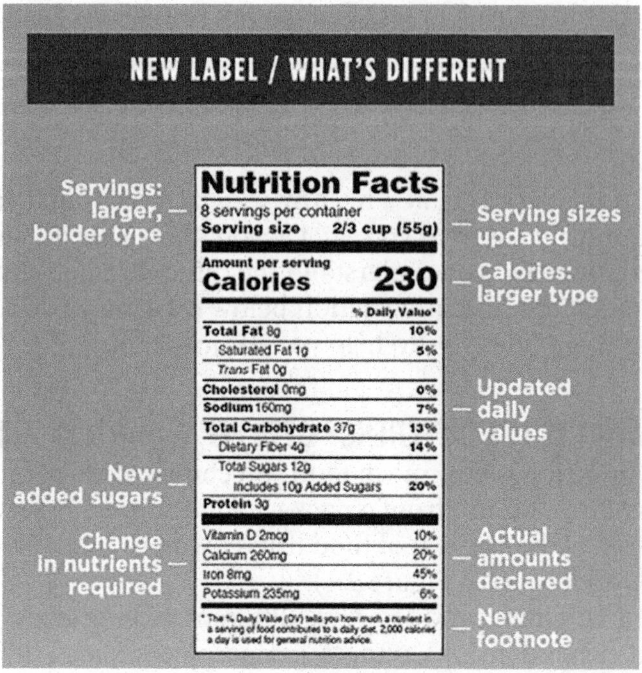
NEW LABEL / WHAT'S DIFFERENT
Servings: larger, bolder type
New: added sugars
Change in nutrients required
Nutrition Facts
8 servings per container
Serving size 2/3 cup (55g)
Amount per serving
Calories 230
% Daily Value*
Total Fat 8g 10%
Saturated Fat 1g 5%
Trans Fat 0g
Cholesterol 0mg 0%
Sodium 160mg 7%
Total Carbohydrate 37g 13%
Dietary Fiber 4g 14%
Total Sugars 12g
Includes 10g Added Sugars 20%
Protein 3g
Vitamin D 2mcg 10%
Calcium 260mg 20%
Iron 8mg 45%
Potassium 235mg 6%
Serving sizes updated
Calories: larger type
Updated daily values
Actual amounts declared
New footnote

Figure 2.1. Updated Nutrition Facts Label
(Source: U.S. Food and Drug Administration (FDA).)

servings or 1 1/3 cups, you need to double the number of calories and nutrients listed on the food label to know how much you are really getting. For example, if you eat two servings of this product, you are taking in 460 calories:

230 calories per serving x two servings eaten = 460 calories

HOW MUCH SHOULD YOU EAT?

How many calories you need each day to lose weight or maintain your weight depends on your age, weight, metabolism, whether you are male or female, how active you are, and other factors. For example, a 150-pound woman who burns a lot of calories through intense physical activity, such as fast running, several times a week will need more calories than a woman about the same size who only goes for a short walk once a week.

Portion Sizes and Servings

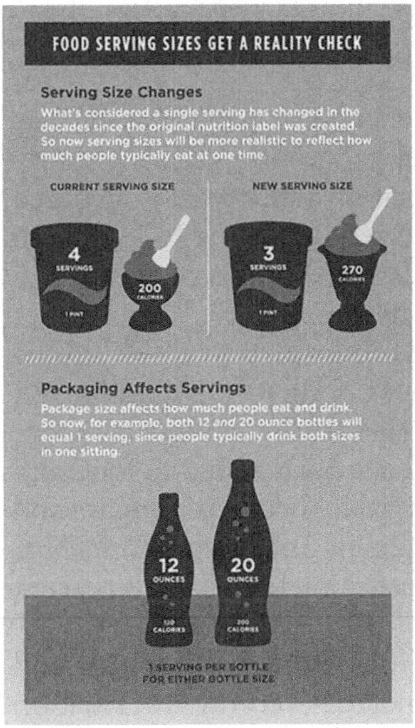

Figure 2.2. The FDA Serving Size Changes *(Source: U.S. Food and Drug Administration (FDA).)*

The *Dietary Guidelines for Americans (DGA) 2015-2020* can give you an idea of how many calories you may need each day based on your age, sex, and physical activity level. Use the body weight planner tool (www.niddk.nih.gov/health-information/weight-management/body-weight-planner) to make your own calorie and physical activity plan to help you reach and maintain your goal weight.

HOW CAN THE NUTRITION FACTS FOOD LABEL HELP ME?

The U.S. Food and Drug Administration's (FDA) food label is printed on most packaged foods. The food label is a quick way to find the number of calories and nutrients in a certain amount of food. For example, reading food labels tells you how many calories and how much fat, protein, sodium, and other ingredients are in one food serving. Many packaged foods contain more than a single serving. The updated food label lists the number of calories in one serving size in larger print than before so it is easier to see.

Other Helpful Facts on the Food Label

The food label has other useful information about what is included in one food serving. For example, one serving on the food label in Figure 2.1 has 1 gram of saturated fat and 0 grams of trans fat, a type of fat that is unhealthy for your heart.

The updated food label also includes information about "added sugars." Added sugars include table sugar, or sucrose, including beet and cane sugars; corn syrup; honey; malt syrup; and other sweeteners, such as fructose or glucose, that have been added to food and beverages. Fruit and milk contain naturally occurring sugars and are not included in the label as added sugars. The *Dietary Guidelines for Americans 2015-2020* calls for consuming less than 10 percent of calories daily from added sugars.

Because Americans do not always get enough vitamin D and potassium, the updated food label includes serving information for both of these nutrients. Since a lack of vitamin A and vitamin C in the general population is rare, these nutrients are no longer included on the food label. However, food makers may include them if they choose.

HOW CAN YOU KEEP TRACK OF HOW MUCH YOU EAT?

In addition to checking food labels for calories per serving, keeping track of what you eat – as well as when, where, why, and how much you eat – may help you manage your food portions. Create a food tracker on your cell phone, calendar, or computer to record the information. You also could download apps that are available for mobile devices to help you track how much you eat – and how much physical activity you get – each day.

The Sample Food Tracker shows what a 1-day page of a food tracker might look like. In the example, the person chose fairly healthy portions for breakfast and lunch and ate to satisfy hunger. The person also ate five cookies in the afternoon out of boredom rather than hunger.

By 8 p.m., the person was very hungry and ate large portions of high-fat, high-calorie food at a social event. An early evening snack of a piece of fruit and four ounces of fat-free or low-fat yogurt might have prevented overeating less healthy food later. The number of calories for the day totaled 2,916, which is more than most people need. Taking in too many calories may lead to weight gain over time.

If, like the person in the food tracker example, you eat even when you are not hungry, try doing something else instead. For instance, call or visit a friend. Or, if you are at work, take a break and walk around the block, if work and schedule permit. If you cannot distract yourself from food, try a healthy option, such as a piece of fruit or a stick of low-fat string cheese.

HOW CAN YOU MANAGE FOOD PORTIONS AT HOME?

You do not need to measure and count everything you eat or drink for the rest of your life. You may only want to do this long enough to learn typical serving and portion sizes. Try these ideas to help manage portions at home:

- Take one serving according to the food label and eat it off a plate instead of straight out of the box or bag.
- Avoid eating in front of the TV, while driving or walking, or while you are busy with other activities.
- Focus on what you are eating, chew your food well, and fully enjoy the smell and taste of your food.
- Eat slowly so your brain can get the message that your stomach is full, which may take at least 15 minutes.
- Use smaller dishes, bowls, and glasses so that you eat and drink less.
- Eat fewer high-fat, high-calorie foods, such as desserts, chips, sauces, and prepackaged snacks.
- Freeze food you would not serve or eat right away, if you make too much. That way, you would not be tempted to finish the whole batch. If you freeze leftovers in single- or family-sized servings, you will have ready-made meals for another day.

Table 2.1. Sample Food Tracker

Time	Food	Amount	Place	Hunger/ Reason	Estimated Calories
8 a.m.	Coffee, Black	6 fl. oz.			2
	Banana	1 medium	Home	Slightly hungry	105
	Low-fat yogurt	1 cup			250
1 p.m.	Grilled cheese sandwich				281
	Apple	1 medium	Work	Hungry	72
	Potato chips	Single -serving bag, 1 ounce			152
	Water	16 fl. oz.			-
3 p.m.	Chocolate -chip cookies	5 medium -sized	Work	Not hungry/ Bored	345
8 p.m.	Mini chicken drumsticks with hot pepper sauce	4			312
	Taco salad	3 cups in fried flour tortilla with beans and cheese	Restaurant/ Out with friends	Very hungry	586
	Chocolate cheesecake	1 piece, 1/12 of 9-inch cake			479
	Soft drink	12 fl. oz.			136

Table 2.1. Continued

Time	Food	Amount	Place	Hunger/ Reason	Estimated Calories
	Latte	Espresso coffee with whole milk, 16 ounces			196
				Total Calories	2,916

Through your tracker, you may become aware of when and why you consume less healthy foods and drinks. The tracker may help you make different choices in the future.

- Eat meals at regular times. Leaving hours between meals or skipping meals altogether may cause you to overeat later in the day.
- Buy snacks, such as fruit or single-serving, prepackaged foods, that are lower in calories. If you buy bigger bags or boxes of snacks, divide the items into single-serve packages right away so you are not tempted to overeat.

HOW CAN YOU MANAGE PORTIONS WHEN EATING OUT?

Although it may be easier to manage your portions when you cook and eat at home, most people eat out from time to time – and some people eat out often. Try these tips to keep your food portions in check when you are away from home:

- Share a meal with a friend, or take half of it home
- Avoid all-you-can-eat buffets
- Order one or two healthy appetizers or side dishes instead of a whole meal. Options include steamed or grilled – instead of fried – seafood or chicken, a salad with dressing on the side, or roasted vegetables.
- Ask to have the bread basket or chips removed from the table
- If you have a choice, pick the small-sized – rather than large-sized – drink, salad, or frozen yogurt

- Stop eating and drinking when you are full. Put down your fork and glass, and focus on enjoying the setting and your company for the rest of the meal.

Is Getting More Food for Your Money Always a Good Value?

Have you noticed that it costs only a few cents more to get the large fries or soft drinks instead of the regular or small size? Although getting the super-sized meal for a little extra money may seem like a good deal, you end up with more calories than you need for your body to stay healthy. Before you buy your next "value meal combo," be sure you are making the best choice for your wallet and your health.

HOW CAN YOU MANAGE PORTIONS AND EAT WELL WHEN MONEY IS TIGHT?

Eating healthier does not have to cost a lot of money. For instance:

- Buy fresh fruit and vegetables when they are in season. Check out a local farmers market for fresh, local produce if there is one in your community. Be sure to compare prices, as produce at some farmer's markets cost more than the grocery store. Buy only as much as you will use to avoid having to throw away spoiled food.
- Match portion sizes to serving sizes. To get the most from the money you spend on packaged foods, try eating no more than the serving sizes listed on food labels. Eating no more than a serving size may also help you better manage your fat, sugar, salt, and calories.

Remember...

Too many calories can affect your weight and health. Along with choosing a healthy variety of foods and reducing the total calories you take in through eating and drinking, pay attention to the size of your portions. Sticking with healthy foods and drinks and managing your portions may help you eat just enough for yourself.

Section 2.2 | **Food Exchange Lists**

This section includes text excerpted from "Food Exchange Lists," National Heart, Lung, and Blood Institute (NHLBI), March 15, 2006. Reviewed May 2021.

You can use the American Dietetic Association's (ADA) food exchange lists to check out serving sizes for each group of foods and to see what other food choices are available for each group of foods.

Vegetables contain 25 calories and 5 grams of carbohydrates. One serving equals:

Table 2.2. Vegetables

Measurement	**Ingredient**
½ C	Cooked vegetables (carrots, broccoli, zucchini, cabbage, etc.)
1 C	Raw vegetables or salad greens
½ C	Vegetable juice

If you are hungry, eat more fresh or steamed vegetables.

Fat-free and very low-fat milk contains 90 calories per serving. One serving equals:

Table 2.3. Fat-Free and Very Low-Fat Milk

Measurement	**Ingredient**
1 C	Milk, fat-free or 1% fat
¾ C	Yogurt, plain nonfat or low fat
1 C	Yogurt, artificially sweetened

Very lean protein choices have 35 calories and 1 gram of fat per serving. One serving equals:

Table 2.4. Very Lean Protein

Measurement	Ingredient
1 oz	Turkey breast or chicken breast, skin removed
1 oz	Fish fillet (flounder, sole, scrod, cod, etc.)
1 oz	Canned tuna in water
1 oz	Shellfish (clams, lobster, scallop, shrimp)
¾ C	Cottage cheese, nonfat or low fat
2	Egg whites
¼ C	Egg substitute
1 oz	Fat-free cheese
½ C	Beans, cooked (black beans, kidney, chickpeas or lentils): count as 1 starch/bread and 1 very lean protein

Fruits contain 15 grams of carbohydrate and 60 calories. One serving equals:

Table 2.5. Fruits

Measurement	Ingredient
1 small	Apple, banana, orange, nectarine
1 med.	Fresh peach
1	Kiwi
½	Grapefruit
½	Mango
1 C	Fresh berries (strawberries, raspberries, or blueberries)
1 C	Fresh melon cubes
1⁄8th	Honeydew melon
4 oz	Unsweetened juice
4 tsp	Jelly or jam

Portion Sizes and Servings

Lean protein choices have 55 calories and 2–3 grams of fat per serving. One serving equals:

Table 2.6. Lean Protein

Measurement	Ingredient
1 oz	Chicken – dark meat, skin removed
1 oz	Turkey – dark meat, skin removed
1 oz	Salmon, swordfish, herring
1 oz	Lean beef (flank steak, London broil, tenderloin, roast beef)*
1 oz	Veal, roast or lean chop*
1 oz	Lamb, roast or lean chop*
1 oz	Pork, tenderloin or fresh ham*
1 oz	Low-fat cheese (with 3 g or less of fat per ounce)
1 oz	Low-fat luncheon meats (with 3 g or less of fat per ounce)
¼ C	4.5% cottage cheese
2 med.	Sardines

**Limit to 1–2 times per week*

Medium-fat proteins have 75 calories and 5 grams of fat per serving. One serving equals:

Table 2.7. Medium-Fat Proteins

Measurement	Ingredient
1 oz	Beef (any prime cut), corned beef, ground beef**
1 oz	Porkchop
1	Whole egg (medium)**
1 oz	Mozzarella cheese

Table 2.7. Continued

Measurement	Ingredient
¼ C	Ricotta cheese
4 oz	Tofu (**Note:** This is a heart-healthy choice.)

"Choose these very infrequently

Starches contain 15 grams of carbohydrate and 80 calories per serving. One serving equals:

Table 2.8. Starches

Measurement	Ingredient
1 slice	Bread (white, pumpernickel, whole wheat, rye)
2 slices	Reduced-calorie or "lite" bread
¼ (1 oz)	Bagel (varies)
½	English muffin
½	Hamburger bun
¾ C	Cold cereal
1/3 C	Rice, brown or white, cooked
1/3 C	Barley or couscous, cooked
1/3 C	Legumes (dried beans, peas or lentils), cooked
½ C	Pasta, cooked
½ C	Bulgar, cooked
½ C	Corn, sweet potato, or green peas
3 oz	Baked sweet or white potato
¾ oz	Pretzels
3 C	Popcorn, hot air-popped or microwave (80% light)

Fats contain 45 calories and 5 grams of fat per serving. One serving equals:

Table 2.9. Fats

Measurement	**Ingredient**
1 tsp	Oil (vegetable, corn, canola, olive, etc.)
1 tsp	Butter
1 tsp	Stick margarine
1 tsp	Mayonnaise
1 Tbsp	Reduced-fat margarine or mayonnaise
1 Tbsp	Salad dressing
1 Tbsp	Cream cheese
2 Tbsp	Lite cream cheese
1/8th	Avocado
8 large	Black olives
10 large	Stuffed green olives
1 slice	Bacon

Section 2.3 | **Calories on the Menu**

This section includes text excerpted from "Calories on the Menu," U.S. Food and Drug Administration (FDA), May 8, 2019.

For the average adult, eating one meal away from home each week translates to roughly 2 extra pounds each year. Over the course of 5 years, that is 10 extra pounds.

Calorie labeling on menus can help you make informed and healthful decisions about meals and snacks. So, beginning May 7, 2018, calories were listed on many menus and menu boards of restaurants and other food establishments that are part of a chain of 20 or more locations. This helps you know your options and make it easier to eat healthy when eating out.

Here are steps for making dining out choices that are healthy and delicious:

- Find out your calorie needs
- Look for calorie and nutrition information
- Make the best choice for you

FIND OUT YOUR CALORIE NEEDS

Knowing your calorie needs is important to managing your daily food and beverage choices. You can use 2,000 calories a day as a guide, but your calorie needs may vary based on your age, sex, and physical activity level. To find out your specific calorie needs, use the (www.fda.gov/media/112972/download).

LOOK FOR CALORIE AND NUTRITION INFORMATION

You may have noticed calorie information on some menus or menu boards. Or maybe you have seen nutrition information on restaurant websites or on phone apps. This information can help you make an informed and healthful meal and snack choices.

Where Will You See the Calories?

Calories are listed next to the name or price of the food or beverage on menus and menu boards, including drive-thru windows, and maybe at the following types of chains:

- Chain restaurants
- Chain coffee shops
- Bakeries
- Ice cream shops
- Self-service food locations, such as buffets and salad bars
- Movie theaters
- Amusement parks
- Grocery/convenience stores

Where Will You Not See Calorie Information?

- Foods sold at deli counters and typically intended for further preparation

- Foods purchased in bulk in grocery stores, such as loaves of bread from the bakery section
- Bottles of liquor displayed behind a bar
- Food in transportation vehicles, such as food trucks, airplanes, and trains
- Food on menus in elementary, middle, and high schools that are part of the U.S. Department of Agriculture's National School Lunch Program (NSLP)
- Restaurants and other establishments that are not part of a chain of 20 or more

What about Meals with Multiple Options?

When a menu item is available in different flavors or varieties (e.g., vanilla and chocolate ice cream), or includes an entrée with your choice of side items, such as a sandwich that comes with either chips, side salad, or fruit, the calorie amounts will be shown as follows:

- Two choices
    - Calories are separated by a slash (e.g., 250/350 calories)
- Three or more choices
    - Calories are shown in a range (e.g., 150–300 calories)

MAKE THE BEST CHOICE FOR YOU

Eating healthy comes down to personal choices. Try these tips to help you make the best choices for yourself and your family.

- Comparing calorie and nutrition information can help you make better decisions before you order.
- Side dishes can add many calories to a meal. Steamed, grilled, or broiled vegetables and fruit are often lower-calorie options. With calorie information, you can make the best choice for yourself.
- Calorie information can help you decide how much to enjoy now and how much to save for later.
- Asking for sauces or salad dressings on the side lets you choose how much to use.

- Foods described with words like creamy, fried, breaded, battered, or buttered are typically higher in calories than foods described as baked, roasted, steamed, grilled, or broiled. Use the calorie information to help you make the choice that is right for you.
- Calories from beverages can add up quickly. With calorie information, you can find lower-calorie options.

Chapter 3 | **Food Labels**

Chapter Contents

Section 3.1 | How to Understand and Use the Nutrition Facts Label

This section includes text excerpted from "How to Understand and Use the Nutrition Facts Label," U.S. Food and Drug Administration (FDA), March 11, 2020.

People look at food labels for a variety of reasons. But, whatever the reason, many consumers would like to know how to use this information more effectively and easily. The following label-reading skills are intended to make it easier for you to use the Nutrition Facts labels to make quick, informed food decisions to help you choose a healthy diet.

NUTRITION FACTS PANEL: AN OVERVIEW
SERVING INFORMATION
#1 on Sample Label

4 servings per container, serving size 1 cup (227g)

When looking at the Nutrition Facts label, first take a look at the number of servings in the package (servings per container) and the serving size. Serving sizes are standardized to make it easier to compare similar foods; they are provided in familiar units, such as cups or pieces, followed by the metric amount, for example the number of grams (g). The serving size reflects the amount that people typically eat or drink. It is not a recommendation of how much you should eat or drink.

It is important to realize that all the nutrient amounts are shown on the label, including the number of calories, refer to the size of the serving. Pay attention to the serving size, especially how many servings there are in the food package. For example, you might ask yourself if you are consuming ½ serving, 1 serving, or more. In the sample label, one serving of lasagna equals 1 cup. If you ate two cups, you would be consuming two servings. That is two times the calories and nutrients shown in the sample label, so you would need to double the nutrient and calorie amounts, as well as the percent Daily Values (DVs), to see what you are getting in two servings.

Table 3.1. Serving Information of Lasagna

Example				
	One Serving of Lasagna	**%DV**	**Two Serving of Lasagna**	**%DV**
Serving Size	1 cup		2 cups	
Calories	280		560	
Total Fat	9g	12%	18g	24%
Saturated Fat	4.5g	23%	9g	46%
Trans Fat	0g		0g	
Cholesterol	35mg	12%	70mg	24%
Sodium	850mg	37%	1700mg	74%
Total Carbohydrate	34g	12%	68g	24%
Dietary Fiber	4g	14%	8g	29%
Total Sugars	6g		12g	
Added Sugars	0g	0%	0g	0%
Protein	15g		30g	
Vitamin D	0mcg	0%	0mcg	0%
Calcium	320mg	25%	640mg	50%
Iron	1.6mg	8%	3.2mg	20%
Potassium	510mg	10%	1020mg	20%

CALORIES
#2 on Sample Label

Amount per serving calories 280

Calories provide a measure of how much energy you get from a serving of this food. In the example, there are 280 calories in one serving of lasagna. What if you ate the entire package? Then, you would consume 4 servings or 1,120 calories.

To achieve or maintain a healthy body weight, balance the number of calories you eat and drink with the number of calories your body uses. 2,000 calories a day is used as a general guide for nutrition advice. Your calorie needs may be higher or lower and vary depending on your age, sex, height, weight, and physical activity level.

Remember: The number of servings you consume determines the number of calories you actually eat. Eating too many calories per day is linked to overweight and obesity.

NUTRIENTS
#3 on Sample Label

This shows you some key nutrients that impact your health. You can use the label to support your personal dietary needs – look for foods that contain more of the nutrients you want to get more of and less of the nutrients you may want to limit.

- Nutrients to get less saturated fat, sodium, and added sugars

Saturated fat, sodium, and added sugars are nutrients listed on the label that may be associated with adverse health effects – and Americans generally consume too much of them, according to the recommended limits for these nutrients. They are identified as nutrients to get less of. Eating too much saturated fat and sodium, for example, is associated with an increased risk of developing some health conditions, such as cardiovascular disease and high blood pressure. Consuming too many added sugars can make it hard to meet important nutrient needs while staying within calorie limits.

THE PERCENT DAILY VALUE
#4 on Sample Label

The percent DV is the percentage of the Daily Value for each nutrient in a serving of the food. The Daily Values are reference amounts (expressed in grams, milligrams, or micrograms) of nutrients to consume or not to exceed each day.

The percent DV shows how much a nutrient in a serving of food contributes to a total daily diet.

Total Fat 9g	**12%**
Saturated Fat 4.5g	**23%**
Trans Fat 0g	
Cholesterol 35mg	**12%**
Sodium 850mg	**37%**
Total Carbohydrate 34g	**12%**
Dietary Fiber 4g	**14%**
Total Sugars 6g	
Includes 0g Added Sugars	**0%**
Protein 15g	
Vitamin D 0mcg	0%
Calcium 320mg	25%
Iron 1.6mg	8%
Potassium 510mg	10%

Figure 3.1. Nutrients

The percent DV helps you determine if a serving of food is high or low in a nutrient.

Do you need to know how to calculate percentages to use the percent DV? No, because the label (the percent DV) does the math for you! It helps you interpret the nutrient numbers (grams, milligrams, or micrograms) by putting them all on the same scale for the day (0-100 percent DV). The percent DV column does not add up vertically to 100 percent. Instead, the percent DV is the percentage of the Daily Value for each nutrient in a serving of the food. It can tell you if a serving of food is high or low in a nutrient and whether a serving of the food contributes a lot, or a little, to your daily diet for each nutrient.

Note: Some nutrients on the Nutrition Facts label, such as total sugars and *trans* fat, do not have a percent DV.

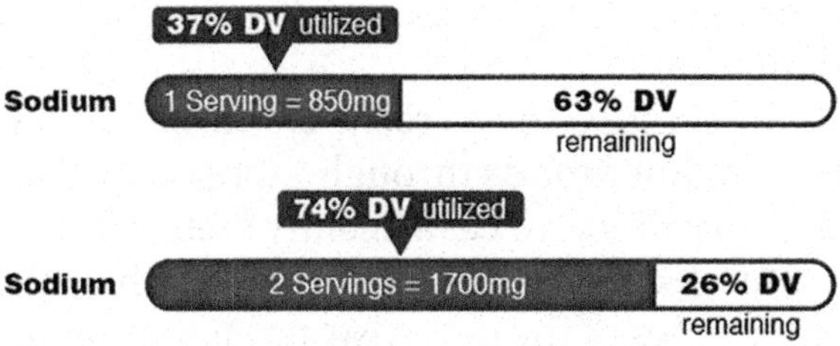

Figure 3.2. Sodium Bars

General Guide to Percent Daily Value

- 5 percent DV or less of a nutrient per serving is considered low.
- 20 percent DV or more of a nutrient per serving is considered high.

More often, choose foods that are:

- Higher in percent DV for dietary fiber, vitamin D, calcium, iron, and potassium.
- Lower in percent DV for saturated fat, sodium, and added sugars.

Example: Look at the amount of sodium in one serving listed on the sample nutrition label. Is percent DV of 37 percent contributing a lot or a little to your diet? Check the general guide to percent DV. This product contains 37 percent DV for sodium, which shows that this is a high sodium product (it has more than 20 percent DV for sodium). If you consumed 2 servings, that would provide 74 percent of the DV for sodium – nearly three-quarters of an entire day's worth of sodium.

Compare foods: Use percent DV to compare food products (remember to make sure the serving size is the same) and more often choose products that are higher in nutrients you want to get more of and lower in nutrients you want to get less of.

Understand nutrient content claims: Use percent DV to help distinguish one claim from another, such as "light," "low," and "reduced." Simply compare percent DVs in each food product to see which one is higher or lower in a particular nutrient. There is no need to memorize definitions.

Dietary trade-offs: You can use the percent DV to help you make dietary trade-offs with other foods throughout the day. You do not have to give up a favorite food to eat a healthy diet. When a food you like is high in saturated fat, balance it with foods that are low in saturated fat at other times of the day. Also, pay attention to how much you eat during the entire day, so that the total amount of saturated fat, as well as other nutrients you want to limit, stays below 100 percent DV.

HOW THE DAILY VALUES RELATE TO THE PERCENT DAILY VALUES

Look at the example below for another way to see how the Daily Values (DVs) relate to the percent DVs and dietary guidance. For each nutrient listed in the table, there is a DV, a percent DV, and dietary advice or a goal. If you follow this dietary advice, you will stay within public-health experts' recommended upper or lower limits for the nutrients listed, based on a 2,000-calorie daily diet.

EXAMPLES OF DAILY VALUES VERSUS PERCENT DAILY VALUES

Table 3.2. Based on a 2,000 Calorie Diet

Nutrient	DV	%DV	Goal
Saturated Fat	20g	Equals 100% DV	Less than
Sodium	2,300mg	Equals 100% DV	Less than
Dietary Fiber	28g	Equals 100% DV	At least
Added Sugars	50g	Equals 100% DV	Less than
Vitamin D	20mcg	Equals 100% DV	At least
Calcium	1,300mg	Equals 100% DV	At least
Iron	18mg	Equals 100% DV	At least
Potassium	4,700mg	Equals 100% DV	At least

Upper Limit – Eat "Less Than"...

Upper limit means it is recommended that you stay below or eat "less than" the Daily Value nutrient amounts listed per day. For example, the DV for saturated fat is 20g. This amount is 100 percent DV for this nutrient. What is the goal or dietary advice? To eat "less than" 20 g or 100 percent DV each day.

Lower Limit – Eat "At Least"...

The DV for dietary fiber is 28g, which is 100 percent DV. This means it is recommended that you eat "at least" this amount of dietary fiber on most days.

NUTRIENTS WITHOUT A PERCENT DAILY VALUE: *TRANS* FATS, PROTEIN, AND TOTAL SUGARS:

Note that *trans* fat and total Sugars do not list a percent DV on the Nutrition Facts label. Protein only lists a percent DV in specific situations listed below

TRANS FAT

Experts could not provide a reference value for *trans* fat nor any other information that the FDA believes is sufficient to establish a Daily Value.

According to the *Dietary Guidelines for Americans*, there is evidence that diets higher in *trans* fat are associated with increased blood levels of low-density lipoprotein (LDL or "bad") cholesterol – which, in turn, are associated with an increased risk of developing cardiovascular disease. Note: Most uses of artificial *trans* fat in the U.S. food supply have been phased out as of 2018.

PROTEIN

A percent DV is required to be listed if a claim is made for protein, such as "high in protein." The percent DV for protein must also be listed on the label if the product is intended for infants and children under 4 years of age. However, if the product is intended for the general population 4 years of age and older and a claim is not made about protein on the label, the percent DV for protein is not required.

Current scientific evidence indicates that protein intake is not a public-health concern for adults and children over 4 years of age in the United States.

TOTAL SUGARS

No daily reference value has been established for total sugars because no recommendations have been made for the total amount to eat in a day. Keep in mind that the total sugars listed on the Nutrition Facts label include naturally occurring sugars (such as those in fruit and milk) as well as added sugars.

Section 3.2 | **Understanding Claims on Food Labels**

This section includes text excerpted from "Label Claims for Conventional Foods and Dietary Supplements," U.S. Food and Drug Administration (FDA), June 19, 2018.

Among the claims that can be used on food and dietary supplement, labels are three categories of claims that are defined by statute and/or the U.S. Food and Drug Administration (FDA) regulations: health claims, nutrient content claims, and structure/function claims.

HEALTH CLAIMS

Health claims describe a relationship between a food substance (a food, food component, or dietary supplement ingredient), and a reduced risk of a disease or health-related condition. There are three ways in which the FDA exercises its oversight in determining which health claims may be used on a label or in labeling for a conventional food or dietary supplement:

1. The 1990 Nutrition Labeling and Education Act (NLEA) provides for the FDA to issue regulations authorizing health claims for foods and dietary

supplements after reviewing and evaluating the scientific evidence, either in response to a health claim petition or on its own initiative.

2. The 1997 U.S. Food and Drug Administration Modernization Act (FDAMA) provides for health claims based on an authoritative statement of the National Academy of Sciences (NAS) or a scientific body of the U.S. government with responsibility for public-health protection or nutrition research; such claims may be used 120 days after a health claim notification has been submitted to the FDA, unless the agency has informed the notifier that the notification does not include all the required information.
3. As described in the FDA's guidance entitled Interim Procedures for Qualified Health Claims in the Labeling of Conventional Human Food and Human Dietary Supplements, the agency reviews petitions for qualified health claims where the quality and strength of the scientific evidence falls below that required for the FDA to issue an authorizing regulation. If the FDA finds that the evidence supporting the proposed claim is credible and the claim can be qualified to prevent it from misleading consumers, the agency issues a letter of enforcement discretion specifying the qualifying language that should accompany the claim and describing the circumstances under which it intends to exercise enforcement discretion for use of the claim in food labeling.

A "health claim" by definition has two essential components:

1. A substance (whether a food, food component or dietary ingredient)
2. A disease or health-related condition. A statement lacking either one of these components does not meet the regulatory definition of a health claim. For example, statements that address the role of dietary patterns or of general categories of foods (e.g., fruits and vegetables) in maintaining good health are considered to be dietary

guidance rather than health claims. Dietary guidance statements used on food labels must be truthful and nonmisleading. Statements that address a role of a specific substance in maintaining normal healthy structures or functions of the body are considered to be structure/function claims.

NLEA Authorized Health Claims

The Nutrition Labeling and Education Act of 1990 (NLEA) provides for the use in food labeling of health claims that characterize a relationship between a food, a food component, or dietary ingredient and risk of a disease (e.g., "adequate calcium throughout life may reduce the risk of osteoporosis"), provided the claims meet certain criteria and are authorized by an FDA regulation. The FDA authorizes these types of health claims based on an extensive review of the scientific literature, generally as a result of the submission of a health claim petition, using the significant scientific agreement standard to determine whether the substance/disease relationship is well established.

Health Claims Based on Authoritative Statements

The U.S. Food and Drug Administration Modernization Act of 1997 (FDAMA) provides a second way for the use of a health claim in food labeling to be authorized. Under FDAMA, a new health claim can be authorized by submitting a notification to the FDA of a claim based on an "authoritative statement" from certain scientific bodies of the U.S. government or the National Academy of Sciences. The FDA has issued guidance on how a firm can submit such notifications and make use of authoritative statement-based health claims. This guidance can be found at the notification of a health claim or nutrient content claim based on an authoritative statement of a scientific body. The FDAMA does not include dietary supplements in the provisions for health claims based on authoritative statements. Consequently, this method of oversight for health claims cannot be used for dietary supplements at this time.

Qualified Health Claims

The FDA's interim procedures for qualified health claims in the labeling of conventional human food and human dietary supplements describe the agency's process for considering petitions for the use of a qualified health claim in food labeling. When there is emerging evidence for a relationship between a food substance (a food, food component, or dietary ingredient) and reduced risk of a disease or health-related condition, but the evidence is not well enough established to meet the significant scientific agreement standard required for the FDA to issue an authorizing regulation, the qualified health claim petition process provides a mechanism to request that the FDA review the scientific evidence and exercise enforcement discretion to permit the use of the qualified claim in food labeling. If, after evaluating the quality and strength of the totality of the scientific evidence, the FDA finds that credible evidence supports the claim, the agency issues a letter outlining the circumstances under which it intends to consider the exercise of enforcement discretion for use of the claim in food labeling. Qualifying language is included as part of the claim to indicate that the evidence supporting the claim is limited. Although the FDA's letters of enforcement discretion are issued to the petitioner requesting the qualified health claim, the qualified claims are available for use on any food or dietary supplement product meeting the enforcement discretion conditions specified in the letter. The FDA has issued guidance on interim procedures for qualified health claims. Qualified health claim petitions that are submitted to the FDA will be available for public review and comment.

NUTRIENT CONTENT CLAIMS

The Nutrition Labeling and Education Act of 1990 (NLEA) permits the use of label claims that characterize the level of a nutrient in a food (i.e., nutrient content claims) if they have been authorized by the FDA and are made in accordance with the FDA's authorizing regulations. Nutrient content claims describe the level of a nutrient in the product, using terms such as free, high, and low, or they compare the level of a nutrient in a food to that of another food, using terms such as more, reduced, and lite. An accurate quantitative statement (e.g., 200 mg of sodium) that does not otherwise "characterize" the nutrient level may be used to describe the amount of a nutrient present. However, a statement such as "only 200 mg of sodium" characterizes the level of sodium by implying that it is low.

Therefore, the food would have to meet the nutritional criteria for a "low" nutrient content claim or carry a disclosure statement that it does not qualify for the claim (e.g., "not a low sodium food"). The requirements that govern the use of nutrient content claims help ensure that descriptive terms, such as high or low, are used consistently for all types of food products and are thus meaningful to consumers. Healthy is an implied nutrient content claim that characterizes a food as having "healthy" levels of total fat, saturated fat, cholesterol, and sodium, as defined in the regulation authorizing the use of the claim.

Percentage claims for dietary supplements are another category of nutrient content claims. These claims are used to describe the percentage level of a dietary ingredient in a dietary supplement and may refer to dietary ingredients for which there is no established Daily Value, provided that the claim is accompanied by a statement of the amount of the dietary ingredient per serving. Examples include simple percentage statements such as "40 percent omega-3 fatty acids, 10 mg per capsule," and comparative percentage claims, for example, "twice the omega-3 fatty acids per capsule (80 mg) as in 100 mg of menhaden oil (40 mg)."

STRUCTURE OR FUNCTION CLAIMS AND RELATED DIETARY SUPPLEMENT CLAIMS

Structure/function claims have historically appeared on the labels of conventional foods and dietary supplements as well as drugs. The Dietary Supplement Health and Education Act of 1994 (DSHEA) established some special regulatory requirements and procedures for using structure/function claims and two related types of dietary supplement labeling claims, claims of general well-being and claims related to a nutrient deficiency disease. Structure/function claims may describe the role of a nutrient or dietary ingredient intended to affect the normal structure or function of the human body, for example, "calcium builds strong bones." In addition, they may characterize the means by which a nutrient or dietary ingredient acts to maintain such structure or function, for example, "fiber maintains bowel regularity," or "antioxidants maintain cell integrity."

General well-being claims describe general well-being from consumption of a nutrient or dietary ingredient. Nutrient deficiency disease claims describe a benefit related to a nutrient deficiency disease (such as vitamin C and scurvy), but such claims are allowed only if they also say how widespread the disease is in the United States. These three types of claims are not preapproved by the FDA, but the manufacturer must have substantiation that the claim is truthful and not misleading and must submit a notification with the text of the claim to the FDA no later than 30 days after marketing the dietary supplement with the claim. If a dietary supplement label includes such a claim, it must state in a "disclaimer" that the FDA has not evaluated the claim. The disclaimer must also state that the dietary supplement product is not intended to "diagnose, treat, cure or prevent any disease," because only a drug can legally make such a claim. Structure/function claims may not explicitly or implicitly link the claimed effect of the nutrient or dietary ingredient to a disease or state of health leading to disease.

Structure/function claims for conventional foods focus on effects derived from nutritive value, while structure/function claims for dietary supplements may focus on nonnutritive as well as nutritive effects. The FDA does not require conventional food manufacturers to notify the FDA about their structure/function claims, and disclaimers are not required for claims on conventional foods.

Section 3.3 | **Changes to the Nutrition Facts Label**

This section includes text excerpted from "Changes to the Nutrition Facts Label," U.S. Food and Drug Administration (FDA), February 10, 2021.

The Nutrition Facts label on packaged foods was updated in 2016 to reflect updated scientific information, including information about the link between diet and chronic diseases, such as obesity and heart disease. The updated label makes it easier for consumers to make better-informed food choices. The updated label appears on the majority of food packages. Manufacturers with $10 million or more in annual sales were required to update their labels by January 1, 2020; manufacturers with less than $10 million in annual food sales were required to update their labels by January 1, 2021. Manufacturers of most single-ingredient sugars, such as honey and maple syrup, and certain cranberry products have until July 1, 2021, to make the changes. The compliance dates are still in place, but the FDA is working cooperatively with manufacturers to meet the new Nutrition Facts label requirements.

NEW LABEL
Highlights of the Updated Label
FEATURES A REFRESHED DESIGN

- The "iconic" look of the label remains, but we made important updates to ensure consumers have access to the information they need to make informed decisions about the foods they eat. These changes include increasing the type size for "calories," "servings per container," and the "serving size" declaration, and bolding the number of calories and the "serving size" declaration to highlight this information.
- Manufacturers must declare the actual amount, in addition to percent Daily Value (percent DV) of vitamin D, calcium, iron, and potassium. They can voluntarily declare the gram amount for other vitamins and minerals.
- The footnote now better explains what percent Daily Value means. It reads: "*The % Daily Value tells you how much

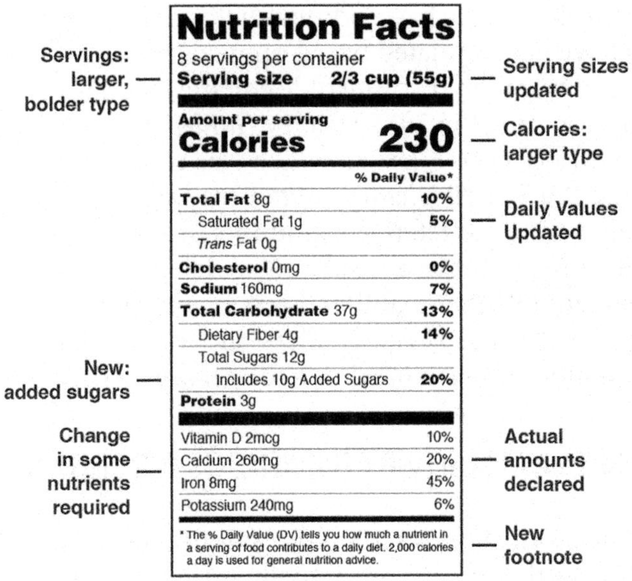
Nutrition Facts
8 servings per container
Serving size 2/3 cup (55g)
Amount per serving
Calories 230
% Daily Value*
Total Fat 8g 10%
Saturated Fat 1g 5%
Trans Fat 0g
Cholesterol 0mg 0%
Sodium 160mg 7%
Total Carbohydrate 37g 13%
Dietary Fiber 4g 14%
Total Sugars 12g
Includes 10g Added Sugars 20%
Protein 3g
Vitamin D 2mcg 10%
Calcium 260mg 20%
Iron 8mg 45%
Potassium 240mg 6%
* The % Daily Value (DV) tells you how much a nutrient in a serving of food contributes to a daily diet. 2,000 calories a day is used for general nutrition advice.
Servings: larger, bolder type
New: added sugars
Change in some nutrients required
Serving sizes updated
Calories: larger type
Daily Values Updated
Actual amounts declared
New footnote

Figure 3.3. New Nutrition Facts Label

a nutrient in a serving of food contributes to a daily diet. 2,000 calories a day is used for general nutrition advice."

REFLECTS UPDATED INFORMATION ABOUT NUTRIENTS

- "Added sugars," in grams and as percent Daily Value, must be included on the label. There are different labeling requirements for single-ingredient sugars.
- The list of nutrients that are required or permitted to be declared is being updated. Vitamin D and potassium are required on the label. Calcium and iron will continue to be required. Vitamins A and C are no longer required but can be included on a voluntary basis.
- While continuing to require "total fat," "saturated fat," and "*trans* fat" on the label, "calories from fat" was removed because research shows the type of fat is more important than the amount.

- Daily values for nutrients such as sodium, dietary fiber, and vitamin D have been updated based on newer scientific evidence from the Institute of Medicine (IOM) and other reports such as the *2015 Dietary Guidelines Advisory Committee (DGAC) Report,* which was used in developing the *2015-2020 Dietary Guidelines for Americans.* Daily values are reference amounts of nutrients to consume or not to exceed and are used to calculate the percent DV that manufacturers include on the label. The percent DV helps consumers understand the nutrition information in the context of a total daily diet.

UPDATED SERVING SIZES AND LABELING REQUIREMENTS FOR CERTAIN PACKAGE SIZES

- By law, serving sizes must be based on the amounts of foods and beverages that people are actually eating, not what they should be eating. How much people eat and drink has changed since the previous serving size requirements were published in 1993. For example, the reference amount used to set a serving of ice cream was previously 1/2 cup but is now 2/3 cup. The reference amount used to set a serving of soda changed from 8 ounces to 12 ounces.
- Package size affects what people eat. So for packages that are between one and two servings, such as a 20-ounce soda or a 15-ounce can of soup, the calories and other nutrients are required to be labeled as one serving because people typically consume it in one sitting.
- For certain products that are larger than a single serving but that could be consumed in one sitting or multiple sittings, manufacturers have to provide "dual column" labels to indicate the number of calories and nutrients on both a "per serving" and "per package/" "per unit" basis. Examples would be a 24-ounce bottle of soda or a pint of ice cream. With dual-column labels available, people can more easily understand how many calories and nutrients they are getting if they eat or drink the entire package/unit at one time.

Chapter 4 | **Healthy Use of Dietary Supplements**

Chapter Contents

Section 4.1 | Dietary Supplements: What You Need to Know

This section includes text excerpted from "What You Need to Know," Office of Dietary Supplements (ODS), National Institutes of Health (NIH), September 3, 2020.

Many adults and children in the United States take one or more vitamins or other dietary supplements. In addition to vitamins, dietary supplements can contain minerals, herbs or other botanicals, amino acids, enzymes, and many other ingredients. Dietary supplements come in a variety of forms, including tablets, capsules, gummies, and powders, as well as drinks and energy bars. Popular supplements include vitamins D and B_{12}; minerals, such as calcium and iron; herbs such as echinacea and garlic; and products, such as glucosamine, probiotics, and fish oils.

THE DIETARY SUPPLEMENT LABEL

Dietary supplements include ingredients such as vitamins, minerals, herbs, amino acids, and enzymes. Dietary supplements are marketed in forms such as tablets, capsules, soft gels, gel caps, powders, and liquids.

EFFECTIVENESS

Some dietary supplements can help you get adequate amounts of essential nutrients if you do not eat a nutritious variety of foods. However, supplements cannot take the place of the variety of foods that are important to a healthy diet.

Some dietary supplements can improve overall health and help manage some health conditions. For example:

- Calcium and vitamin D help keep bones strong and reduce bone loss.
- Folic acid decreases the risk of certain birth defects.
- Omega-3 fatty acids from fish oils might help some people with heart disease.
- A combination of vitamins C and E, zinc, copper, lutein, and zeaxanthin (known as "AREDS") may slow

down further vision loss in people with age-related macular degeneration (AMD).

Many other supplements need more study to determine if they have value. The U.S. Food and Drug Administration (FDA) does not determine whether dietary supplements are effective before they are marketed.

SAFETY AND RISK

Many supplements contain active ingredients that can have strong effects in the body. Always be alert to the possibility of a bad reaction, especially when taking a new product.

You are most likely to have side effects from dietary supplements if you take them at high doses or instead of prescribed medicines, or if you take many different supplements. Some supplements can increase the risk of bleeding or, if taken before surgery, can change your response to anesthesia. Supplements can also interact with some medicines in ways that might cause problems. Here are a few examples:

- Vitamin K can reduce the ability of the blood thinner warfarin to prevent blood from clotting.
- St. John's wort can speed the breakdown of many medicines and reduce their effectiveness (including some antidepressants, birth control pills, heart medications, anti-HIV medications, and transplant drugs).
- Antioxidant supplements, such as vitamins C and E, might reduce the effectiveness of some types of cancer chemotherapy.

Manufacturers may add vitamins, minerals, and other supplement ingredients to foods you eat, especially breakfast cereals and beverages. As a result, you may get more of these ingredients than you think, and more might not be better. Taking more than you need costs more and might also raise your risk of side effects. For example, too much vitamin A can cause headaches and liver damage, reduce bone strength, and cause birth defects. Excess iron causes nausea and vomiting and may damage the liver and other organs.

Be cautious about taking dietary supplements if you are pregnant or nursing. Also, be careful about giving supplements to a child, unless recommended by their healthcare provider. Many supplements have not been well tested for safety in pregnant women, nursing mothers, or children.

If you think that you have had a bad reaction to a dietary supplement, let your healthcare provider know. She or he may report your experience to the FDA. You may also submit a report directly to the FDA by calling 800-FDA-1088. You should also report your reaction to the manufacturer by using the contact information on the product label.

QUALITY

The FDA has established good manufacturing practices (GMPs) that companies must follow to help ensure the identity, purity, strength, and composition of their dietary supplements. These GMPs can prevent adding the wrong ingredient (or too much or too little of the correct ingredient) and reduce the chance of contamination or improper packaging and labeling of a product. The FDA periodically inspects facilities that manufacture supplements.

Several independent organizations offer quality testing and allow products that pass these tests to display a seal of quality assurance that indicates the product was properly manufactured, contains the ingredients listed on the label, and does not contain harmful levels of contaminants. These seals do not guarantee that a product is safe or effective. Organizations that offer quality testing include:*

- ConsumerLab.com
- NSF International
- U.S. Pharmacopeia

*Any mention of a specific company, organization, or service does not represent an endorsement by the Office of Dietary Supplements (ODS).

TALK WITH YOUR HEALTHCARE PROVIDERS

Tell your healthcare providers (including doctors, dentists, pharmacists, and dietitians) about any dietary supplements you are taking. They can help you determine which supplements, if any, might be valuable for you.

Keep a complete record of any dietary supplements and medicines you take. The ODS website has a useful form, "My Dietary Supplement and Medicine Record," that you can print and fill out at home. For each product, note the name, the dose you take, how often you take it, and the reason for use. You can share this record with your healthcare providers to discuss what is best for your overall health.

KEEP IN MIND

Dietary supplement labels must include name and location information for the manufacturer or distributor.

If you want to know more about the product that you are taking, check with the manufacturer or distributor about:

- Information to support the claims of the product
- Information on the safety and effectiveness of the ingredients in the product

HOW CAN YOU BE A SMART SUPPLEMENT SHOPPER?

- Consult your healthcare provider before taking dietary supplements to treat a health condition.
- Get your healthcare provider's approval before taking dietary supplements in place of, or in combination with, prescribed medicines.
- If you are scheduled to have any type of surgical procedure, talk with your healthcare provider about any supplements you take.
- Keep in mind the term "natural" does not always mean safe. Some all-natural botanical products, for example, comfrey and kava, can harm the liver. A dietary supplement's safety depends on many things, such as its chemical makeup, how it works in the body, how it is prepared, and the amount you take.

- Before taking any dietary supplement, use the information sources listed in this brochure and talk to your healthcare providers to answer these questions:
  - What are its potential benefits for me?
  - Does it have any safety risks?
  - What is the proper dose to take?
  - How, when, and for how long should I take it?

FEDERAL REGULATION OF DIETARY SUPPLEMENTS

Dietary supplements are not medicines and are not intended to treat, diagnose, mitigate, prevent, or cure diseases. The FDA is the federal agency that oversees both supplements and medicines, but the FDA regulations for dietary supplements are different from those for prescription or over-the-counter medicines.

Medicines must be approved by the FDA before they can be sold or marketed. Supplements do not require this approval. Supplement companies are responsible for having evidence that their products are safe, and the label claims are truthful and not misleading. However, as long as the product does not contain a "new dietary ingredient" (one introduced since October 15, 1994), the company does not have to provide this safety evidence to the FDA before the product is marketed.

Dietary supplement labels may include certain types of health-related claims. Manufacturers are permitted to say, for example, that a supplement promotes health or supports a body function (such as immunity or heart health). These claims must be followed by the words, "This statement has not been evaluated by the FDA. This product is not intended to diagnose, treat, cure, or prevent any disease."

Manufacturers must follow good manufacturing practices (GMPs) to ensure the identity, purity, strength, and composition of their products. If the FDA finds a dietary supplement to be unsafe, it may remove the product from the Marketplace or ask the manufacturer to voluntarily recall the product.

The FDA monitors the Marketplace for potential illegal products that may be unsafe or make false or misleading claims. The Federal Trade Commission (FTC), which monitors product advertising, also requires information about a supplement product to be truthful and not misleading.

The federal government can take legal action against companies and websites that sell dietary supplements when the companies make false or deceptive statements about their products, if they promote them as treatments or cures for diseases, or if their products are unsafe.

Section 4.2 | Safety Tips for Dietary Supplement Users

This section includes text excerpted from "Tips for Dietary Supplement Users," U.S. Food and Drug Administration (FDA), February 23, 2018.

MAKING INFORMED DECISIONS AND EVALUATING INFORMATION

The U.S. Food and Drug Administration (FDA), as well as health professionals and their organizations, receive many inquiries each year from consumers seeking health-related information, especially about dietary supplements. Clearly, people choosing to supplement their diets with herbals, vitamins, minerals, or other substances want to know more about the products they choose so that they can make informed decisions about them. The choice to use a dietary supplement can be a wise decision that provides health benefits. However, under certain circumstances, these products may be unnecessary for good health or they may even create unexpected risks.

Given the abundance and conflicting nature of information now available about dietary supplements, you may need help to sort the reliable information from the questionable. Below are tips and resources that will help you be a savvy dietary supplement user. The principles underlying these tips are similar to those principles a savvy consumer would use for any product.

- Basic points to consider
- Tips on searching the web for information on dietary supplements
- More tips and to-do's

Note: Links to nonfederal government organizations found on this site are provided solely as a service to consumers and do not represent an FDA endorsement of these organizations or their products.

Basic Points to Consider

DO YOU NEED TO THINK ABOUT YOUR TOTAL DIET?

Yes. Dietary supplements are intended to supplement the diets of some people, but not to replace the balance of the variety of foods important to a healthy diet. While you need enough nutrients, too much of some nutrients can cause problems. You can find information on the functions and potential benefits of vitamins and minerals, as well as upper safe limits for nutrients at the National Academy of Sciences (NAS) website (www.nasonline.org).

SHOULD YOU CHECK WITH YOUR DOCTOR OR HEALTHCARE PROVIDER BEFORE USING A SUPPLEMENT?

This is a good idea, especially for certain population groups. Dietary supplements may not be risk-free under certain circumstances. If you are pregnant, nursing a baby, or have a chronic medical condition, such as diabetes, hypertension, or heart disease, be sure to consult your doctor or pharmacist before purchasing or taking any supplement. While vitamin and mineral supplements are widely used and generally considered safe for children, you may wish to check with your doctor or pharmacist before giving these or any other dietary supplements to your child. If you plan to use a dietary supplement in place of drugs or in combination with any drug, tell your healthcare provider first. Many supplements contain active ingredients that have strong biological effects and their safety is not always assured in all users. If you have certain health conditions and take these products, you may be placing yourself at risk.

SOME SUPPLEMENTS MAY INTERACT WITH PRESCRIPTION AND OVER-THE-COUNTER (OTC) MEDICINES

Taking a combination of supplements or using these products together with medications (whether prescription or OTC drugs) could under certain circumstances produce adverse effects, some of which could be life-threatening. Be alert to advisories about these products, whether taken alone or in combination. For example: Coumadin (a prescription medicine), ginkgo biloba (an herbal supplement), aspirin (an OTC drug) and vitamin E (a vitamin supplement) can each thin the blood, and taking any of these products together can increase the potential for internal bleeding. Combining St. John's wort with certain human immunodeficiency virus (HIV) drugs significantly reduces their effectiveness. St. John's wort may also reduce the effectiveness of prescription drugs for heart disease, depression, seizures, certain cancers or oral contraceptives.

SOME SUPPLEMENTS CAN HAVE UNWANTED EFFECTS DURING SURGERY

It is important to fully inform your doctor about the vitamins, minerals, herbals, or any other supplements you are taking, especially before elective surgery. You may be asked to stop taking these products at least two to three weeks ahead of the procedure to avoid potentially dangerous supplement/drug interactions – such as changes in heart rate, blood pressure and increased bleeding – that could adversely affect the outcome of your surgery.

ADVERSE EFFECTS FROM THE USE OF DIETARY SUPPLEMENTS SHOULD BE REPORTED TO MEDWATCH

You, your healthcare provider, or anyone may directly report to the FDA if you believe it is related to the use of any dietary supplement product, by calling the FDA at 800-FDA-1088 (800-332-1088), by fax at 800-FDA-0178 (800-332-0178), or reporting a serious adverse event or illness online. The FDA would like to know whenever you think a product caused you a serious problem, even if you are not sure that the product was the cause, and even if you do not visit a doctor or clinic. In addition to communicating with the FDA online or by phone, you may use the MedWatch form available from the FDA website (www.fda.gov/downloads/aboutfda/reportsmanualsforms/forms/ucm163919.pdf).

WHO IS RESPONSIBLE FOR ENSURING THE SAFETY AND EFFICACY OF DIETARY SUPPLEMENTS?

Under the law, manufacturers of dietary supplements are responsible for making sure their products are safe before they go to market. They are also responsible for determining that the claims on their labels are accurate and truthful. Dietary supplement products are not reviewed by the government before they are marketed, but the FDA has the responsibility to take action against any unsafe dietary supplement product that reaches the market. If the FDA can prove that claims on marketed dietary supplement products are false and misleading, the agency may take action also against products with such claims.

Tips on Searching the Web for Information on Dietary Supplements

When searching on the web, try using directory sites of respected organizations, rather than doing blind searches with a search engine. Ask yourself the following questions:

WHO OPERATES THE SITE

Is the site run by the government, a university, or a reputable medical or health-related association (e.g., American Medical Association (AMA), American Diabetes Association (ADA), American Heart Association (AHA), National Institutes of Health (NIH), National Academy of Sciences (NAS), or U.S. Food and Drug Administration (FDA))? Is the information written or reviewed by qualified health professionals, experts in the field, academia, government, or the medical community?

WHAT IS THE PURPOSE OF THE SITE?

Is the purpose of the site to objectively educate the public or just to sell a product? Be aware of practitioners or organizations whose main interest is in marketing products, either directly or through sites with which they are linked. Commercial sites should clearly distinguish scientific information from advertisements. Most nonprofit and government sites contain no advertising, and access to the site and materials offered are usually free.

WHAT IS THE SOURCE OF THE INFORMATION AND DOES IT HAVE ANY REFERENCES?

Has the study been reviewed by recognized scientific experts and published in reputable peer-reviewed scientific journals, such as the *New England Journal of Medicine?* Does the information say "some studies show..." or does it state where the study is listed so that you can check the authenticity of the references? For example, can the study be found in the U.S. National Library of Medicine's (NLM) database of literature citations (PubMed).

IS THE INFORMATION CURRENT?

Check the date when the material was posted or updated. Often new research or other findings are not reflected in old material, for example, side effects or interactions with other products or new evidence that might have changed earlier thinking. Ideally, health and medical sites should be updated frequently.

HOW RELIABLE IS THE INTERNET OR E-MAIL SOLICITATIONS?

While the Internet is a rich source of health information, it is also an easy vehicle for spreading myths, hoaxes, and rumors about alleged news, studies, products or findings. To avoid falling prey to such hoaxes, be skeptical and watch out for overly emphatic language with uppercase letters and lots of exclamation points!!!! Beware of such phrases such as: "This is not a hoax" or "Send this to everyone you know."

More Tips and To-Do's

ASK YOURSELF: DOES IT SOUND TOO GOOD TO BE TRUE?

Do the claims for the product seem exaggerated or unrealistic? Are there simplistic conclusions being drawn from a complex study to sell a product? While the web can be a valuable source of accurate, reliable information, it also has a wealth of misinformation that may not be obvious. Learn to distinguish hype from evidence-based science. Nonsensical lingo can sound very convincing. Also, be skeptical about anecdotal information from persons who have no formal training in nutrition or botanicals, or from personal testimonials (e.g., from store employees, friends, or online chat rooms and message boards) about incredible benefits or results obtained from using a product. Question these people on their training and knowledge in nutrition or medicine.

THINK TWICE ABOUT CHASING THE LATEST HEADLINE

Sound health advice is generally based on a body of research, not a single study. Be wary of results claiming a "quick fix" that depart from previous research and scientific beliefs. Keep in mind science does not proceed by dramatic breakthroughs, but by taking many small steps, slowly building towards a consensus. Furthermore, news stories, about the latest scientific study, especially those on TV or radio, are often too brief to include important details that may apply to you or allow you to make an informed decision.

CHECK YOUR ASSUMPTIONS ABOUT THE FOLLOWING

- #1 Questionable assumption. "Even if a product may not help me, it at least would not hurt me." It is best not to assume that this will always be true. When consumed in high enough amounts, for a long enough time, or in combination with certain other substances, all chemicals can be toxic, including nutrients, plant components, and other biologically active ingredients.
- #2 Questionable assumption. "When I see the term "natural," it means that a product is healthful and safe." Consumers can be misled if they assume this term assures wholesomeness, or that these food-like substances necessarily have milder effects, which makes them safer to use than drugs. The term "natural" on labels is not well defined and is sometimes used ambiguously to imply unsubstantiated benefits or safety. For example, many weight-loss products claim to be "natural" or "herbal" but this does not necessarily make them safe. Their ingredients may interact with drugs or may be dangerous for people with certain medical conditions.

- #3 Questionable assumption. "A product is safe when there is no cautionary information on the product label." Dietary supplement manufacturers may not necessarily include warnings about potential adverse effects on the labels of their products. If consumers want to know about the safety of a specific dietary supplement, they should contact the manufacturer of that brand directly. It is the manufacturer's responsibility to determine that the supplement manufacturer produces or distributes is safe and that there is substantiated evidence that the label claims are truthful and not misleading.
- #4 Questionable assumption. "A recall of a harmful product guarantees that all such harmful products will be immediately and completely removed from the Marketplace." A product recall of a dietary supplement is voluntary and while many manufacturers do their best, a recall does not necessarily remove all harmful products from the Marketplace.

CONTACT THE MANUFACTURER FOR MORE INFORMATION ABOUT THE SPECIFIC PRODUCT THAT YOU ARE PURCHASING

If you cannot tell whether the product you are purchasing meets the same standards as those used in the research studies you read about, check with the manufacturer or distributor. Ask to speak to someone who can address your questions, some of which may include:

1. What information does the firm have to substantiate the claims made for the product? Be aware that sometimes firms supply so-called proof of their claims by citing undocumented reports from satisfied consumers, or "internal" graphs and charts that could be mistaken for evidence-based research.
2. Does the firm have information to share about tests it has conducted on the safety or efficacy of the ingredients in the product?

3. Does the firm have a quality control system in place to determine if the product actually contains what is stated on the label and is free of contaminants?
4. Has the firm received any adverse events reports from consumers using their products?

Section 4.3 | **Probiotics: What You Need to Know**

This section includes text excerpted from "Probiotics: What You Need to Know," National Center for Complementary and Integrative Health (NCCIH), August 2019.

WHAT ARE PROBIOTICS?

Probiotics are live microorganisms that are intended to have health benefits. Products sold as probiotics include foods (such as yogurt), dietary supplements, and products that are not used orally, such as skin creams.

Although people often think of bacteria and other microorganisms as harmful "germs," many microorganisms help our bodies function properly. For example, bacteria that are normally present in our intestines help digest food, destroy disease-causing microorganisms, and produce vitamins. Large numbers of microorganisms live on and in our bodies. Many of the microorganisms in probiotic products are the same as or similar to microorganisms that naturally live in our bodies.

What Types of Bacteria Are in Probiotics?

Probiotics may contain a variety of microorganisms. The most common are bacteria that belong to groups called "*Lactobacillus*" and "*Bifidobacterium*." Other bacteria may also be used as probiotics, and so may yeasts such as *Saccharomyces boulardii*.

Different types of probiotics may have different effects. For example, if a specific kind of *Lactobacillus* helps prevent an illness, that does not necessarily mean that another kind of *Lactobacillus* or any of the *Bifidobacterium* probiotics would do the same thing.

Are Prebiotics the Same as Probiotics?

No, prebiotics are not the same as probiotics. Prebiotics are nondigestible food components that selectively stimulate the growth or activity of desirable microorganisms.

How Popular Are Probiotics?

The 2012 National Health Interview Survey (NHIS) showed that about 4 million (1.6 percent) U.S. adults had used probiotics or prebiotics in the past 30 days. Among adults, probiotics or prebiotics were the third most commonly used dietary supplement other than vitamins and minerals. The use of probiotics by adults quadrupled between 2007 and 2012. The 2012 NHIS also showed that 300,000 children age 4 to 17 (0.5 percent) had used probiotics or prebiotics in the 30 days before the survey.

How Might Probiotics Work?

Probiotics may have a variety of effects in the body, and different probiotics may act in different ways.

Probiotics might:

- Help your body maintain a healthy community of microorganisms or help your body's community of microorganisms return to a healthy condition after being disturbed
- Produce substances that have desirable effects
- Influence your body's immune response

How Are Probiotics Regulated in the United States?

Government regulation of probiotics in the United States is complex. Depending on a probiotic product's intended use, the U.S. Food and Drug Administration (FDA) might regulate it as a dietary supplement, a food ingredient, or a drug.

Many probiotics are sold as dietary supplements, which do not require the FDA approval before they are marketed. Dietary supplement labels may make claims about how the product affects the structure or function of the body without the FDA approval, but they are not allowed to make health claims, such as saying the supplement lowers your risk of getting a disease, without the FDA's consent.

If a probiotic is going to be marketed as a drug for treatment of a disease or disorder, it has to meet stricter requirements. It must be proven safe and effective for its intended use through clinical trials and be approved by the FDA before it can be sold.

Learning about the Microbiome

The community of microorganisms that lives on us and in us is called the "microbiome," and it is a hot topic for research. The Human Microbiome Project, supported by the National Institutes of Health (NIH) from 2007–2016, played a key role in this research by mapping the normal bacteria that live in and on the healthy human body. With this understanding of a normal microbiome as the basis, researchers around the world, including many supported by NIH, are now exploring the links between changes in the microbiome and various diseases. They are also developing new therapeutic approaches designed to modify the microbiome to treat disease and support health.

The National Center for Complementary and Integrative Health (NCCIH) is among the many agencies funding research on the microbiome. Researchers supported by NCCIH are studying the interactions between components of food and microorganisms in the digestive tract. The focus is on the ways in which diet-microbiome interactions may lead to the production of substances with beneficial health effects.

WHAT THE SCIENCE SAYS ABOUT THE EFFECTIVENESS OF PROBIOTICS

A great deal of research has been done on probiotics, but much remains to be learned about whether they are helpful and safe for various health conditions.

Probiotics have shown promise for a variety of health purposes, including prevention of antibiotic-associated diarrhea (including diarrhea caused by *Clostridium difficile*), prevention of necrotizing enterocolitis and sepsis in premature infants, treatment of infant colic, treatment of periodontal disease, and induction or maintenance of remission in ulcerative colitis.

However, in most instances, we still do not know which probiotics are helpful and which are not. We also do not know how much of the probiotic people would have to take or who would be most likely to benefit. Even for the conditions that have been studied the most, researchers are still working toward finding the answers to these questions.

The following sections summarize the research on probiotics for some of the conditions for which they have been studied.

GASTROINTESTINAL CONDITIONS

- Antibiotic-associated diarrhea
- *Clostridium difficile* infection
- Constipation
- Diarrhea caused by cancer treatment
- Diverticular disease
- Inflammatory bowel disease
- Irritable bowel syndrome
- Traveler's diarrhea

CONDITIONS IN INFANTS

- Infant colic
- Necrotizing enterocolitis
- Sepsis in infants

DENTAL DISORDERS

- Dental caries (tooth decay)
- Periodontal diseases (gum disease)

CONDITIONS RELATED TO ALLERGY

- Allergic rhinitis (hay fever)
- Asthma
- Atopic dermatitis

OTHER CONDITIONS

- Acne
- Hepatic encephalopathy
- Upper respiratory infections
- Urinary tract infections

Can Probiotics Be Harmful?

- Probiotics have an extensive history of apparently safe use, particularly in healthy people. However, few studies have looked at the safety of probiotics in detail, so there is a lack of solid information on the frequency and severity of side effects.
- The risk of harmful effects from probiotics is greater in people with severe illnesses or compromised immune systems. When probiotics are being considered for high-risk individuals, such as premature infants or seriously ill hospital patients, the potential risks of probiotics should be carefully weighed against their benefits.
- Possible harmful effects of probiotics include infections, production of harmful substances by the probiotic microorganisms, and transfer of antibiotic resistance genes from probiotic microorganisms to other microorganisms in the digestive tract.
- Some probiotic products have been reported to contain microorganisms other than those listed on the label. In some instances, these contaminants may pose serious health risks.

Part 2 | **The Elements of Good Nutrition**

Chapter 5 | Carbohydrates

WHAT ARE THE DIFFERENT TYPES OF CARBOHYDRATES?

Carbohydrates are found primarily in plant foods; the exception is dairy products, which contain milk sugar (lactose). Total carbohydrate on the Nutrition Facts label includes:

- **Dietary fiber** is a type of carbohydrate made up of many sugar molecules linked together in such a way that it cannot be easily digested in the small intestine. Dietary fiber can increase the frequency of bowel movements, lower blood glucose and cholesterol levels, and reduce calorie intake.
- **Total sugars** include sugars that are naturally present in food and added sugars, which include sugars that are added during the processing of foods (such as sucrose or dextrose), foods packaged as sweeteners (such as table sugar), sugars from syrups and honey, and sugars from concentrated fruit or vegetable juices. Sugars are the smallest type of carbohydrate and are easily digested and absorbed by the body.
- **Sugar alcohols** are a type of carbohydrate that chemically has characteristics of both sugars and alcohols but are not completely absorbed by the body – providing a sweet taste with fewer calories per gram than sugar.

WHERE ARE THEY FOUND?

- **Dietary fiber** includes naturally occurring fibers in plants (such as beans, fruits, nuts, peas, vegetables,

This chapter contains text excerpted from "Interactive Nutrition Facts Label – Total Carbohydrate," U.S. Food and Drug Administration (FDA), March 2020.

seeds, whole grains, and foods made with whole-grain ingredients) and certain isolated or synthetic non-digestible carbohydrates added to food that the U.S. Food and Drug Administration has determined have beneficial physiological effects to human health.

- **Total sugars** include sugars found naturally in foods such as dairy products, fruits, and vegetables and added sugars often found in foods such as baked goods, desserts, sugar-sweetened beverages, and sweets.
- **Sugar alcohols** are found naturally in small amounts in a variety of fruits and vegetables and are also commercially produced and added as reduced-calorie sweeteners to foods (such as chewing gum, baked goods, desserts, frostings, and sweets).

WHAT DO THEY DO?

Carbohydrates provide calories, or "energy," for the body. Each gram of carbohydrate provides 4 calories. The human body breaks down carbohydrates into glucose. Glucose in the blood (often referred to as "blood sugar") is the primary energy source for the body's cells, tissues, and organs (such as the brain and muscles). Glucose can be used immediately or stored in the liver and muscles for later use.

HEALTH FACTS

- Most Americans exceed the recommended limits for added sugars in the diet. There is evidence that diets characterized, in part, by lower consumption of sugar-sweetened foods and beverages relative to less healthy dietary patterns are associated with a reduced risk of developing cardiovascular disease. Diets higher in all sugars can also increase the risk of developing dental cavities. The *Dietary Guidelines for Americans* recommend limiting calories from added sugars to less than 10 percent of total calories per day (e.g., 200 calories or 50 grams per day of added sugars based on a 2,000 calorie daily diet).

- Many Americans also do not get the recommended amount of dietary fiber. Diets higher in dietary fiber can increase the frequency of bowel movements and can reduce the risk of developing cardiovascular disease. The *Dietary Guidelines for Americans 2020-2025* recommend consuming a variety of foods that are good sources of dietary fiber, consuming at least half of grains as whole grains, and limiting the intake of refined grains and products made with refined grains.

ACTION STEPS
For Monitoring Total Carbohydrate in Your Diet

Use the Nutrition Facts label as a tool for monitoring the consumption of total carbohydrates. The Nutrition Facts label on food and beverage packages shows the amount in grams (g) of total carbohydrate and the percent Daily Value (percent DV) of total carbohydrate per serving of the food.

The Nutrition Facts label also lists the types of carbohydrates that make up the total carbohydrate in a product. This includes the amount in grams (g) per serving of dietary fiber, total sugars, and added sugars; as well as the percent DV of dietary fiber and added sugars. Food manufacturers may also voluntarily list the amount in grams (g) per serving of soluble dietary fiber, insoluble dietary fiber, and sugar alcohols. The Daily Value for total carbohydrates is 275 g per day. This is based on a 2,000 calorie daily diet – your Daily Value may be higher or lower depending on your calorie needs.

- When comparing and choosing foods, look at the percent DV of total carbohydrate. And remember:
  - 5 percent DV or less of total carbohydrate per serving is considered low.
  - 20 percent DV or more of total carbohydrate per serving is considered high.
- Try whole grains (such as brown rice, bulgur, couscous, and quinoa) as side dishes and switch from refined to whole-grain versions of commonly consumed foods (such as breads, cereals, pasta, and rice). Also, look for options that are lower in added sugars, saturated fats,

and/or sodium, such as bread instead of croissants; English muffins instead of biscuits; and plain popcorn instead of buttered.

- Choose whole fruit (fresh, frozen, dried, and canned in 100 percent fruit juice) as snacks and desserts and use fruit to top foods such as cereal, yogurt, oatmeal, and pancakes.
- Keep raw, cut-up vegetables handy for quick snacks – choose colorful dark green, orange, and red vegetables (such as broccoli florets, carrots, and red peppers).
- Add beans and peas or unsalted nuts and seeds to salads, soups, and side dishes. These are also great sources of dietary fiber and protein.
- Try unsweetened or no-sugar-added versions of fruit sauces (such as applesauce) and plain, fat-free, or 1 percent low-fat yogurt.
- More often, choose beverages such as water and fat-free or 1 percent low-fat milk. Less often, choose beverages that are high in calories but have few or no beneficial nutrients, such as energy drinks, fruit drinks, soft drinks, and sports drinks.
- Consume smaller portions of foods and beverages that are higher in added sugars or consume them less often.

Chapter 6 | **Protein**

Protein is found in foods from both plants and animals. Protein is made up of hundreds or thousands of smaller units, called "amino acids," which are linked to one another in long chains. The sequence of amino acids determines each protein's unique structure and its specific function. There are 20 different amino acids that can be combined to make every type of protein in the body. These amino acids fall into two categories:

- Essential amino acids are required for normal body functioning, but they cannot be made by the body and must be obtained from food. Of the 20 amino acids, 9 are considered essential.
- Nonessential amino acids can be made by the body from essential amino acids consumed in food or in the normal breakdown of body proteins. Of the 20 amino acids, 11 are considered nonessential.

WHERE IS IT FOUND?

Protein is found in a variety of foods, including:

- Beans and peas
- Dairy products (such as milk, cheese, and yogurt)
- Eggs
- Meats and poultry
- Nuts and seeds
- Seafood (fish and shellfish)

This chapter contains text excerpted from the following sources: Text in this chapter begins with excerpts from "Interactive Nutrition Facts Label – Protein," U.S. Food and Drug Administration (FDA), March 2020; Text under the heading "Facts That You Should Know" is excerpted from "Protein Foods," MyPlate, U.S. Department of Agriculture (USDA), December 31, 2020.

- Soy products
- Whole grains and vegetables (these generally provide less protein than is found in other sources)

WHAT DOES IT DO?

Protein provides calories, or "energy" for the body. Each gram of protein provides 4 calories.

- Protein is a component of every cell in the human body and is necessary for proper growth and development, especially during childhood, adolescence, and pregnancy.
- Protein helps your body build and repair cells and body tissue.
- Protein is a major part of your skin, hair, nails, muscle, bone, and internal organs. Protein is also found in almost all body fluids.
- Protein is important for many body processes, such as blood clotting, fluid balance, immune response, vision, and production of hormones, antibodies, and enzymes.

HEALTH FACTS

- Most Americans get the recommended amounts of protein to meet their needs. However, many individuals do not eat enough seafood and dairy products.
- According to the *Dietary Guidelines for Americans*, there is evidence that diets lower in meats and processed meats and processed poultry are associated with a reduced risk of developing cardiovascular disease in adults.
- The *Dietary Guidelines for Americans* recommend eating a variety of protein foods from both plant and animal sources. The guidelines also note that while processed meats and poultry are sources of sodium and saturated fat, they can be included in a healthy diet when consumed within recommended limits for total calories, sodium, saturated fat, and added sugars.

PROTEIN: A CLOSER LOOK

Dietary proteins are not all the same. They are made up of different combinations of amino acids and are characterized according to how many of the essential amino acids they provide.

- Complete proteins contain all of the essential amino acids in adequate amounts. Animal foods (such as dairy products, eggs, meats, poultry, and seafood) and soy are complete protein sources.
- Incomplete proteins are missing, or do not have enough of, one or more of the essential amino acids, making the protein imbalanced. Most plant foods (such as beans, grains, nuts, peas, seeds, and vegetables) are incomplete protein sources.
- Complementary proteins are two or more incomplete protein sources that, when eaten in combination (at the same meal or during the same day), compensate for each other's lack of amino acids. For example, grains are low in the amino acid lysine, while beans and nuts (legumes) are low in the amino acid methionine. When grains and legumes are eaten together (such as rice and beans or peanut butter on whole-wheat bread), they form a complete protein.

ACTION STEPS: FOR MONITORING PROTEIN IN YOUR DIET

Use the Nutrition Facts label as a tool for monitoring consumption of protein, and choosing protein foods that are lower in saturated fat. The Nutrition Facts label on food and beverage packages shows the amount in grams (g) of protein per serving of the food. Protein generally has no percent Daily Value (percent DV) listed on the label, so use the number of grams (g) as a guide. Food manufacturers may voluntarily list the percent DV of protein per serving on the Nutrition Facts label, but they are required to list the percent DV of protein if a statement is made on the package labeling about the health effects or the amount of protein (e.g., "high" or "low") contained in the food.

The Daily Value for protein is 50 g per day. This is based on a 2,000 calorie daily diet – your Daily Value may be higher or lower depending on your calorie needs.

- When comparing and choosing foods, look at the percent DV of protein (if listed). And remember:
  - 5 percent DV or less of protein per serving is considered low.
  - 20 percent DV or more of protein per serving is considered high.
- Choose a variety of protein foods, such as beans and peas, eggs, fat-free or 1 percent low-fat dairy products, lean meats and poultry, seafood, soy products, and unsalted nuts and seeds.
- Choose seafood and plant sources of protein (such as beans and peas, tofu and other soy products, and unsalted nuts and seeds) in place of some meats and poultry.
- Add beans and peas to salads, soups, and side dishes – or serve them as a main dish.
- Substitute fat-free or 1 percent low-fat dairy products and fortified plant-based beverages (such as soy, rice, and almond) for whole and 2 percent reduced-fat dairy products.
- Select fresh meats, poultry, and seafood, rather than processed varieties.
- Trim or drain fat from meats before or after cooking and remove poultry skin before eating.
- Try baking, broiling, grilling, or steaming. These cooking methods do not add extra fat.

FACTS THAT YOU SHOULD KNOW

- Most Americans get enough protein in their diets but may need to make leaner and more varied selections of the foods in the protein foods group. These recommended choices include lean meats, seafood, and plant-based proteins such as dried peas and beans, and nuts.
- The amount of food an adult needs from the protein foods group depends on age, sex, and level of physical activity. The recommended amount varies between 5- to 7-ounce equivalents per day.

Protein

- Packaged and prepared meat, poultry, and seafood products are common sources of sodium (salt). Sodium is added to packaged foods during processing such as in curing meat, enhancing flavor, or as a preservative.
- Beans, peas, and lentils can be counted in either food group because they contain nutrients that are similar to foods in the protein foods group (protein, iron, and zinc) and the vegetable group (fiber, potassium, and folate). Because of their high nutrient content, consuming dried beans, peas, and lentils is recommended for everyone, including people who also eat meat, poultry, and seafood regularly.
- Vegetarian choices in the protein foods group include nuts, nut butter, soy products such as tofu and veggie burgers, and beans, peas, and lentils.
- Nuts and seeds are good sources of protein, dietary fiber, minerals, and vitamin E.
- Eating canned fish with bones, such as sardines or anchovies, provides you with calcium. Because the bones are soft, they are edible.
- Eat seafood in place of meat or poultry twice a week. You should select a variety of seafood and include some that are higher in oils and low in mercury, such as salmon, trout, and herring.
- Do not wash or rinse raw meat or poultry before you cook it. Washing can cause bacteria found on the surface of meat or poultry to be spread to ready-to-eat foods, kitchen utensils, and counter surfaces. This is called cross-contamination. Cooking (baking, broiling, boiling, and grilling) to the right temperature kills the bacteria.

Chapter 7 | Dietary Fats

Chapter Contents

Section 7.1 | Dietary Fats: An Overview

This section includes text excerpted from "The Skinny on Fat," *NIH News in Health*, National Institutes of Health (NIH), March 2019.

Fat is an essential nutrient for our bodies. It provides energy. It helps our guts absorb certain vitamins from foods. But, what types of fat should you be eating? Are there any you should avoid?

Recommendations about dietary fat have shifted over the last two decades. From the 1970s through the 1990s, nutrition researchers emphasized eating a low-fat diet.

This was largely because of concerns about saturated fats, explains Dr. Alice H. Lichtenstein, who studies diet and heart health at Tufts University. Saturated fat that is in the bloodstream raises the levels of LDL cholesterol – the "bad" cholesterol. This in turn raises the risk of heart disease.

But, when people started following low-fat diets, they did not only cut saturated fats but in many cases, they replaced healthy unsaturated fats with processed carbohydrates, explains Lichtenstein.

"Initially, when we recommended cutting total fat we did not anticipate people would replace it with fat-free foods, like cookies, crackers, and ice cream, made with refined grains and sugar," says Lichtenstein. "It is what we refer to as an unanticipated consequence."

As scientists have learned, those replacement calories matter. Studies have shown that replacing saturated fat with unsaturated fat reduces the risk of heart disease. However, replacing saturated fat with simple carbohydrates, such as added sugar and white bread, does not.

"There is still this misconception that eating fat – any kind of fat – is bad. That it will lead to heart attacks or weight gain. That is not true. People really should be encouraged to eat healthy fats," says Dr. Frank Sacks, a nutrition expert at Harvard University.

HEALTHY FATS

Research has shown that unsaturated fats are good for you. These fats come mostly from plant sources. Cooking oils that are liquid at room temperatures, such as canola, peanut, safflower, soybean, and olive oil, contain mostly unsaturated fat. Nuts, seeds, and avocados are also good sources. Fatty fish – such as salmon, sardines, and herring – are rich in unsaturated fats, too.

Large studies have found that replacing saturated fats in your diet with unsaturated fats can reduce your risk of heart disease by about the same amount as cholesterol-lowering drugs.

People should actively make unsaturated fats a part of their diet, Sacks says. You do not need to avoid healthy fats to lose weight, he adds.

In an NIH-funded study Sacks led, called the "pounds lost trial," people who ate higher-fat or lower-fat diets had similar rates of weight loss. They were also successful at keeping the weight off.

"Low-fat diets have the same effect on body weight gain or weight loss as higher-fat diets, or higher-protein diets," he explains. "For weight loss, it's about getting a handle on whatever foods in your diet are giving you excess calories."

REPLACING BAD FATS

So are there fats you should avoid? Only a few years ago, doctors still had to advise people to avoid so-called "*trans* fats" in their diets. These largely manufactured fats could be found in things like margarine and many processed foods. They have been shown to raise the risk of heart disease.

Since 2015, the U.S. Food and Drug Administration (FDA) has taken steps to remove artificial *trans* fats from the food supply. Most *trans* fats now in food come from the small amounts found naturally in animal products, like meat and butter.

Experts already recommend that people limit their intake of animal fats. "So that takes care of those *trans* fats as well," Lichtenstein says.

As for saturated fat, it is complicated. Not all of the saturated fat in the bloodstream comes from the saturated fat that we eat, explains Dr. Ronald Krauss, who studies cholesterol at the UCSF Benioff Children's Hospital Oakland. Instead, it is produced when the body breaks down simple carbohydrates and sugars. That is one reason why replacing saturated fat in the diet with simple carbohydrates does not reduce the risk of heart disease.

Nutrition experts still recommend that people minimize the amount of saturated fat in the diet. But, researchers are now looking at whether the type of food that saturated fat is found in matters. For example, the influence of plant-based saturated fats, such as those in coconut and palm oil, is still unclear and being researched further.

Studies suggest that some full-fat dairy products, such as yogurt, may actually have benefits for the heart, Krauss says.

Krauss and his colleagues recently ran a small study looking at the effects of replacing some of the sugar allowed in the DASH diet with saturated dairy fats. The DASH diet was developed by NIH to help lower blood pressure.

Participants who ate saturated dairy fat instead of sugar had less fat called "triglycerides" in their bloodstream. The higher-fat diet was also as effective at lowering blood pressure as the standard DASH diet.

INDIVIDUAL NEEDS

Researchers know that there are big differences in how people's bodies react to different types and amounts of fat. But, they still do not know why. Studies have found that genes are not likely responsible, Sacks explains.

Lichtenstein and Krauss are both studying how the microbes that live in the gut interact with dietary fats. The makeup of the microbiome – all the microorganisms that normally live in the body, mainly in the gut – can differ widely between people.

It may turn out that different types of gut bacteria produce different compounds from fats. These compounds could then affect the body in different ways, Lichtenstein explains. Or different types of fats could promote the growth of different bacteria in the gut, which may then have varying effects on health.

"We just don't know yet, but there is tremendous interest in trying to understand the role of the gut microbiome in human health," she says.

If there is one thing that the research has shown, it is that the science of diets is very complex. Experts have moved away from focusing on single nutrients – such as fat – by themselves. Instead,

Sacks says, researchers now talk about healthy dietary patterns: ways of eating that take all aspects of the diet into account.

Section 7.2 | Types of Fats

This section includes text excerpted from "What Are the Types of Fat?" U.S. Department of Veterans Affairs (VA), March 22, 2014. Reviewed May 2021.

Most foods contain several different kinds of fat. Some are better for your health than others. It is wise to choose healthier types of fat, and enjoy them in moderation. Keep in mind that even healthier fats contain calories and should be used sparingly for weight management. Here is some information about healthy and harmful dietary fats. The four major types of fats are:

- Monounsaturated fats
- Polyunsaturated fats
- Saturated fats
- *Trans* fats

Monounsaturated and polyunsaturated fats are known as "healthy fats" because they are good for your heart, cholesterol levels, and overall health. These fats tend to be "liquid" at room temperature. Consider beneficial polyunsaturated fats containing omega-3 fatty acids found in fatty fish, flaxseed, and walnuts.

HEALTHY DIETARY FATS

Tips for increasing healthy fats in your diet:

- Cook with olive oil.
- Plan snacks of nuts or olives.
- Eat more avocados.
- Dress your own salads instead of using commercial dressings.

Table 7.1. Healthy Fats

Monounsaturated Fat	**Polyunsaturated Fat**
Olive oil	Soybean oil
Canola oil	Corn oil
Sunflower oil	Safflower oil
Peanut oil	Walnuts
Olives	Sunflower, sesame, and pumpkin seeds; flaxseed
Nuts (almonds, peanuts, hazelnuts, macadamia nuts, pecans, cashews)	Fatty fish (salmon, tuna, mackerel, herring, trout, anchovies, sardines, and eel)
Avocados	Soymilk
Peanut butter	Tofu

HARMFUL DIETARY FATS

Tips for decreasing harmful fats in your diet:

- Read food labels and avoid *trans* fats and hydrogenated/ partially hydrogenated oils.
- Avoid fried products.
- Avoid fast food.
- When eating out, ask that foods be prepared with olive oil.

Saturated fats and *trans* fats are known as the "harmful fats." They increase your risk of disease and elevate cholesterol. Saturated fats tend to be solid at room temperature, but they are also found in liquid tropical oils (palm and coconut). *Trans* fats (partially hydrogenated or hydrogenated fats) are oils that have been modified for longer shelf life. *Trans* fats are very bad for you. No amount of *trans* fats is healthy.

Table 7.2. Unhealthy Fats

Saturated Fat	***Trans* Fat**
High-fat cuts of meat (beef, lamb, pork)	Commercially baked pastries, cookies, doughnuts, muffins, cakes, pizza dough, pie crusts
Chicken with the skin	Packaged snack foods (crackers, microwave popcorn, chips)
Whole-fat dairy products (cream/milk)	Stick margarine
Butter	Vegetable shortening
Palm and coconut oil (snack foods, nondairy creamers, whipped toppings)	Fried foods (French fries, fried chicken, chicken nuggets, breaded fish)
Ice cream	Candy bars
Cheese	Premixed products (cake mix, pancake mix, chocolate drink mix)

Section 7.3 | **Omega-3 Supplements**

This section includes text excerpted from "Omega-3 Fatty Acids," Office of Dietary Supplements (ODS), National Institutes of Health (NIH), March 22, 2021.

WHAT ARE OMEGA-3 FATTY ACIDS AND WHAT DO THEY DO?

Omega-3 fatty acids are found in foods, such as fish and flaxseed, and in dietary supplements, such as fish oil.

The three main omega-3 fatty acids are alpha-linolenic acid (ALA), eicosapentaenoic acid (EPA), and docosahexaenoic acid (DHA). ALA is found mainly in plant oils such as flaxseed, soybean, and canola oils. DHA and EPA are found in fish and other seafood.

ALA is an essential fatty acid, meaning that your body cannot make it, so you must get it from the foods and beverages you consume. Your body can convert some ALA into EPA and then to DHA, but only in very small amounts. Therefore, getting EPA and DHA from foods (and dietary supplements if you take them) is the only practical way to increase levels of these omega-3 fatty acids in your body.

Omega-3s are important components of the membranes that surround each cell in your body. DHA levels are especially high in retina (eye), brain, and sperm cells. Omega-3s also provide calories to give your body energy and have many functions in your heart, blood vessels, lungs, immune system, and endocrine system (the network of hormone-producing glands).

HOW MUCH OMEGA-3S DO YOU NEED?

Experts have not established recommended amounts for omega-3 fatty acids, except for ALA. Average daily recommended amounts for ALA are listed below in grams (g). The amount you need depends on your age and sex.

Table 7.3. Omega-3s Required in Each Stages of Life

Life Stage	Recommended Amount of ALA
Birth to 12 months*	0.5 g
Children 1–3 years	0.7 g
Children 4–8 years	0.9 g
Boys 9–13 years	1.2 g
Girls 9–13 years	1.0 g
Teen boys 14–18 years	1.6 g
Teen girls 14–18 years	1.1 g
Men	1.6 g
Women	1.1 g
Pregnant teens and women	1.4 g
Breastfeeding teens and women	1.3 g

**As total omega-3s. All other values are for ALA alone.*

WHAT FOODS PROVIDE OMEGA-3S

Omega-3s are found naturally in some foods and are added to some fortified foods. You can get adequate amounts of omega-3s by eating a variety of foods, including the following:

- Fish and other seafood (especially cold-water fatty fish, such as salmon, mackerel, tuna, herring, and sardines)
- Nuts and seeds (such as flaxseed, chia seeds, and walnuts)
- Plant oils (such as flaxseed oil, soybean oil, and canola oil)
- Fortified foods (such as certain brands of eggs, yogurt, juices, milk, soy beverages, and infant formulas)

WHAT KINDS OF OMEGA-3 DIETARY SUPPLEMENTS ARE AVAILABLE?

Omega-3 dietary supplements include fish oil, krill oil, cod liver oil, and algal oil (a vegetarian source that comes from algae). They provide a wide range of doses and forms of omega-3s.

ARE YOU GETTING ENOUGH OMEGA-3S?

Most people in the United States get enough ALA from the foods they eat. They also get small amounts of eicosapentaenoic acid (EPA) and docosahexaenoic acid (DHA). Recommended amounts of EPA and DHA have not been established.

WHAT HAPPENS IF YOU DO NOT GET ENOUGH OMEGA-3S?

A deficiency of omega-3s can cause rough, scaly skin and a red, swollen, itchy rash. Omega-3 deficiency is very rare in the United States.

WHAT ARE SOME EFFECTS OF OMEGA-3S ON HEALTH?

Scientists are studying omega-3s to understand how they affect health. People who eat fish and other seafood have a lower risk of several chronic diseases. But, it is not clear whether these health benefits come from simply eating these foods or from the omega-3s in these foods. Below are some examples of what the researchers have shown.

Cardiovascular Disease

Many studies show that eating fatty fish and other types of seafood as part of a healthy eating pattern helps keep your heart healthy and helps protect you from some heart problems. Getting more EPA and DHA from foods or dietary supplements lowers triglyceride levels, for example.

The American Heart Association (AHA) recommends eating one to two servings of seafood per week to reduce your risk of some heart problems, especially if you consume seafood in place of less healthy foods. For people with heart disease, the AHA recommends consuming about 1 g per day EPA plus DHA, preferably from oily fish, but supplements are an option under the guidance of a healthcare provider. The AHA does not recommend omega-3 supplements for people who do not have a high risk of cardiovascular disease (CVD).

Infant Health and Development

During pregnancy and breastfeeding, eating 8 to 12 ounces per week of fish and other seafood may improve your baby's health. However, it is important to choose fish that are higher in EPA and DHA and lower in mercury. Examples are salmon, herring, sardines, and trout. It is not clear whether taking dietary supplements containing EPA and DHA during pregnancy or breastfeeding affects a baby's health or development. However, some studies show that taking these supplements may slightly increase a baby's weight at birth and the length of time the baby is in the womb, both of which may be beneficial. Breast milk contains DHA. Most commercial infant formulas also contain DHA.

Cancer Prevention

Some studies suggest that people who get more omega-3s from foods and dietary supplements may have a lower risk of breast cancer and perhaps colorectal cancer. But, a large clinical trial found that omega-3 supplements did not reduce the overall risk of cancer, or the risk of breast, prostate, or colorectal cancers. Other clinical trials in progress will help clarify whether omega-3s affect cancer risk.

Alzheimer Disease, Dementia, and Cognitive Function

Some – but not all – research shows that people who consume more omega-3s from food such as fish may have a lower risk of developing Alzheimer disease (AD), dementia, and other problems with cognitive function. More study of the effects of omega-3s on the brain is needed.

Age-Related Macular Degeneration

Age-related macular degeneration (AMD) is a major cause of vision loss among older adults. Studies suggest that people who get higher amounts of omega-3s from the foods they eat may have a lower risk of developing AMD. But, once someone has AMD, taking omega-3 supplements does not keep the disease from getting worse or slow down vision loss.

Dry Eye Disease

Dry eye disease occurs when tears do not provide enough moisture, causing eye discomfort and vision problems. Some studies show that getting more omega-3s from foods or supplements – mainly EPA and DHA – helps relieve symptoms of dry eye disease. But a large, recent study found that the symptoms of people with dry eye disease who took fish oil supplements of 2,000 mg EPA plus 1,000 mg DHA daily for 1 year did not improve any more than those who took a placebo (a dummy pill). More research on the effects of omega-3s on dry eye disease is needed.

Rheumatoid Arthritis

Rheumatoid arthritis (RA) causes chronic pain, swelling, stiffness, and loss of function in the joints. Some clinical trials have shown that taking omega-3 supplements may help manage RA when taken together with standard RA medications and other treatments. For example, people with RA who take omega-3 supplements may need less pain-relief medication, but it is not clear if the supplements reduce joint pain, swelling, or morning stiffness.

Other Conditions

Researchers are studying whether taking omega-3 dietary supplements may help lessen some of the symptoms of attention deficit hyperactivity disorder (ADHD), childhood allergies, and cystic fibrosis (CF). But, more research is needed to fully understand the potential benefits of omega-3s for these and other conditions.

CAN OMEGA-3S BE HARMFUL?

The U.S. Food and Drug Administration (FDA) recommends consuming no more than 3 g/day of EPA and DHA combined, including up to 2 g/day from dietary supplements. Higher doses are sometimes used to lower triglycerides, but anyone taking omega-3s for this purpose should be under the care of a healthcare provider because these doses could cause bleeding problems and possibly affect immune function. Any side effects from taking omega-3 supplements in smaller amounts are usually mild. They include an unpleasant taste in the mouth, bad breath, heartburn, nausea, stomach discomfort, diarrhea, headache, and smelly sweat.

ARE THERE ANY INTERACTIONS WITH OMEGA-3S THAT YOU SHOULD KNOW ABOUT?

Omega-3 dietary supplements may interact with the medications you take. For example, high doses of omega-3s may cause bleeding problems when taken with warfarin (Coumadin®) or other anticoagulant medicines.

Talk with your healthcare provider about possible interactions between omega-3 supplements and your medications.

OMEGA-3S AND HEALTHFUL EATING

People should get most of their nutrients from food, advises the federal government's *Dietary Guidelines for Americans* (health.gov/our-work/food-nutrition/previous-dietary-guidelines/2015). Foods contain vitamins, minerals, dietary fiber, and other substances that benefit health. In some cases, fortified foods and dietary supplements may provide nutrients that otherwise may be consumed in less-than-recommended amounts.

Chapter 8 | **Dietary Fiber**

Diets higher in dietary fiber can increase the frequency of bowel movements and can reduce the risk of developing cardiovascular disease (CVD).

Dietary fiber is a type of carbohydrate made up of many sugar molecules linked together. But, unlike other carbohydrates, dietary fiber is bound together in such a way that it cannot be easily digested in the small intestine.

There are two types of dietary fiber:

- Soluble dietary fiber dissolves in water to form a thick gel-like substance in the stomach. It is broken down by bacteria in the large intestine and provides some calories.
- Insoluble dietary fiber does not dissolve in water and may pass through the gastrointestinal tract (GIT) relatively intact and, therefore, is not a source of calories.

WHERE IS DIETARY FIBER FOUND

Naturally occurring dietary fiber is found in a variety of foods, including:

- Beans and peas
- Fruits
- Nuts
- Seeds
- Vegetables
- Wheat bran

This chapter contains text excerpted from the following sources: Text in this chapter begins with excerpts from "Interactive Nutrition Facts Label – Dietary Fiber," U.S. Food and Drug Administration (FDA), March 2020; Text under the heading "Food Sources of Dietary Fiber" is excerpted from "Food Sources of Dietary Fiber," *Dietary Guidelines for Americans* (*DGA*), U.S. Department of Agriculture (USDA), December 29, 2020.

- Whole grains (such as whole oats, brown rice, popcorn, and quinoa) and foods made with whole grain ingredients (such as breads, cereals, crackers, and pasta)

WHAT DIETARY FIBER DOES

- **Soluble dietary fiber** can interfere with the absorption of dietary fat and cholesterol. This, in turn, can help lower low-density lipoprotein (LDL or "bad") cholesterol levels in the blood. Soluble fiber can also slow digestion and the rate at which carbohydrates and other nutrients are absorbed into the bloodstream. This can help control the level of blood glucose (often referred to as "blood sugar") by preventing rapid rises in blood glucose following a meal.
- **Insoluble dietary fiber** can speed up the movement of food and waste through the digestive system.
- **Soluble and insoluble dietary fiber** can make you feel full, which may lower your calorie intake if you eat less and stay satisfied longer.

HEALTH FACTS OF DIETARY FIBER

- Many Americans do not get the recommended amount of dietary fiber. Dietary fiber is considered a "nutrient of public-health concern" because low intakes are associated with potential health risks.
- Diets higher in dietary fiber can increase the frequency of bowel movements and can reduce the risk of developing cardiovascular disease.
- The *Dietary Guidelines for Americans* recommend consuming a variety of foods that are good sources of dietary fiber. The guidelines also recommend consuming at least half of grains as whole grains and limiting the intake of refined grains and products made with refined grains.
- Dietary Fiber on the Nutrition Facts label includes naturally occurring fibers in plants and certain isolated

or synthetic nondigestible carbohydrates added to food that the U.S. Food and Drug Administration (FDA) has determined have beneficial physiological effects on human health. These isolated or synthetic nondigestible carbohydrates include: alginate, arabinoxylan, beta-glucan soluble fiber, cellulose, cross-linked phosphorylated RS4, galactooligosaccharide, glucomannan, guar gum, high amylose starch (resistant starch 2), hydroxypropylmethylcellulose, inulin, and inulin-type fructans, locust bean gum, mixed plant cell wall fibers (a broad category that includes fibers, such as sugar cane fiber and apple fiber, among many others), pectin, polydextrose, psyllium husk, and resistant maltodextrin/dextrin.

ACTION STEPS FOR INCREASING DIETARY FIBER IN YOUR DIET

Use the Nutrition Facts label as a tool for increasing the consumption of dietary fiber. The Nutrition Facts label on food and beverage packages shows the amount in grams (g) and the percentage Daily Value (percent DV) of dietary fiber per serving of the food. Food manufacturers may voluntarily list the amount in grams (g) per serving of soluble dietary fiber and insoluble dietary fiber on the Nutrition Facts label (under Dietary Fiber), but they are required to list soluble dietary fiber and/or insoluble dietary fiber if a statement is made on the package labeling about their health effects or the amount (e.g., "high" or "low") contained in the food.

The Daily Value for dietary fiber is 28 g per day. This is based on a 2,000 calorie daily diet – your Daily Value may be higher or lower depending on your calorie needs:

- Compare and choose foods to get 100 percent DV of dietary fiber on most days. And remember:
  - 5 percent DV or less of dietary fiber per serving is considered low.
  - 20 percent DV or more of dietary fiber per serving is considered high.
- Look for whole grains on the ingredient list on a food package. Some examples of whole grain ingredients

are barley, brown rice, buckwheat, bulgur, millet, oatmeal, quinoa, rolled oats, whole grain corn, whole grain sorghum, whole oats, whole rye, and whole wheat.

- **Tip:** Ingredients are listed in descending order by weight – the closer an ingredient is to the beginning of the list, the more of that ingredient is in the food.
- Try whole grains (such as brown rice, bulgur, couscous, and quinoa) as side dishes and switch from refined to whole-grain versions of commonly consumed foods (such as bread, cereals, pasta, and rice).
- Limit refined grains and products made with refined grains (such as cakes, cookies, chips, and crackers), which can be high in added sugars, saturated fat, and/or sodium and are common sources of excess calories.
- Start your day with a bowl of whole-grain breakfast cereal (such as bran or oatmeal) that is high in dietary fiber and low in added sugars. Top your cereal with fruit for sweetness and even more fiber!
- Choose whole fruit (fresh, frozen, dried, and canned in 100 percent fruit juice) as snacks and desserts and add fruits to salads and side dishes.
- Keep raw, cut-up vegetables handy for quick snacks. Choose colorful dark green, orange, and red vegetables, such as broccoli florets, carrots, and red peppers.
- Add beans (such as garbanzo, kidney, or pinto), lentils, and peas to salads, soups, and side dishes – or serve them as a main dish.
- Try unsalted nuts and seeds in place of some meats and poultry.

FOOD SOURCES OF DIETARY FIBER

Larger Portions and Smaller Portions

Dietary fiber: Nutrient-dense[a] Food and Beverage Sources, Amounts of Dietary Fiber and Energy per Standard Portion

DIETARY FIBER VALUE FOR LARGER PORTIONS

Table 8.1. Grains

Food[bc]	**Standard Portion**[d]	**Calories**	**Fiber (g)**
Ready-to-eat cereal, high fiber, unsweetened	1/2 cup	62	14
Ready-to-eat cereal, whole grain kernels	1/2 cup	209	7.5
Ready-to-eat cereal, wheat, shredded	1 cup	172	6.2
Popcorn	3 cups	169	5.8
Ready-to-eat cereal, bran flakes	3/4 cup	98	5.5
Bulgur, cooked	1/2 cup	76	4.1
Spelt, cooked	1/2 cup	123	3.8
Teff, cooked	1/2 cup	128	3.6
Barley, pearled, cooked	1/2 cup	97	3
Ready-to-eat cereal, toasted oat	1 cup	111	3
Oat bran	1/2 cup	44	2.9
Crackers, whole wheat	1 ounce	122	2.9
Chapati or roti, whole wheat	1 ounce	85	2.8
Tortillas, whole wheat	1 ounce	88	2.8

[a]All foods listed are assumed to be in nutrient-dense forms; lean or low-fat and prepared with minimal added sugars, saturated fat, or sodium.

[b]Some fortified foods and beverages are included. Other fortified options may exist on the market, but not all fortified foods are nutrient dense. For example, some foods with added sugars may be fortified and would not be examples in the lists provided here.

[c]Some foods or beverages are not appropriate for all ages, (e.g., nuts, popcorn), particularly young children for whom some foods could be a choking hazard.

[d]Portions listed are not recommended serving sizes. Two lists – in standard and smaller portions – are provided for each dietary component. Standard portions provide at least 2.8 g of dietary fiber. Smaller portions are generally one half of a standard portion.

*(**Source:** U.S. Department of Agriculture (USDA), Agricultural Research Service (ARS). FoodData Central (FDC), 2019.)*

Table 8.2. Vegetables

Food[bc]	Standard Portion[d]	Calories	Fiber (g)
Artichoke, cooked	1 cup	89	9.6
Navy beans, cooked	1/2 cup	128	9.6
Small white beans, cooked	1/2 cup	127	9.3
Yellow beans, cooked	1/2 cup	128	9.2
Lima beans, cooked	1 cup	209	9.2
Green peas, cooked	1 cup	134	8.8
Adzuki beans, cooked	1/2 cup	147	8.4
French beans, cooked	1/2 cup	114	8.3
Split peas, cooked	1/2 cup	116	8.2
Breadfruit, cooked	1 cup	170	8
Lentils, cooked	1/2 cup	115	7.8
Lupini beans, cooked	1/2 cup	115	7.8
Mung beans, cooked	1/2 cup	106	7.7
Black turtle beans, cooked	1/2 cup	120	7.7
Pinto beans, cooked	1/2 cup	123	7.7
Cranberry (roman) beans, cooked	1/2 cup	121	7.6
Black beans, cooked	1/2 cup	114	7.5
Fufu, cooked	1 cup	398	7.4
Pumpkin, canned	1 cup	83	7.1
Taro root (dasheen or yautia), cooked	1 cup	187	6.7
Brussels sprouts, cooked	1 cup	65	6.4
Chickpeas (garbanzo beans), cooked	1/2 cup	135	6.3
Sweet potato, cooked	1 cup	190	6.3
Great northern beans, cooked	1/2 cup	105	6.2

Table 8.2. Continued

Food[bc]	**Standard Portion**[d]	**Calories**	**Fiber (g)**
Parsnips, cooked	1 cup	110	6.2
Nettles, cooked	1 cup	37	6.1
Jicama, raw	1 cup	46	5.9
Winter squash, cooked	1 cup	76	5.7
Pigeon peas, cooked	1/2 cup	102	5.7
Kidney beans, cooked	1/2 cup	113	5.7
White beans, cooked	1/2 cup	125	5.7
Black-eyed peas, dried and cooked	1/2 cup	99	5.6
Cowpeas, dried and cooked	1/2 cup	99	5.6
Yam, cooked	1 cup	158	5.3
Broccoli, cooked	1 cup	54	5.2
Tree fern, cooked	1 cup	56	5.2
Luffa gourd, cooked	1 cup	100	5.2
Soybeans, cooked	1/2 cup	148	5.2
Turnip greens, cooked	1 cup	29	5
Drumstick pods (moringa), cooked	1 cup	42	5
Avocado	1/2 cup	120	5
Cauliflower, cooked	1 cup	34	4.9
Kohlrabi, raw	1 cup	36	4.9
Carrots, cooked	1 cup	54	4.8
Collard greens, cooked	1 cup	63	4.8
Kale, cooked	1 cup	43	4.7
Fava beans, cooked	1/2 cup	94	4.6
Chayote (mirliton), cooked	1 cup	38	4.5

Table 8.2. Continued

Food[bc]	Standard Portion[d]	Calories	Fiber (g)
Snow peas, cooked	1 cup	67	4.5
Pink beans, cooked	1/2 cup	126	4.5
Spinach, cooked	1 cup	41	4.3
Escarole, cooked	1 cup	22	4.2
Beet greens, cooked	1 cup	39	4.2
Salsify, cooked	1 cup	92	4.2
Cabbage, savoy, cooked	1 cup	35	4.1
Cabbage, red, cooked	1 cup	41	4.1
Wax beans, snap, cooked	1 cup	44	4.1
Edamame, cooked	1/2 cup	94	4.1
Okra, cooked	1 cup	36	4
Green beans, snap, cooked	1 cup	44	4
Hominy, canned	1 cup	115	4
Corn, cooked	1 cup	134	4
Potato, baked, with skin	1 medium	161	3.9
Lambsquarters, cooked	1 cup	58	3.8
Lotus root, cooked	1 cup	108	3.8
Swiss chard, cooked	1 cup	35	3.7
Mustard spinach, cooked	1 cup	29	3.6
Carrots, raw	1 cup	52	3.6
Hearts of palm, canned	1 cup	41	3.5
Mushrooms, cooked	1 cup	44	3.4
Bamboo shoots, raw	1 cup	41	3.3
Yardlong beans, cooked	1/2 cup	101	3.3

Table 8.2. Continued

Food[bc]	Standard Portion[d]	Calories	Fiber (g)
Turnip, cooked	1 cup	34	3.1
Red bell pepper, raw	1 cup	39	3.1
Rutabaga, cooked	1 cup	51	3.1
Plantains, cooked	1 cup	215	3.1
Nopales, cooked	1 cup	22	3
Dandelion greens, cooked	1 cup	35	3
Cassava (yucca), cooked	1 cup	267	3
Asparagus, cooked	1 cup	32	2.9
Taro leaves, cooked	1 cup	35	2.9
Onions, cooked	1 cup	92	2.9
Cabbage, cooked	1 cup	34	2.8
Mustard greens, cooked	1 cup	36	2.8
Beets, cooked	1 cup	49	2.8
Celeriac, raw	1 cup	66	2.8

[a]*All foods listed are assumed to be in nutrient-dense forms; lean or low-fat and prepared with minimal added sugars, saturated fat, or sodium.*
[b]*Some fortified foods and beverages are included. Other fortified options may exist on the market, but not all fortified foods are nutrient dense. For example, some foods with added sugars may be fortified and would not be examples in the lists provided here.*
[c]*Some foods or beverages are not appropriate for all ages, (e.g., nuts, popcorn), particularly young children for whom some foods could be a choking hazard.*
[d]*Portions listed are not recommended serving sizes. Two lists – in standard and smaller portions – are provided for each dietary component. Standard portions provide at least 2.8 g of dietary fiber. Smaller portions are generally one half of a standard portion.*
*(**Source:** U.S. Department of Agriculture (USDA), Agricultural Research Service (ARS). FoodData Central (FDC), 2019.).*

Table 8.3. Fruits

Food[bc]	Standard Portion[d]	Calories	Fiber (g)
Sapote or Sapodilla	1 cup	217	9.5
Durian	1 cup	357	9.2
Guava	1 cup	112	8.9
Nance	1 cup	82	8.4
Raspberries	1 cup	64	8
Loganberries	1 cup	81	7.8
Blackberries	1 cup	62	7.6
Soursop	1 cup	148	7.4
Boysenberries	1 cup	66	7
Gooseberries	1 cup	66	6.5
Pear, Asian	1 medium	75	6.5
Blueberries, wild	1 cup	80	6.2
Passionfruit	1/4 cup	57	6.1
Persimmon	1 fruit	118	6
Pear	1 medium	103	5.5
Kiwifruit	1 cup	110	5.4
Grapefruit	1 fruit	130	5
Apple, with skin	1 medium	104	4.8
Cherimoya	1 cup	120	4.8
Durian	1/2 cup	179	4.6
Starfruit	1 cup	41	3.7
Orange	1 medium	73	3.7
Figs, dried	1/4 cup	93	3.7
Blueberries	1 cup	84	3.6

Table 8.3. Continued

Food[bc]	Standard Portion[d]	Calories	Fiber (g)
Pomegranate seeds	1/2 cup	72	3.5
Mandarin orange	1 cup	103	3.5
Tangerine (tangelo)	1 cup	103	3.5
Pears, dried	1/4 cup	118	3.4
Peaches, dried	1/4 cup	96	3.3
Banana	1 medium	112	3.2
Apricots	1 cup	74	3.1
Prunes or dried plum	1/4 cup	105	3.1
Strawberries	1 cup	49	3
Dates	1/4 cup	104	3
Blueberries, dried	1/4 cup	127	3
Cherries	1 cup	87	2.9

[a]All foods listed are assumed to be in nutrient-dense forms; lean or low-fat and prepared with minimal added sugars, saturated fat, or sodium.
[b]Some fortified foods and beverages are included. Other fortified options may exist on the market, but not all fortified foods are nutrient dense. For example, some foods with added sugars may be fortified and would not be examples in the lists provided here.
[c]Some foods or beverages are not appropriate for all ages, (e.g., nuts, popcorn), particularly young children for whom some foods could be a choking hazard.
[d]Portions listed are not recommended serving sizes. Two lists – in standard and smaller portions – are provided for each dietary component. Standard portions provide at least 2.8 g of dietary fiber. Smaller portions are generally one half of a standard portion.
*(**Source:** U.S. Department of Agriculture (USDA), Agricultural Research Service (ARS). FoodData Central (FDC), 2019.)*

Table 8.4. Protein Foods

Food[bc]	Standard Portion[d]	Calories	Fiber (g)
Wocas, yellow pond lily seeds	1 ounce	102	5.4
Pumpkin seeds, whole	1 ounce	126	5.2

Table 8.4. Continued

Food[bc]	Standard Portion[d]	Calories	Fiber (g)
Coconut	1 ounce	187	4.6
Chia seeds	1 Tbsp	58	4.1
Almonds	1 ounce	164	3.5
Chestnuts	1 ounce	106	3.3
Sunflower seeds	1 ounce	165	3.1
Pine nuts	1 ounce	178	3
Pistachio nuts	1 ounce	162	2.9
Flax seeds	1 Tbsp	55	2.8
Hazelnuts (filberts)	1 ounce	178	2.8

[a]All foods listed are assumed to be in nutrient-dense forms; lean or low-fat and prepared with minimal added sugars, saturated fat, or sodium.

[b]Some fortified foods and beverages are included. Other fortified options may exist on the market, but not all fortified foods are nutrient dense. For example, some foods with added sugars may be fortified and would not be examples in the lists provided here.

[c]Some foods or beverages are not appropriate for all ages, (e.g., nuts, popcorn), particularly young children for whom some foods could be a choking hazard.

[d]Portions listed are not recommended serving sizes. Two lists – in standard and smaller portions – are provided for each dietary component. Standard portions provide at least 2.8 g of dietary fiber. Smaller portions are generally one half of a standard portion.

*(**Source:** Source: U.S. Department of Agriculture (USDA), Agricultural Research Service (ARS). FoodData Central (FDC), 2019.)*

DIETARY FIBER VALUE FOR SMALLER PORTIONS

Dietary Fiber: Nutrient-densea Food and Beverage Sources, Amounts of Dietary Fiber and Energy per Smaller Portion

Table 8.5. Value of Grains in Smaller Portions

Food[bc]	Standard Portion[d]	Calories	Fiber (g)
Ready-to-eat cereal, high fiber, unsweetened	1/4 cup	31	7
Ready-to-eat cereal, whole grain kernels	1/4 cup	105	3.8
Ready-to-eat cereal, wheat, shredded	1/2 cup	86	3.1
Bulgur, cooked	1/4 cup	38	2.1

Table 8.5. Continued

Food[bc]	Standard Portion[d]	Calories	Fiber (g)
Spelt, cooked	1/4 cup	62	1.9
Ready-to-eat cereal, bran flakes	1/4 cup	33	1.8
Teff, cooked	1/4 cup	64	1.8
Barley, pearled, cooked	1/4 cup	49	1.5
Ready-to-eat cereal, toasted oat	1/2 cup	56	1.5
Oat bran	1/4 cup	22	1.5
Crackers, whole wheat	1/2 ounce	61	1.5
Chapati or roti, whole wheat	1/2 ounce	43	1.4
Tortillas, whole wheat	1/2 ounce	44	1.4

[a]All foods listed are assumed to be in nutrient-dense forms; lean or low fat and prepared with minimal added sugars, saturated fat, or sodium.

[b]Some fortified foods and beverages are included. Other fortified options may exist on the market, but not all fortified foods are nutrient dense. For example, some foods with added sugars may be fortified and would not be examples in the lists provided here.

[c]Some foods or beverages are not appropriate for all ages, (e.g., nuts, popcorn), particularly young children for whom some foods could be a choking hazard.

[d]Portions listed are not recommended serving sizes. Two lists – in "standard" and "smaller" portions – are provided for each dietary component. Standard portions provide at least 2.8 g of dietary fiber. Smaller portions are generally one half of a standard portion.

*(**Source:** U.S. Department of Agriculture (USDA), Agricultural Research Service (ARS). FoodData Central (FDC), 2019.)*

Table 8.6. Value of Vegetables in Smaller Portions

Food[bc]	Standard Portion[d]	Calories	Fiber (g)
Artichoke, cooked	1/2 cup	45	4.8
Navy beans, cooked	1/4 cup	64	4.8
Small white beans, cooked	1/4 cup	64	4.7
Yellow beans, cooked	1/4 cup	64	4.6
Lima beans, cooked	1/2 cup	105	4.6
Green peas, cooked	1/2 cup	67	4.4
Adzuki beans, cooked	1/4 cup	74	4.2

Table 8.6. Continued

Food[bc]	Standard Portion[d]	Calories	Fiber (g)
French beans, cooked	1/4 cup	57	4.2
Split peas, cooked	1/4 cup	58	4.1
Breadfruit, cooked	1/2 cup	85	4
Lentils, cooked	1/4 cup	58	3.9
Lupini beans, cooked	1/4 cup	58	3.9
Mung beans, cooked	1/4 cup	53	3.9
Black turtle beans, cooked	1/4 cup	60	3.9
Pinto beans, cooked	1/4 cup	62	3.9
Cranberry (roman) beans, cooked	1/4 cup	61	3.8
Black beans, cooked	1/4 cup	57	3.8
Fufu, cooked	1/2 cup	199	3.7
Pumpkin, canned	1/2 cup	42	3.6
Taro root (dasheen or yautia), cooked	1/2 cup	94	3.4
Brussels sprouts, cooked	1/2 cup	33	3.2
Sweet potato, cooked	1/2 cup	95	3.2
Chickpeas (garbanzo beans), cooked	1/4 cup	68	3.2
Great northern beans, cooked	1/4 cup	53	3.1
Parsnips, cooked	1/2 cup	55	3.1
Nettles, cooked	1/2 cup	19	3.1
Jicama, raw	1/2 cup	23	3
Winter squash, cooked	1/2 cup	38	2.9
Pigeon peas, cooked	1/4 cup	51	2.9
Kidney beans, cooked	1/4 cup	57	2.9

Table 8.6. Continued

Food[bc]	Standard Portion[d]	Calories	Fiber (g)
White beans, cooked	1/4 cup	63	2.9
Cowpeas, dried and cooked	1/4 cup	50	2.8
Black-eyed peas, dried and cooked	1/4 cup	50	2.8
Yam, cooked	1/2 cup	79	2.7
Broccoli, cooked	1/2 cup	27	2.6
Tree fern, cooked	1/2 cup	28	2.6
Luffa gourd, cooked	1/2 cup	50	2.6
Soybeans, cooked	1/4 cup	74	2.6
Turnip greens, cooked	1/2 cup	15	2.5
Drumstick pods (moringa), cooked	1/2 cup	21	2.5
Avocado	1/4 cup	60	2.5
Cauliflower, cooked	1/2 cup	17	2.5
Kohlrabi, raw	1/2 cup	18	2.5
Kale, cooked	1/2 cup	22	2.4
Carrots, cooked	1/2 cup	27	2.4
Collard greens, cooked	1/2 cup	32	2.4
Fava beans, cooked	1/4 cup	47	2.3
Chayote (mirliton), cooked	1/2 cup	19	2.3
Snow peas, cooked	1/2 cup	34	2.3
Pink beans, cooked	1/4 cup	63	2.3
Spinach, cooked	1/2 cup	21	2.2
Escarole, cooked	1/2 cup	11	2.1
Beet greens, cooked	1/2 cup	20	2.1
Wax beans, snap, cooked	1/2 cup	22	2.1

Table 8.6. Continued

Food[bc]	Standard Portion[d]	Calories	Fiber (g)
Salsify, cooked	1/2 cup	46	2.1
Edamame, cooked	1/4 cup	47	2.1
Cabbage, savoy, cooked	1/2 cup	18	2.1
Cabbage, red, cooked	1/2 cup	21	2.1
Okra, cooked	1/2 cup	18	2
Green beans, snap, cooked	1/2 cup	22	2
Hominy, canned	1/2 cup	58	2
Corn, cooked	1/2 cup	67	2
Potato, baked, with skin	1/2 medium	81	2
Swiss chard, cooked	1/2 cup	18	1.9
Lambsquarters, cooked	1/2 cup	29	1.9
Lotus root, cooked	1/2 cup	54	1.9
Mustard spinach, cooked	1/2 cup	15	1.8
Carrots, raw	1/2 cup	26	1.8
Hearts of palm, canned	1/2 cup	21	1.8
Mushrooms, cooked	1/2 cup	22	1.7
Yardlong beans, cooked	1/4 cup	51	1.7
Bamboo shoots, raw	1/2 cup	21	1.7
Plantains, cooked	1/2 cup	108	1.6
Turnip, cooked	1/2 cup	17	1.6
Red bell pepper, raw	1/2 cup	20	1.6
Rutabaga, cooked	1/2 cup	26	1.6
Nopales, cooked	1/2 cup	11	1.5
Dandelion greens, cooked	1/2 cup	18	1.5

Table 8.6. Continued

Food[bc]	Standard Portion[d]	Calories	Fiber (g)
Cassava (yucca), cooked	1/2 cup	134	1.5
Asparagus, cooked	1/2 cup	16	1.5
Taro leaves, cooked	1/2 cup	18	1.5
Onions, cooked	1/2 cup	46	1.5
Cabbage, cooked	1/2 cup	17	1.4
Mustard greens, cooked	1/2 cup	18	1.4
Beets, cooked	1/2 cup	25	1.4
Celeriac, raw	1/2 cup	33	1.4

[a]All foods listed are assumed to be in nutrient-dense forms; lean or low fat and prepared with minimal added sugars, saturated fat, or sodium.
[b]Some fortified foods and beverages are included. Other fortified options may exist on the market, but not all fortified foods are nutrient dense. For example, some foods with added sugars may be fortified and would not be examples in the lists provided here.
[c]Some foods or beverages are not appropriate for all ages, (e.g., nuts, popcorn), particularly young children for whom some foods could be a choking hazard.
[d]Portions listed are not recommended serving sizes. Two lists – in "standard" and "smaller" portions – are provided for each dietary component. Standard portions provide at least 2.8 g of dietary fiber. Smaller portions are generally one half of a standard portion.
*(**Source:** U.S. Department of Agriculture (USDA), Agricultural Research Service (ARS). FoodData Central (FDC), 2019.)*

Table 8.7. Value of Fruits in Smaller Portions

Food[bc]	Standard Portiond	Calories	Fiber (g)
Sapote or Sapodilla	1/2 cup	109	4.8
Durian	1/2 cup	179	4.6
Guava	1/2 cup	56	4.5
Nance	1/2 cup	41	4.2
Raspberries	1/2 cup	32	4
Loganberries	1/2 cup	41	3.9
Blackberries	1/2 cup	31	3.8

Table 8.7. Continued

Food[bc]	Standard Portion[d]	Calories	Fiber (g)
Soursop	1/2 cup	74	3.7
Boysenberries	1/2 cup	33	3.5
Gooseberries	1/2 cup	33	3.3
Pear, Asian	1/2 medium	38	3.3
Passionfruit	1/8 cup	29	3.1
Blueberries, wild	1/2 cup	40	3.1
Persimmon	1/2 fruit	59	3
Pear	1/2 medium	52	2.8
Kiwifruit	1/2 cup	55	2.7
Grapefruit	1/2 fruit	65	2.5
Apple, with skin	1/2 medium	52	2.4
Cherimoya	1/2 cup	60	2.4
Durian	1/4 cup	90	2.3
Starfruit	1/2 cup	21	1.9
Figs, dried	1/8 cup	47	1.9
Orange	1/2 medium	37	1.9
Blueberries	1/2 cup	42	1.8
Mandarin orange	1/2 cup	52	1.8
Tangerine (tangelo)	1/2 cup	52	1.8
Pomegranate seeds	1/4 cup	36	1.8
Pears, dried	1/8 cup	59	1.7
Peaches, dried	1/8 cup	48	1.7
Banana	1/2 medium	56	1.6
Apricots	1/2 cup	37	1.6

Table 8.7. Continued

Food[bc]	Standard Portiond	Calories	Fiber (g)
Prunes or dried plum	1/8 cup	53	1.6
Strawberries	1/2 cup	25	1.5
Dates	1/8 cup	52	1.5
Blueberries, dried	1/8 cup	64	1.5
Cherries	1/2 cup	44	1.5

[a]All foods listed are assumed to be in nutrient-dense forms; lean or low fat and prepared with minimal added sugars, saturated fat, or sodium.
[b]Some fortified foods and beverages are included. Other fortified options may exist on the market, but not all fortified foods are nutrient dense. For example, some foods with added sugars may be fortified and would not be examples in the lists provided here.
[c]Some foods or beverages are not appropriate for all ages, (e.g., nuts, popcorn), particularly young children for whom some foods could be a choking hazard.
[d]Portions listed are not recommended serving sizes. Two lists – in "standard" and "smaller" portions – are provided for each dietary component. Standard portions provide at least 2.8 g of dietary fiber. Smaller portions are generally one half of a standard portion.
*(**Source:** U.S. Department of Agriculture (USDA), Agricultural Research Service (ARS). FoodData Central (FDC), 2019.)*

Table 8.8. Value of Vegetables in Smaller Portions

Food[bc]	Standard Portion[d]	Calories	Fiber (g)
Wocas, yellow pond lily seeds	1/2 ounce	51	2.7
Pumpkin seeds, whole	1/2 ounce	63	2.6
Coconut	1/2 ounce	94	2.3
Almonds	1/2 ounce	82	1.8
Chestnuts	1/2 ounce	53	1.7
Sunflower seeds	1/2 ounce	83	1.6
Pine nuts	1/2 ounce	89	1.5
Pistachio nuts	1/2 ounce	81	1.5
Chia seeds	1 teaspoon	19	1.4

Table 8.8. Continued

Food[bc]	Standard Portion[d]	Calories	Fiber (g)
Hazelnuts (filberts)	1/2 ounce	89	1.4
Flax seeds	1 teaspoon	18	0.9

[a]*All foods listed are assumed to be in nutrient-dense forms; lean or low fat and prepared with minimal added sugars, saturated fat, or sodium.*

[b]*Some fortified foods and beverages are included. Other fortified options may exist on the market, but not all fortified foods are nutrient dense. For example, some foods with added sugars may be fortified and would not be examples in the lists provided here.*

[c]*Some foods or beverages are not appropriate for all ages, (e.g., nuts, popcorn), particularly young children for whom some foods could be a choking hazard.*

[d]*Portions listed are not recommended serving sizes. Two lists – in "standard" and "smaller" portions – are provided for each dietary component. Standard portions provide at least 2.8 g of dietary fiber. Smaller portions are generally one half of a standard portion.*

*(**Source:** U.S. Department of Agriculture (USDA), Agricultural Research Service (ARS). FoodData Central (FDC), 2019.)*

Chapter 9 | **Fluids and Hydration**

Drinking enough water every day is good for overall health. As plain drinking water has zero calories, it can also help with managing body weight and reducing caloric intake when substituted for drinks with calories, such as regular soda. Drinking water can prevent dehydration, a condition that can cause unclear thinking, mood change, body overheat, constipation, and kidney stones.

WATER CONSUMPTION EVERYDAY FOR ADULTS AND YOUTH

- Daily fluid intake (total water) is defined as the amount of water consumed from foods, plain drinking water, and other beverages. Daily fluid intake recommendations vary by age, sex, pregnancy, and breastfeeding status.
- Although there is no recommendation for how much plain water adults and youth should drink daily, there are recommendations for daily total water intake that can be obtained from a variety of beverages and foods.
- Although daily fluid intake can come from food and beverages, plain drinking water is one good way of getting fluids as it has zero calories.

This chapter contains text excerpted from the following sources: Text in this chapter begins with excerpts from "Get the Facts: Drinking Water and Intake," Centers for Disease Control and Prevention (CDC), December 3, 2020; Text under the heading "Importance of Water" is excerpted from "Water and Healthier Drinks," Centers for Disease Control and Prevention (CDC), January 12, 2021.

PLAIN WATER CONSUMPTION

- In 2005–2010, United States youth drank an average of 15 ounces of water and in 2011–2014, United States adults drank an average of 39 ounces of water on a given day.
- Among U.S. youth, plain water intake is lower in younger children, non-Hispanic Black, Mexican American.
- Among U.S. adults, plain water intake is lower in older adults, lower-income adults, and those with lower education.
- U.S. adolescents who drink less water tended to drink less milk, eat fewer fruits and vegetables, drink more sugar-sweetened beverages, and get less physical activity.

IMPORTANCE OF WATER

Water helps your body:

- Keep a normal temperature
- Lubricate and cushion joints
- Protect your spinal cord and other sensitive tissues
- Get rid of wastes through urination, perspiration, and bowel movements

Your body needs more water when you are:

- In hot climates
- More physically active
- Running a fever
- Having diarrhea or vomiting

Most of your fluid needs are met through the water and beverages you drink. You can get some fluids through the foods that you eat – especially foods with high water content, such as many fruits and vegetables.

Chapter 10 | Vitamins

Chapter Contents

Section 10.1 | Vitamin A

This section contains text excerpted from the following sources: Text in this section begins with excerpts from "Vitamin A," MedlinePlus, National Institutes of Health (NIH), April 6, 2021; Text beginning with the heading "What Is Vitamin A and What Does It Do?" is excerpted from "Vitamin A," Office of Dietary Supplements (ODS), National Institutes of Health (NIH), January 14, 2021.

Vitamins are substances that your body needs to grow and develop normally. Vitamin A plays a role in your:

- Vision
- Bone growth
- Reproduction
- Cell functions
- Immune system

Vitamin A is an antioxidant. It can come from plant or animal sources. Plant sources include colorful fruits and vegetables. Animal sources include liver and whole milk. Vitamin A is also added to foods such as cereals.

Vegetarians, young children, and alcoholics may need extra Vitamin A. You might also need more if you have certain conditions, such as liver diseases, cystic fibrosis (CF), and Crohn disease. Check with your healthcare provider to see if you need to take vitamin A supplements.

WHAT IS VITAMIN A AND WHAT DOES IT DO?

Vitamin A is a fat-soluble vitamin that is naturally present in many foods. Vitamin A is important for normal vision, the immune system, and reproduction. Vitamin A also helps the heart, lungs, kidneys, and other organs work properly.

There are two different types of vitamin A. The first type, preformed vitamin A, is found in meat, poultry, fish, and dairy products. The second type, provitamin A, is found in fruits, vegetables, and other plant-based products. The most common type of provitamin A in foods and dietary supplements is beta-carotene.

HOW MUCH VITAMIN A DO YOU NEED?

The amount of vitamin A you need depends on your age and sex. Average daily recommended amounts are listed below in micrograms (mcg) of retinol activity equivalents (RAEs).

Table 10.1. Recommended Vitamin A Amounts

Life Stage	Recommended Amount
Birth to 6 months	400 mcg RAE
Infants 7–12 months	500 mcg RAE
Children 1–3 years	300 mcg RAE
Children 4–8 years	400 mcg RAE
Children 9–13 years	600 mcg RAE
Teen boys 14–18 years	900 mcg RAE
Teen girls 14–18 years	700 mcg RAE
Adult men	900 mcg RAE
Adult women	700 mcg RAE
Pregnant teens	750 mcg RAE
Pregnant women	770 mcg RAE
Breastfeeding teens	1,200 mcg RAE
Breastfeeding women	1,300 mcg RAE

WHAT FOODS PROVIDE VITAMIN A

Vitamin A is found naturally in many foods and is added to some foods, such as milk and cereal. You can get recommended amounts of vitamin A by eating a variety of foods, including the following:

- Beef liver and other organ meats (but these foods are also high in cholesterol, so limit the amount you eat)
- Some types of fish, such as salmon
- Green leafy vegetables and other green, orange, and yellow vegetables, such as broccoli, carrots, and squash
- Fruits, including cantaloupe, apricots, and mangoes

- Dairy products, which are among the major sources of vitamin A for Americans
- Fortified breakfast cereals

WHAT KINDS OF VITAMIN A DIETARY SUPPLEMENTS ARE AVAILABLE?

Vitamin A is available in dietary supplements, usually in the form of retinyl acetate or retinyl palmitate (preformed vitamin A), beta-carotene (provitamin A), or a combination of preformed and provitamin A. Most multivitamin-mineral supplements contain vitamin A. Dietary supplements that contain only vitamin A are also available.

ARE YOU GETTING ENOUGH VITAMIN A?

Most people in the United States get enough vitamin A from the foods they eat, and vitamin A deficiency is rare. However, certain groups of people are more likely than others to have trouble getting enough vitamin A:

- Premature infants, who often have low levels of vitamin A in their first year
- Infants, young children, pregnant women, and breastfeeding women in developing countries
- People with cystic fibrosis (CF)

WHAT HAPPENS IF YOU DO NOT GET ENOUGH VITAMIN A

Vitamin A deficiency is rare in the United States, although it is common in many developing countries. The most common symptom of vitamin A deficiency in young children and pregnant women is an eye condition called "xerophthalmia." Xerophthalmia is the inability to see in low light, and it can lead to blindness if it is not treated.

WHAT ARE SOME EFFECTS OF VITAMIN A ON HEALTH?

Scientists are studying vitamin A to understand how it affects health. Here are some examples of what this research has shown.

Cancer

People who eat a lot of foods containing beta-carotene might have a lower risk of certain kinds of cancer, such as lung cancer or prostate cancer. But, studies to date have not shown that vitamin A or beta-carotene supplements can help prevent cancer or lower the chances of dying from this disease. In fact, studies show that smokers who take high doses of beta-carotene supplements have an increased risk of lung cancer.

Age-Related Macular Degeneration

Age-related macular degeneration (AMD), or the loss of central vision as people age, is one of the most common causes of vision loss in older people. Among people with AMD who are at high risk of developing advanced AMD, a supplement containing antioxidants, zinc, and copper with or without beta-carotene has shown promise for slowing down the rate of vision loss.

Measles

When children with vitamin A deficiency (which is rare in North America) get measles, the disease tends to be more severe. In these children, taking supplements with high doses of vitamin A can shorten the fever and diarrhea caused by measles. These supplements can also lower the risk of death in children with measles who live in developing countries where vitamin A deficiency is common.

CAN VITAMIN A BE HARMFUL?

Yes, high intakes of some forms of vitamin A can be harmful.

Getting too much preformed vitamin A (usually from supplements or certain medicines) can cause dizziness, nausea, headaches, coma, and even death. High intakes of preformed vitamin A in pregnant women can also cause birth defects in their babies. Women who might be pregnant should not take high doses of vitamin A supplements.

Consuming high amounts of beta-carotene or other forms of provitamin A can turn the skin yellow-orange, but this condition is harmless. High intakes of beta-carotene do not cause birth defects

Table 10.2. Daily Upper Limits for Preformed Vitamin A

Ages	Upper Limit
Birth to 12 months	600 mcg
Children 1–3 years	600 mcg
Children 4–8 years	900 mcg
Children 9–13 years	1,700 mcg
Teens 14–18 years	2,800 mcg
Adults 19 years and older	3,000 mcg

or the other more serious effects caused by getting too much preformed vitamin A.

The daily upper limits for preformed vitamin A include intakes from all sources – food, beverages, and supplements – and are listed below. These levels do not apply to people who are taking vitamin A for medical reasons under the care of a doctor. Upper limits for beta-carotene and other forms of provitamin A have not been established.

DOES VITAMIN A INTERACT WITH MEDICATIONS OR OTHER DIETARY SUPPLEMENTS?

Yes, vitamin A supplements can interact or interfere with medicines you take. Here are several examples:

- Orlistat (Alli®, Xenical®), a weight-loss drug, can decrease the absorption of vitamin A, causing low blood levels in some people.
- Several synthetic forms of vitamin A are used in prescription medicines. Examples are the psoriasis treatment acitretin (Soriatane®) and bexarotene (Targretin®), used to treat the skin effects of T-cell lymphoma. Taking these medicines in combination with a vitamin A supplement can cause dangerously high levels of vitamin A in the blood.

Tell your doctor, pharmacist, and other healthcare providers about any dietary supplements and medicines you take. They can tell you if those dietary supplements might interact or interfere with your prescription or over-the-counter (OTC) medicines or if the medicines might interfere with how your body absorbs, uses, or breaks down nutrients.

Section 10.2 | Vitamin B

This section contains text excerpted from the following sources: Text under the heading "Thiamin" is excerpted from "Thiamin – Fact Sheet for Consumers," Office of Dietary Supplements (ODS), National Institutes of Health (NIH), March 22, 2021; Text under the heading "Riboflavin" is excerpted from "Riboflavin – Fact Sheet for Consumers," Office of Dietary Supplements (ODS), National Institutes of Health (NIH), January 13, 2021; Text under the heading "Vitamin B6" is excerpted from "Vitamin B6 – Fact Sheet for Consumers," Office of Dietary Supplements (ODS), National Institutes of Health (NIH), March 22, 2021; Text under the heading "Vitamin B12" is excerpted from "Vitamin B12 – Fact Sheet for Consumers," Office of Dietary Supplements (ODS), National Institutes of Health (NIH), January 15, 2021.

THIAMIN

What Is Thiamin and What Does It Do?

Thiamin (also called "vitamin B1") helps turn the food you eat into the energy you need. Thiamin is important for the growth, development, and function of the cells in your body.

How Much Thiamin Do You Need?

The amount of thiamin you need depends on your age and sex. Average daily recommended amounts are listed below in milligrams (mg).

What Foods Provide Thiamin?

Thiamin is found naturally in many foods and is added to some fortified foods. You can get recommended amounts of thiamin by eating a variety of foods, including the following:

- Whole grains and fortified bread, cereal, pasta, and rice
- Meat (especially pork) and fish

Table 10.3. Recommended Thiamin Amounts

Life Stage	Recommended Amount
Birth to 6 months	0.2 mg
Infants 7–12 months	0.3 mg
Children 1–3 years	0.5 mg
Children 4–8 years	0.6 mg
Children 9–13 years	0.9 mg
Teen boys 14–18 years	1.2 mg
Teen girls 14–18 years	1.0 mg
Men	1.2 mg
Women	1.1 mg
Pregnant teens and women	1.4 mg
Breastfeeding teens and women	1.4 mg

- Legumes (such as black beans and soybeans), seeds, and nuts

What Kinds of Thiamin Dietary Supplements Are Available?

Thiamin is found in multivitamin/multimineral supplements, in B-complex dietary supplements, and in supplements containing only thiamin. Common forms of thiamin in dietary supplements are thiamin mononitrate and thiamin hydrochloride. Some supplements use a synthetic form of thiamin called "benfotiamine."

Are You Getting Enough Thiamin?

Most people in the United States get enough thiamin from the foods they eat. Thiamin deficiency is rare in this country. However, certain groups of people are more likely than others to have trouble getting enough thiamin:

- People with alcohol dependence
- Older individuals

- People with HIV/AIDS
- People with diabetes
- People who have had bariatric surgery

Talk with your healthcare provider(s) about thiamin and other dietary supplements to help you determine which, if any, might be valuable for you.

What Happens If You Do Not Get Enough Thiamin

You can develop thiamin deficiency if you do not get enough thiamin in the foods you eat or if your body eliminates too much or absorbs too little thiamin.

Thiamin deficiency can cause loss of weight and appetite, confusion, memory loss, muscle weakness, and heart problems. Severe thiamin deficiency leads to a disease called "beriberi" with the added symptoms of tingling and numbness in the feet and hands, loss of muscle, and poor reflexes. Beriberi is not common in the United States and other developed countries.

A more common example of thiamin deficiency in the United States is Wernicke-Korsakoff syndrome, which mostly affects people with alcoholism. It causes tingling and numbness in the hands and feet, severe memory loss, disorientation, and confusion.

What Are Some Effects of Thiamin on Health?

Scientists are studying thiamin to better understand how it affects health. Here are some examples of what this research has shown.

DIABETES

People with diabetes often have low levels of thiamin in their blood. Scientists are studying whether thiamin supplements can improve blood sugar levels and glucose tolerance in people with type 2 diabetes. They are also studying whether benfotiamine (a synthetic form of thiamin) supplements can help with nerve damage caused by diabetes.

HEART FAILURE

Many people with heart failure have low levels of thiamin. Scientists are studying whether thiamin supplements might help people with heart failure.

ALZHEIMER DISEASE

Scientists are studying the possibility that thiamin deficiency could affect the dementia of Alzheimer disease (AD). Whether thiamin supplements may help mental function in people with AD needs further study.

Can Thiamin Be Harmful?

Thiamin has not been shown to cause any harm.

Are There Any Interactions with Thiamin That You Should Know About?

Yes. Some medicines can lower thiamin levels in the body. Here are a couple of examples:

- Furosemide (Lasix®), which is used to treat high blood pressure and swelling caused by excess fluid in the body
- Fluorouracil (5-fluorouracil and Adrucil®), which is used in chemotherapy treatments for some types of cancer

Tell your doctor, pharmacist, and other healthcare providers about any dietary supplements and prescription or over-the-counter (OTC) medicines you take. They can tell you if the dietary supplements might interact with your medicines or if the medicines might interfere with how your body absorbs, uses, or breaks down nutrients such as thiamin.

RIBOFLAVIN

What Is Riboflavin and What Does It Do?

Riboflavin (also called "vitamin B_2") is important for the growth, development, and function of the cells in your body. It also helps turn the food you eat into the energy you need.

Table 10.4. Recommended Riboflavin Amounts

Life Stage	Recommended Amount
Birth to 6 months	0.3 mg
Infants 7–12 months	0.4 mg
Children 1–3 years	0.5 mg
Children 4–8 years	0.6 mg
Children 9–13 years	0.9 mg
Teen boys 14–18 years	1.3 mg
Teen girls 14–18 years	1.0 mg
Men	1.3 mg
Women	1.1 mg
Pregnant teens and women	1.4 mg
Breastfeeding teens and women	1.6 mg

How Much Riboflavin Do You Need?

The amount of riboflavin you need depends on your age and sex. Average daily recommended amounts are listed below in milligrams (mg).

What Foods Provide Riboflavin

Riboflavin is found naturally in some foods and is added to many fortified foods. You can get recommended amounts of riboflavin by eating a variety of foods, including the following:

- Eggs, organ meats (such as kidneys and liver), lean meats, and low-fat milk
- Green vegetables (such as asparagus, broccoli, and spinach)
- Fortified cereals, bread, and grain products

What Kinds of Riboflavin Dietary Supplements Are Available?

Riboflavin is found in multivitamin/multimineral supplements, in B-complex dietary supplements, and in supplements containing only riboflavin. Some supplements have much more than the recommended amounts of riboflavin, but your body cannot absorb more than about 27 mg at a time.

Are You Getting Enough Riboflavin?

Most people in the U.S. get enough riboflavin from the foods they eat and deficiencies are very rare. However, certain groups of people are more likely than others to have trouble getting enough riboflavin:

- Athletes who are vegetarians (especially strict vegetarians who avoid dairy foods and eggs)
- Pregnant women and breastfeeding women and their babies
- People who are vegan
- People who do not eat dairy foods
- People with a genetic disorder called "riboflavin transporter deficiency." This disorder prevents the body from properly absorbing and using riboflavin, causing riboflavin deficiency.

What Happens If You Do Not Get Enough Riboflavin

You can develop riboflavin deficiency if you do not get enough riboflavin in the foods you eat, or if you have certain diseases or hormone disorders.

Riboflavin deficiency can cause skin disorders, sores at the corners of your mouth, swollen and cracked lips, hair loss, sore throat, liver disorders, and problems with your reproductive and nervous systems.

Severe, long-term riboflavin deficiency causes a shortage of red blood cells (anemia), which makes you feel weak and tired. It also causes clouding of the lens in your eyes (cataracts), which affects your vision.

What Is an Effect of Riboflavin Supplements on Health?

Scientists are studying riboflavin to better understand how it affects health. Here is an example of what this research has shown.

MIGRAINE HEADACHE

Some studies show that riboflavin supplements might help prevent migraine headaches, but other studies do not. Riboflavin supplements usually have very few side effects, so some medical experts recommend trying riboflavin, under the guidance of a healthcare provider, for preventing migraines.

Can Riboflavin Be Harmful?

Riboflavin has not been shown to cause any harm.

Does Riboflavin Interact with Medications or Other Dietary Supplements?

Riboflavin is not known to interact with any medications. But, it is always important to tell your doctor, pharmacist, and other healthcare providers about any dietary supplements and prescription or OTC medicines you take. They can tell you if the dietary supplements might interact with your medicines or if the medicines might interfere with how your body absorbs, uses, or breaks down nutrients.

VITAMIN B_6

What Is Vitamin B_6 and What Does It Do?

Vitamin B_6 is a vitamin that is naturally present in many foods. The body needs vitamin B_6 for more than 100 enzyme reactions involved in metabolism. Vitamin B_6 is also involved in brain development during pregnancy and infancy as well as immune function.

How Much Vitamin B_6 Do You Need?

The amount of vitamin B_6 you need depends on your age. Average daily recommended amounts are listed below in milligrams (mg).

What Foods Provide Vitamin B_6

Vitamin B_6 is found naturally in many foods and is added to other foods.

Table 10.5. Recommended Vitamin B_6 Amounts

Life Stage	Recommended Amount
Birth to 6 months	0.1 mg
Infants 7–12 months	0.3 mg
Children 1–3 years	0.5 mg
Children 4–8 years	0.6 mg
Children 9–13 years	1.0 mg
Teens 14–18 years (boys)	1.3 mg
Teens 14–18 years (girls)	1.2 mg
Adults 19–50 years	1.3 mg
Adults 51+ years (men)	1.7 mg
Adults 51+ years (women)	1.5 mg
Pregnant teens and women	1.9 mg
Breastfeeding teens and women	2 mg

You can get recommended amounts of vitamin B_6 by eating a variety of foods, including the following:

- Poultry, fish, and organ meats, all rich in vitamin B_6
- Potatoes and other starchy vegetables, which are some of the major sources of vitamin B_6 for Americans
- Fruit (other than citrus), which are also among the major sources of vitamin B_6 for Americans

What Kinds of Vitamin B_6 Dietary Supplements Are Available?

Vitamin B_6 is available in dietary supplements, usually in the form of pyridoxine. Most multivitamin-mineral supplements contain vitamin B_6. Dietary supplements that contain only vitamin B_6, or vitamin B_6 with other B vitamins, are also available.

Are You Getting Enough Vitamin B_6?

Most people in the U.S. get enough vitamin B_6 from the foods they eat. However, certain groups of people are more likely than others to have trouble getting enough vitamin B_6:

- People whose kidneys do not work properly, including people who are on kidney dialysis, and those who have had a kidney transplant
- People with autoimmune disorders, which cause their immune system to mistakenly attack their own healthy tissues. For example, people with rheumatoid arthritis, celiac disease, Crohn disease, ulcerative colitis, or inflammatory bowel disease sometimes have low vitamin B_6 levels.
- People with alcohol dependence

What Happens If You Do Not Get Enough Vitamin B_6

Vitamin B_6 deficiency is uncommon in the United States. People who do not get enough vitamin B_6 can have a range of symptoms, including anemia, itchy rashes, scaly skin on the lips, cracks at the corners of the mouth, and a swollen tongue. Other symptoms of very low vitamin B_6 levels include depression, confusion, and a weak immune system. Infants who do not get enough vitamin B_6 can become irritable or develop extremely sensitive hearing or seizures.

What Are Some Effects of Vitamin B_6 on Health?

Scientists are studying vitamin B_6 to understand how it affects health. Here are some examples of what this research has shown.

CARDIOVASCULAR DISEASE

Some scientists had thought that certain B vitamins (such as folic acid, vitamin B_{12}, and vitamin B_6) might reduce cardiovascular disease (CVD) risk by lowering levels of homocysteine, an amino acid in the blood. Although vitamin B supplements do lower blood homocysteine, research shows that they do not actually reduce the risk or severity of heart disease or stroke.

CANCER

People with low levels of vitamin B_6 in the blood might have a higher risk of certain kinds of cancer, such as colorectal cancer. But, studies to date have not shown that vitamin B_6 supplements can help prevent cancer or lower the chances of dying from this disease.

COGNITIVE FUNCTION

Some research indicates that elderly people who have higher blood levels of vitamin B_6 have better memory. However, taking vitamin B_6 supplements (alone or combined with vitamin B_{12} and/or folic acid) does not seem to improve cognitive function or mood in healthy people or in people with dementia.

PREMENSTRUAL SYNDROME

Scientists are not yet certain about the potential benefits of taking vitamin B_6 for premenstrual syndrome (PMS). But, some studies show that vitamin B_6 supplements could reduce PMS symptoms, including moodiness, irritability, forgetfulness, bloating, and anxiety.

NAUSEA AND VOMITING IN PREGNANCY

At least half of all women experience nausea, vomiting, or both in the first few months of pregnancy. Based on the results of several studies, the American Congress of Obstetricians and Gynecologists (ACOG) recommends taking vitamin B_6 supplements under a doctor's care for nausea and vomiting during pregnancy.

Can Vitamin B_6 Be Harmful?

People almost never get too much vitamin B_6 from food or beverages. But, taking high levels of vitamin B6 from supplements for a year or longer can cause severe nerve damage, leading people to lose control of their bodily movements. The symptoms usually stop when they stop taking the supplements. Other symptoms of too much vitamin B_6 include painful, unsightly skin patches, extreme sensitivity to sunlight, nausea, and heartburn.

Table 10.6. Daily Upper Limits for Vitamin B_6

Life Stage	**Upper Limit**
Birth to 12 months	Not established
Children 1–3 years	30 mg
Children 4–8 years	40 mg
Children 9–13 years	60 mg
Teens 14–18 years	80 mg
Adults	100 mg

The daily upper limits for vitamin B_6 include intakes from all sources – food, beverages, and supplements – and are listed below. These levels do not apply to people who are taking vitamin B_6 for medical reasons under the care of a doctor.

Does Vitamin B_6 Interact with Medications or Other Dietary Supplements?

Yes, vitamin B_6 supplements can interact or interfere with medicines that you take. Here are several examples:

- Vitamin B_6 supplements might interact with cycloserine (Seromycin®), an antibiotic used to treat tuberculosis, and worsen any seizures and nerve cell damage that the drug might cause.
- Taking certain epilepsy drugs could decrease vitamin B_6 levels and reduce the drugs' ability to control seizures.
- Taking theophylline (Aquaphyllin®, Elixophyllin®, Theolair®, Truxophyllin®, and many others) for asthma or another lung disease can reduce vitamin B_6 levels and cause seizures.

Tell your doctor, pharmacist, and other healthcare providers about any dietary supplements and medicines you take. They can tell you if those dietary supplements might interact or interfere with your prescription or OTC medicines or if the medicines might interfere with how your body absorbs, uses, or breaks down nutrients.

VITAMIN B_{12}

What Is Vitamin B_{12} and What Does It Do?

Vitamin B_{12} is a nutrient that helps keep the body's nerve and blood cells healthy and helps make DNA, the genetic material in all cells. Vitamin B_{12} also helps prevent a type of anemia called "megaloblastic anemia" that makes people tired and weak.

Two steps are required for the body to absorb vitamin B_{12} from food. First, hydrochloric acid in the stomach separates vitamin B_{12} from the protein to which vitamin B_{12} is attached in food. After this, vitamin B12 combines with a protein made by the stomach called "intrinsic factor" and is absorbed by the body. Some people have pernicious anemia, a condition in which they cannot make intrinsic factors. As a result, they have trouble absorbing vitamin B_{12} from all foods and dietary supplements.

How Much Vitamin B_{12} Do You Need?

The amount of vitamin B_{12} you need each day depends on your age. Average daily recommended amounts for different ages are listed below in micrograms (mcg):

What Foods Provide Vitamin B_{12}

Vitamin B_{12} is found naturally in a wide variety of animal foods and is added to some fortified foods. Plant foods have no vitamin B_{12} unless they are fortified. You can get recommended amounts of vitamin B_{12} by eating a variety of foods including the following:

- Beef liver and clams, which are the best sources of vitamin B_{12}
- Fish, meat, poultry, eggs, milk, and other dairy products, which also contain vitamin B_{12}
- Some breakfast cereals, nutritional yeasts, and other food products that are fortified with vitamin B_{12}. To find out if vitamin B_{12} has been added to a food product, check the product labels.

Table 10.7. Recommended Vitamin B_{12} Amounts

Life Stage	Recommended Amount
Birth to 6 months	0.4 mcg
Infants 7–12 months	0.5 mcg
Children 1–3 years	0.9 mcg
Children 4–8 years	1.2 mcg
Children 9–13 years	1.8 mcg
Teens 14–18 years	2.4 mcg
Adults	2.4 mcg
Pregnant teens and women	2.6 mcg
Breastfeeding teens and women	2.8 mcg

What Kinds of Vitamin B_{12} Dietary Supplements Are Available?

Vitamin B_{12} is found in almost all multivitamins. Dietary supplements that contain only vitamin B_{12}, or vitamin B_{12} with nutrients such as folic acid and other B vitamins, are also available. Check the Supplement Facts label to determine the amount of vitamin B_{12} provided.

Vitamin B_{12} is also available in sublingual forms (which are dissolved under the tongue). There is no evidence that sublingual forms are better absorbed than pills that are swallowed.

A prescription form of vitamin B_{12} can be administered as a shot. This is usually used to treat vitamin B_{12} deficiency. Vitamin B_{12} is also available as a prescription medication in a nasal gel form that is sprayed into the nose.

Are You Getting Enough Vitamin B_{12}?

Most people in the United States get enough vitamin B_{12} from the foods they eat. But, some people have trouble absorbing vitamin B_{12} from food. As a result, vitamin B_{12} deficiency affects between 1.5 percent and 15 percent of the public. Your doctor can test your vitamin B_{12} level to see if you have a deficiency.

Certain groups may not get enough vitamin B_{12} or have trouble absorbing it:

- Many older adults, who do not have enough hydrochloric acid in their stomach to absorb the vitamin B_{12} naturally present in food. People over 50 should get most of their vitamin B_{12} from fortified foods or dietary supplements because, in most cases, their bodies can absorb vitamin B_{12} from these sources.
- People with pernicious anemia whose bodies do not make the intrinsic factor needed to absorb vitamin B_{12}. Doctors usually treat pernicious anemia with vitamin B_{12} shots, although very high oral doses of vitamin B_{12} might also be effective.
- People who have had gastrointestinal surgery, such as weight loss surgery, or who have digestive disorders, such as celiac disease or Crohn disease. These conditions can decrease the amount of vitamin B_{12} that the body can absorb.
- Some people who eat little or no animal foods such as vegetarians and vegans. Only animal foods have vitamin B_{12} naturally. When pregnant women and women who breastfeed their babies are strict vegetarians or vegans, their babies might also not get enough vitamin B_{12}.

What Happens If You Do Not Get Enough Vitamin B_{12}

Vitamin B_{12} deficiency causes tiredness, weakness, constipation, loss of appetite, weight loss, and megaloblastic anemia. Nerve problems, such as numbness and tingling in the hands and feet, can also occur. Other symptoms of vitamin B_{12} deficiency include problems with balance, depression, confusion, dementia, poor memory, and soreness of the mouth or tongue. Vitamin B_{12} deficiency can damage the nervous system even in people who do not have anemia, so it is important to treat a deficiency as soon as possible.

In infants, signs of a vitamin B_{12} deficiency include failure to thrive, problems with movement, delays in reaching the typical developmental milestones, and megaloblastic anemia.

Large amounts of folic acid can hide a vitamin B_{12} deficiency by correcting megaloblastic anemia, a hallmark of vitamin B_{12} deficiency. But, folic acid does not correct the progressive damage to the nervous system that vitamin B_{12} deficiency also causes. For this reason, healthy adults should not get more than 1,000 mcg of folic acid a day.

What Are Some Effects of Vitamin B_{12} on Health?

Scientists are studying vitamin B_{12} to understand how it affects health. Here are several examples of what this research has shown:

HEART DISEASE

Vitamin B_{12} supplements (along with folic acid and vitamin B_6) do not reduce the risk of getting cardiovascular disease. Scientists had thought that these vitamins might be helpful because they reduce blood levels of homocysteine, a compound linked to an increased risk of having a heart attack or stroke.

DEMENTIA

As they get older, some people develop dementia. These people often have high levels of homocysteine in the blood. Vitamin B_{12} (with folic acid and vitamin B_6) can lower homocysteine levels, but scientists do not know yet whether these vitamins actually help prevent or treat dementia.

ENERGY AND ATHLETIC PERFORMANCE

Advertisements often promote vitamin B_{12} supplements as a way to increase energy or endurance. Except in people with a vitamin B_{12} deficiency, no evidence shows that vitamin B_{12} supplements increase energy or improve athletic performance.

Can Vitamin B_{12} Be Harmful?

Vitamin B_{12} has not been shown to cause any harm.

Does Vitamin B_{12} Interact with Medications or Other Dietary Supplements?

Yes. Vitamin B_{12} can interact or interfere with medicines that you take, and in some cases, medicines can lower vitamin B12 levels in the body. Here are several examples of medicines that can interfere with the body's absorption or use of vitamin B_{12}:

- Chloramphenicol (Chloromycetin®), an antibiotic that is used to treat certain infections
- Proton pump inhibitors, such as omeprazole (Prilosec®) and lansoprazole (Prevacid®), that are used to treat acid reflux and peptic ulcer disease
- Histamine H2 receptor antagonists, such as cimetidine (Tagamet®), famotidine (Pepcid®), and ranitidine (Zantac®), that are used to treat peptic ulcer disease
- Metformin, a drug used to treat diabetes

Tell your doctor, pharmacist, and other healthcare providers about any dietary supplements and medicines you take. They can tell you if those dietary supplements might interact or interfere with your prescription or over-the-counter medicines or if the medicines might interfere with how your body absorbs, uses, or breaks down nutrients.

Section 10.3 | **Vitamin C**

This section includes text excerpted from "Vitamin C – Fact Sheet for Consumers," Office of Dietary Supplements (ODS), National Institutes of Health (NIH), December 22, 2021.

WHAT IS VITAMIN C AND WHAT DOES IT DO?

Vitamin C, also known as "ascorbic acid," is a water-soluble nutrient found in some foods. In the body, it acts as an antioxidant, helping to protect cells from the damage caused by free radicals. Free radicals are compounds formed when our bodies convert the food we eat into energy. People are also exposed to free radicals in the environment from cigarette smoke, air pollution, and ultraviolet (UV) light from the sun.

The body also needs vitamin C to make collagen, a protein required to help heal wounds. In addition, vitamin C improves the absorption of iron from plant-based foods and helps the immune system work properly to protect the body from disease.

HOW MUCH VITAMIN C DO YOU NEED?

The amount of vitamin C you need each day depends on your age. Average daily recommended amounts for different ages are listed below in milligrams (mg).

If you smoke, add 35 mg to the above values to calculate your total daily recommended amount.

WHAT FOODS PROVIDE VITAMIN C

Fruits and vegetables are the best sources of vitamin C. You can get recommended amounts of vitamin C by eating a variety of foods including the following:

- Citrus fruits (such as oranges and grapefruit) and their juices, as well as red and green pepper and kiwifruit) which have a lot of vitamin C
- Other fruits and vegetables – such as broccoli, strawberries, cantaloupe, baked potatoes, and tomatoes – which also have vitamin C
- Some foods and beverages that are fortified with vitamin C. To find out if vitamin C has been added to a food product, check the product labels.

The vitamin C content of food may be reduced by prolonged storage and by cooking. Steaming or microwaving may lessen cooking losses. Fortunately, many of the best food sources of vitamin C, such as fruits and vegetables, are usually eaten raw.

WHAT KINDS OF VITAMIN C DIETARY SUPPLEMENTS ARE AVAILABLE?

Most multivitamins have vitamin C. Vitamin C is also available alone as a dietary supplement or in combination with other

Table 10.8. Recommended Vitamin C Amounts

Life Stage	Recommended Amount
Birth to 6 months	40 mg
Infants 7–12 months	50 mg
Children 1–3 years	15 mg
Children 4–8 years	25 mg
Children 9–13 years	45 mg
Teens 14–18 years (boys)	75 mg
Teens 14–18 years (girls)	65 mg
Adults (men)	90 mg
Adults (women)	75 mg
Pregnant teens	80 mg
Pregnant women	85 mg
Breastfeeding teens	115 mg
Breastfeeding women	120 mg

nutrients. The vitamin C in dietary supplements is usually in the form of ascorbic acid, but some supplements have other forms, such as sodium ascorbate, calcium ascorbate, other mineral ascorbates, and ascorbic acid with bioflavonoids. Research has not shown that any form of vitamin C is better than the other forms.

ARE YOU GETTING ENOUGH VITAMIN C?

Most people in the U.S. get enough vitamin C from foods and beverages. However, certain groups of people are more likely than others to have trouble getting enough vitamin C:

- People who smoke and those who are exposed to secondhand smoke. People who smoke will require an increased amount of vitamin C to repair the damage caused by free radicals. Hence, they need 35 mg more vitamin C per day than nonsmokers.

- Infants who are fed evaporated or boiled cow's milk, because cow's milk has very little vitamin C and heat can destroy vitamin C. Cow's milk is not recommended for infants under one year of age. Breast milk and infant formula have adequate amounts of vitamin C.
- People who eat a very limited variety of food
- People with certain medical conditions such as severe malabsorption, some types of cancer, and kidney disease requiring hemodialysis

WHAT HAPPENS IF YOU DO NOT GET ENOUGH VITAMIN C

Vitamin C deficiency is rare in the United States and Canada. People who get little or no vitamin C (below about 10 mg per day) for many weeks can get scurvy. Scurvy causes fatigue, inflammation of the gums, small red or purple spots on the skin, joint pain, poor wound healing, and corkscrew hairs. Additional signs of scurvy include depression as well as swollen, bleeding gums and loosening or loss of teeth. People with scurvy can also develop anemia. Scurvy is fatal if it is not treated.

WHAT ARE SOME EFFECTS OF VITAMIN C ON HEALTH?

Scientists are studying vitamin C to understand how it affects health. Here are several examples of what this research has shown.

Cancer Prevention and Treatment

People with high intakes of vitamin C from fruits and vegetables might have a lower risk of getting many types of cancer, such as lung, breast, and colon cancer. However, taking vitamin C supplements, with or without other antioxidants, does not seem to protect people from getting cancer.

It is not clear whether taking high doses of vitamin C is helpful as a treatment for cancer. Vitamin C's effects appear to depend on how it is administered to the patient. Oral doses of vitamin C cannot raise blood levels of vitamin C nearly as high as intravenous doses given through injections. A few studies in animals and test tubes indicate that very high blood levels of vitamin C might shrink tumors. But, more research is needed to determine whether high-dose intravenous vitamin C helps treat cancer in people.

Vitamin C dietary supplements and other antioxidants might interact with chemotherapy and radiation therapy for cancer. People being treated for cancer should talk with their oncologist before taking vitamin C or other antioxidant supplements, especially in high doses.

Cardiovascular Disease

People who eat lots of fruits and vegetables seem to have a lower risk of cardiovascular disease. Researchers believe that the antioxidant content of these foods might be partly responsible for this association because oxidative damage is a major cause of cardiovascular disease. However, scientists are not sure whether vitamin C itself, either from food or supplements, helps protect people from cardiovascular disease. It is also not clear whether vitamin C helps prevent cardiovascular disease from getting worse in people who already have it.

Age-Related Macular Degeneration and Cataracts

Age-related macular degeneration (AMD) and cataracts are two of the leading causes of vision loss in older people. Researchers do not believe that vitamin C and other antioxidants affect the risk of getting AMD. However, research suggests that vitamin C combined with other nutrients might help slow AMD progression.

In a large study among older people with AMD who were at high risk of developing advanced AMD, those who took a daily dietary supplement with 500 mg vitamin C, 80 mg zinc, 400 IU vitamin E, 15 mg beta-carotene, and 2 mg copper for about six years had a lower chance of developing advanced AMD. They also had less vision loss than those who did not take the dietary supplement. People who have or are developing the disease might want to talk with their doctor about taking dietary supplements.

The relationship between vitamin C and cataract formation is unclear. Some studies show that people who get more vitamin C from foods have a lower risk of getting cataracts. But, further research is needed to clarify this association and to determine whether vitamin C supplements affect the risk of getting cataracts.

The Common Cold

Although vitamin C has long been a popular remedy for the common cold, research shows that for most people, vitamin C supplements do not reduce the risk of getting the common cold. However, people who take vitamin C supplements regularly might have slightly shorter colds or somewhat milder symptoms when they do have a cold. Using vitamin C supplements after cold symptoms start does not appear to be helpful.

CAN VITAMIN C BE HARMFUL?

Taking too much vitamin C can cause diarrhea, nausea, and stomach cramps. In people with a condition called "hemochromatosis," which causes the body to store too much iron, high doses of vitamin C could worsen iron overload and damage body tissues.

The daily upper limits for vitamin C are listed below:

Table 10.9. Daily Upper Limits for Vitamin C

Life Stage	Upper Limit
Birth to 12 months	Not established
Children 1–3 years	400 mg
Children 4–8 years	650 mg
Children 9–13 years	1,200 mg
Teens 14–18 years	1,800 mg
Adults	2,000 mg

ARE THERE ANY INTERACTIONS WITH VITAMIN C THAT YOU SHOULD KNOW ABOUT?

Vitamin C dietary supplements can interact or interfere with medicines that you take. Here are several examples:

- Vitamin C dietary supplements might interact with cancer treatments, such as chemotherapy and radiation

therapy. It is not clear whether vitamin C might have the unwanted effect of protecting tumor cells from cancer treatments or whether it might help protect normal tissues from getting damaged. If you are being treated for cancer, check with your healthcare provider before taking vitamin C or other antioxidant supplements, especially in high doses.
- In one study, vitamin C plus other antioxidants (such as vitamin E, selenium, and beta-carotene) reduced the heart-protective effects of two drugs taken in combination (a statin and niacin) to control blood-cholesterol levels. It is not known whether this interaction also occurs with other statins. Healthcare providers should monitor lipid levels in people taking both statins and antioxidant supplements.

Tell your doctor, pharmacist, and other healthcare providers about any dietary supplements and medicines you take. They can tell you if those dietary supplements might interact or interfere with your prescription or over-the-counter (OTC) medicines or if the medicines might interfere with how your body absorbs, uses, or breaks down nutrients.

Section 10.4 | **Vitamin D**

This section includes text excerpted from "Vitamin D – Fact Sheet for Consumers," Office of Dietary Supplements (ODS), National Institutes of Health (NIH), March 22, 2021.

WHAT IS VITAMIN D AND WHAT DOES IT DO?

Vitamin D is a nutrient you need for good health. It helps your body absorb calcium, one of the main building blocks for strong bones. Together with calcium, vitamin D helps protect you from developing osteoporosis, a disease that thins and weakens the bones and makes them more likely to break. Your body needs vitamin D for other functions too. Your muscles need it to move, and your nerves need it to carry messages between your brain and your body. Your immune system needs vitamin D to fight off invading bacteria and viruses.

HOW MUCH VITAMIN D DO YOU NEED?

The amount of vitamin D you need each day depends on your age. Average daily recommended amounts are listed below in micrograms (mcg) and International Units (IUs):

Table 10.10. Average Daily Recommended Amounts of Vitamin D

Life Stage	Recommended Amount
Birth to 12 months	10 mcg (400 IU)
Children 1–13 years	15 mcg (600 IU)
Teens 14–18 years	15 mcg (600 IU)
Adults 19–70 years	15 mcg (600 IU)
Adults 71 years and older	20 mcg (800 IU)
Pregnant and breastfeeding teens and women	15 mcg (600 IU)

WHAT FOODS PROVIDE VITAMIN D

Very few foods naturally contain vitamin D. Fortified foods provide most of the vitamin D in the diets of people in the United States. Check the Nutrition Facts label for the amount of vitamin D in a food or beverage.

- Almost all of the Unites States milk supply is fortified with about 3 mcg (120 IU) vitamin D per cup. Many plant-based alternatives such as soy milk, almond milk, and oat milk are similarly fortified. But, foods made from milk, such as cheese and ice cream, are usually not fortified.
- Vitamin D is added to many breakfast cereals and to some brands of orange juice, yogurt, margarine, and other food products.
- Fatty fish (such as trout, salmon, tuna, and mackerel) and fish liver oils are among the best natural sources of vitamin D.

- Beef liver, cheese, and egg yolks have small amounts of vitamin D.
- Mushrooms provide a little vitamin D. Some mushrooms have been exposed to ultraviolet light to increase their vitamin D content.

CAN YOU GET VITAMIN D FROM THE SUN?

Your body makes vitamin D when your bare skin is exposed to the sun. Most people get at least some vitamin D this way. However, clouds, smog, old age, and having dark-colored skin reduce the amount of vitamin D your skin makes. Also, your skin does not make vitamin D from sunlight through a window.

Ultraviolet (UV) radiation from sunshine can cause skin cancer, so it is important to limit how much time you spend in the sun. Although sunscreen limits vitamin D production, health experts recommend using sunscreen with a sun protection factor (SPF) of 15 or more when you are out in the sun for more than a few minutes.

WHAT KINDS OF VITAMIN D DIETARY SUPPLEMENTS ARE AVAILABLE?

Vitamin D is found in multivitamin/multimineral supplements. It is also available in dietary supplements containing only vitamin D or vitamin D combined with a few other nutrients. The two forms of vitamin D in supplements are D2 (ergocalciferol) and D3 (cholecalciferol). Both forms increase vitamin D in your blood, but D3 might raise it higher and for longer than D2. Because vitamin D is fat soluble, it is best absorbed when taken with a meal or snack that includes some fat.

ARE YOU GETTING ENOUGH VITAMIN D?

Because you get vitamin D from food, sunshine, and dietary supplements, one way to know if you are getting enough is a blood test that measures the amount of vitamin D in your blood. In the blood, a form of vitamin D known as “25-hydroxyvitamin D” is measured in either nanomoles per liter (nmol/L) or nanograms per milliliter (ng/mL). One nmol/L is the same as 0.4 ng/mL.

- Levels of 50 nmol/L (20 ng/mL) or above are adequate for most people for bone and overall health.
- Levels below 30 nmol/L (12 ng/mL) are too low and might weaken your bones and affect your health.
- Levels above 125 nmol/L (50 ng/mL) are too high and might cause health problems.

In the United States most people have adequate blood levels of vitamin D. However, almost one out of four people have vitamin D blood levels that are too low or inadequate for bone and overall health.

Some people are more likely than others to have trouble getting enough vitamin D:

- **Breastfed infants.** Breast milk alone does not provide infants with an adequate amount of vitamin D. Breastfed infants should be given a supplement of 10 mcg (400 IU) of vitamin D each day.
- **Older adults.** As you age, your skin's ability to make vitamin D when exposed to sunlight declines.
- People who seldom expose their skin to sunshine because they do not go outside or because they keep their body and head covered. Sunscreen also limits the amount of vitamin D your skin produces.
- **People with dark skin.** The darker your skin, the less vitamin D you make from sunlight exposure.
- People with conditions that limit fat absorption, such as Crohn disease, celiac disease, or ulcerative colitis. This is because the vitamin D you consume is absorbed in the gut along with fat, so if your body has trouble absorbing fat, it will also have trouble absorbing vitamin D.
- People who are obese or have undergone gastric bypass surgery. They may need more vitamin D than other people.

WHAT HAPPENS IF YOU DO NOT GET ENOUGH VITAMIN D

In children, vitamin D deficiency causes rickets, a disease in which the bones become soft, weak, deformed, and painful. In teens and adults, vitamin D deficiency causes osteomalacia, a disorder that causes bone pain and muscle weakness.

WHAT ARE SOME EFFECTS OF VITAMIN D ON HEALTH?

Scientists are studying vitamin D to better understand how it affects health. Here are several examples of what this research has shown:

Bone Health and Osteoporosis

Long-term shortages of vitamin D and calcium cause your bones to become fragile and break more easily. This condition is called "osteoporosis." Millions of older women and men have osteoporosis or are at risk of developing this condition. Muscles are also important for healthy bones because they help maintain balance and prevent falls. A shortage of vitamin D may lead to weak, painful muscles.

Getting recommended amounts of vitamin D and calcium from foods (and supplements, if needed) will help maintain healthy bones and prevent osteoporosis. Taking vitamin D and calcium supplements slightly increases bone strength in older adults, but it is not clear whether they reduce the risk of falling or breaking a bone.

Cancer

Vitamin D does not seem to reduce the risk of developing cancer of the breast, colon, rectum, or lung. It is not clear whether vitamin D affects the risk of prostate cancer or chance of surviving this cancer. Very high blood levels of vitamin D may even increase the risk of pancreatic cancer.

Clinical trials suggest that while vitamin D supplements (with or without calcium) may not affect your risk of getting cancer, they might slightly reduce your risk of dying from this disease. More research is needed to better understand the role that vitamin D plays in cancer prevention and cancer-related death.

Heart Disease

Vitamin D is important for a healthy heart and blood vessels and for normal blood pressure. Some studies show that vitamin D supplements might help reduce blood cholesterol levels and high blood pressure – two of the main risk factors for heart disease. Other studies show no benefits. If you are a person with overweight or obesity, taking vitamin D at doses above 20 mcg (800 IU) per day plus calcium might actually raise your blood pressure. Overall, clinical trials found that vitamin D supplements do not reduce the risk of developing heart disease or dying from it, even if you have low blood levels of the vitamin.

Depression

Vitamin D is needed for your brain to function properly. Some studies have found links between low blood levels of vitamin D and an increased risk of depression. However, clinical trials show that taking vitamin D supplements does not prevent or ease symptoms of depression.

Multiple Sclerosis

People who live near the equator have more sun exposure and higher vitamin D levels. They also rarely develop multiple sclerosis (MS), a disease that affects the nerves that carry messages from the brain to the rest of the body. Many studies find a link between low blood vitamin D levels and the risk of developing MS. However, scientists have not actually studied whether vitamin D supplements can prevent MS. In people who have MS, clinical trials show that taking vitamin D supplements does not keep symptoms from getting worse or coming back.

Type 2 Diabetes

Vitamin D helps your body regulate blood sugar levels. However, clinical trials in people with and without diabetes show that supplemental vitamin D does not improve blood sugar levels, insulin resistance, or hemoglobin A1c levels (the average level of blood sugar over the past three months). Other studies show that vitamin

D supplements do not stop most people with prediabetes from developing diabetes.

Weight Loss

Taking vitamin D supplements or eating foods that are rich in vitamin D does not help you lose weight.

CAN VITAMIN D BE HARMFUL?

Yes, getting too much vitamin D can be harmful. Very high levels of vitamin D in your blood (greater than 375 nmol/L or 150 ng/mL) can cause nausea, vomiting, muscle weakness, confusion, pain, loss of appetite, dehydration, excessive urination and thirst, and kidney stones. Extremely high levels of vitamin D can cause kidney failure, irregular heartbeat, and even death. High levels of vitamin D are almost always caused by consuming excessive amounts of vitamin D from dietary supplements. You cannot get too much vitamin D from sunshine because your skin limits the amount of vitamin D it makes.

The daily upper limits for vitamin D are listed below in micrograms (mcg) and International Units (IU):

Table 10.11. Daily Upper Limits for Vitamin D

Ages	Upper Limit
Birth to 6 months	25 mcg (1,000 IU)
Infants 7–12 months	38 mcg (1,500 IU)
Children 1–3 years	63 mcg (2,500 IU)
Children 4–8 years	75 mcg (3,000 IU)
Children 9–18 years	100 mcg (4,000 IU)
Adults 19 years and older	100 mcg (4,000 IU)
Pregnant and breastfeeding teens and women	100 mcg (4,000 IU)

DOES VITAMIN D INTERACT WITH MEDICATIONS OR OTHER DIETARY SUPPLEMENTS?

Yes, vitamin D supplements may interact with some medicines. Here are several examples:

- Orlistat (Xenical® and alli®) is a weight-loss drug. It can reduce the amount of vitamin D your body absorbs from food and supplements.
- Cholesterol-lowering statins might not work as well if you take high-dose vitamin D supplements. This includes atorvastatin (Lipitor®), lovastatin (Altoprev® and Mevacor®), and simvastatin (FloLipid™ and Zocor®)
- Steroids such as prednisone (Deltasone®, Rayos®, and Sterapred®) can lower your blood levels of vitamin D.
- Thiazide diuretics (such as Hygroton®, Lozol®, and Microzide®) could raise your blood calcium level too high if you take vitamin D supplements.

Tell your doctor, pharmacist, and other healthcare providers about any dietary supplements and prescription or over-the-counter (OTC) medicines you take. They can tell you if the dietary supplements might interact with your medicines. They can also explain whether the medicines you take might interfere with how your body absorbs or uses other nutrients.

Section 10.5 | Vitamin E

This section includes text excerpted from "Vitamin E – Fact Sheet for Consumers," Office of Dietary Supplements (ODS), National Institutes of Health (NIH), March 22, 2021.

WHAT IS VITAMIN E AND WHAT DOES IT DO?

Vitamin E is a fat-soluble nutrient found in many foods. In the body, it acts as an antioxidant, helping to protect cells from the damage caused by free radicals. Free radicals are compounds formed when our bodies convert the food we eat into energy. People are also exposed to free radicals in the environment from cigarette smoke, air pollution, and ultraviolet (UV) light from the sun.

The body also needs vitamin E to boost its immune system so that it can fight off invading bacteria and viruses. It helps to widen blood vessels and keep blood from clotting within them. In addition, cells use vitamin E to interact with each other and to carry out many important functions.

HOW MUCH VITAMIN E DO YOU NEED?

The amount of vitamin E you need each day depends on your age. Average daily recommended amounts are listed below in milligrams (mg).

Table 10.12. Recommended Vitamin E Amounts

Life Stage	Recommended Amount
Birth to 6 months	4 mg
Infants 7–12 months	5 mg
Children 1–3 years	6 mg
Children 4–8 years	7 mg
Children 9–13 years	11 mg
Teens 14–18 years	15 mg
Adults	15 mg
Pregnant teens and women	15 mg
Breastfeeding teens and women	19 mg

WHAT FOODS PROVIDE VITAMIN E

Vitamin E is found naturally in foods and is added to some fortified foods. You can get recommended amounts of vitamin E by eating a variety of foods including the following:

- Vegetable oils such as wheat germ, sunflower, and safflower oils are among the best sources of vitamin E. Corn and soybean oils also provide some vitamin E.
- Nuts (such as peanuts, hazelnuts, and, especially, almonds) and seeds (such as sunflower seeds) are also among the best sources of vitamin E.

- Green vegetables, such as spinach and broccoli, provide some vitamin E.

Food companies add vitamin E to some breakfast cereals, fruit juices, margarines and spreads, and other foods. To find out which ones have vitamin E, check the product labels.

WHAT KINDS OF VITAMIN E DIETARY SUPPLEMENTS ARE AVAILABLE?

Vitamin E supplements come in different amounts and forms. Two main things to consider when choosing a vitamin E supplement are:

- **The amount of vitamin E.** Most once-daily multivitamin-mineral supplements provide about 13.5 mg of vitamin E, whereas vitamin E-only supplements commonly contain 67 mg or more. The doses in most vitamin E-only supplements are much higher than the recommended amounts. Some people take large doses because they believe or hope that doing so will keep them healthy or lower their risk of certain diseases.
- **The form of vitamin E.** Although vitamin E sounds like a single substance, it is actually the name of eight related compounds in food, including alpha-tocopherol. Each form has a different potency or level of activity in the body.

Vitamin E from natural sources is commonly listed as "d-alpha-tocopherol" on food packaging and supplement labels. Synthetic (laboratory-made) vitamin E is commonly listed as "dl-alpha-tocopherol." The natural form is more potent; 1 mg vitamin E = 1 mg d-alpha-tocopherol (natural vitamin E) = 2 mg dl-alpha-tocopherol (synthetic vitamin E).

Some food and dietary supplement labels still list vitamin E in International Units (IUs) rather than mg.

- 1 IU of the natural form of vitamin E is equivalent to 0.67 mg.
- 1 IU of the synthetic form of vitamin E is equivalent to 0.45 mg.

Some vitamin E supplements provide other forms of the vitamin, such as gamma-tocopherol, tocotrienols, and mixed tocopherols. Scientists do not know if any of these forms are superior to alpha-tocopherol in supplements.

ARE YOU GETTING ENOUGH VITAMIN E?

The diets of most Americans provide less than the recommended amounts of vitamin E. Nevertheless, healthy people rarely show any clear signs that they are not getting enough vitamin E.

WHAT HAPPENS IF YOU DO NOT GET ENOUGH VITAMIN E

Vitamin E deficiency is very rare in healthy people. It is almost always linked to certain diseases in which fat is not properly digested or absorbed. Examples include Crohn disease, cystic fibrosis (CF), and certain rare genetic diseases, such as abetalipoproteinemia and ataxia with vitamin E deficiency (AVED). Vitamin E needs some fat for the digestive system to absorb it.

Vitamin E deficiency can cause nerve and muscle damage that results in loss of feeling in the arms and legs, loss of body movement control, muscle weakness, and vision problems. Another sign of deficiency is a weakened immune system.

WHAT ARE SOME EFFECTS OF VITAMIN E ON HEALTH?

Scientists are studying vitamin E to understand how it affects health. Here are several examples of what this research has shown.

Heart Disease

Some studies link higher intakes of vitamin E from supplements to lower chances of developing coronary heart disease (CHD). But, the best research finds no benefit. People in these studies are randomly assigned to take vitamin E or a placebo (dummy pill with no vitamin E or active ingredients) and they do not know which they are taking. Vitamin E supplements do not seem to prevent heart disease, reduce its severity, or affect the risk of death from this disease. Scientists do not know whether high intakes of vitamin E might protect the heart in younger, healthier people who do not have a high risk of heart disease.

Cancer

Most research indicates that vitamin E does not help prevent cancer and may be harmful in some cases. Large doses of vitamin E have not consistently reduced the risk of colon and breast cancer in studies, for example. A large study found that taking vitamin E supplements (180 mg/day [400 IU]) for several years increased the risk of developing prostate cancer in men. Two studies that followed middle-aged men and women for 7 or more years found that extra vitamin E (201–268 mg/day [300–400 IU], on average) did not protect them from any form of cancer. However, one study found a link between the use of vitamin E supplements for 10 years or more and a lower risk of death from bladder cancer.

Vitamin E dietary supplements and other antioxidants might interact with chemotherapy and radiation therapy. People undergoing these treatments should talk with their doctor or oncologist before taking vitamin E or other antioxidant supplements, especially in high doses.

Eye Disorders

Age-related macular degeneration (AMD), or the loss of central vision in older people, and cataracts are among the most common causes of vision loss in older people. The results of research on whether vitamin E can help prevent these conditions are inconsistent. Among people with AMD who were at high risk of developing advanced AMD, a supplement containing large doses of vitamin E combined with other antioxidants, zinc, and copper showed promise for slowing down the rate of vision loss.

Mental Function

Several studies have investigated whether vitamin E supplements might help older adults remain mentally alert and active as well as prevent or slow the decline of mental function and Alzheimer disease (AD). So far, the research provides little evidence that taking vitamin E supplements can help healthy people or people with mild mental functioning problems to maintain brain health.

CAN VITAMIN E BE HARMFUL?

Vitamin E that is naturally present in food and beverages is not harmful and does not need to be limited.

In supplement form, however, high doses of vitamin E might increase the risk of bleeding (by reducing the blood's ability to form clots after a cut or injury) and of serious bleeding in the brain (known as "hemorrhagic stroke"). Because of this risk, the upper limit for adults is 1,000 mg/day for supplements of either natural or synthetic vitamin E. This is equal to 1,500 IU/day for natural vitamin E supplements and 1,100 IU/day for synthetic vitamin E supplements. The upper limits for children are lower than those for adults. Some research suggests that taking vitamin E supplements even below these upper limits might cause harm. In one study, for example, men who took 400 IU (180 mg) of synthetic vitamin E each day for several years had an increased risk of prostate cancer.

ARE THERE ANY INTERACTIONS WITH VITAMIN E THAT YOU SHOULD KNOW ABOUT?

Vitamin E dietary supplements can interact or interfere with certain medicines that you take. Here are some examples:

- Vitamin E can increase the risk of bleeding in people taking anticoagulant or antiplatelet medicines, such as warfarin (Coumadin®).
- In one study, vitamin E plus other antioxidants (such as vitamin C, selenium, and beta-carotene) reduced the heart-protective effects of two drugs taken in combination (a statin and niacin) to affect blood cholesterol levels.
- Taking antioxidant supplements while undergoing chemotherapy or radiation therapy for cancer could alter the effectiveness of these treatments.

Tell your doctor, pharmacist, and other healthcare providers about any dietary supplements and medicines you take. They can tell you if those dietary supplements might interact or interfere with your prescription or over-the-counter (OTC) medicines, or if the medicines might interfere with how your body absorbs, uses, or breaks down nutrients.

Section 10.6 | Vitamin K

This section includes text excerpted from "Vitamin K – Fact Sheet for Consumers," Office of Dietary Supplements (ODS), National Institutes of Health (NIH), March 22, 2021.

WHAT IS VITAMIN K AND WHAT DOES IT DO?

Vitamin K is a nutrient that the body needs to stay healthy. It is important for blood clotting and healthy bones and also has other functions in the body. If you are taking a blood thinner such as warfarin (Coumadin®), it is very important to get about the same amount of vitamin K each day.

HOW MUCH VITAMIN K DO YOU NEED?

The amount of vitamin K you need depends on your age and sex. Average daily recommended amounts are listed below in micrograms (mcg).

Table 10.13. Recommended Vitamin K Amounts

Life Stage	Recommended Amount
Birth to 6 months	2 mcg
7–12 months	2.5 mcg
1–3 years	30 mcg
4–8 years	55 mcg
9–13 years	60 mcg
14–18 years	75 mcg
Adult men 19 years and older	120 mcg

Table 10.13. Continued

Life Stage	Recommended Amount
Adult women 19 years and older	90 mcg
Pregnant or breastfeeding teens	75 mcg
Pregnant or breastfeeding women	90 mcg

WHAT FOODS PROVIDE VITAMIN K

Vitamin K is found naturally in many foods. You can get recommended amounts of vitamin K by eating a variety of foods, including the following:

- Green leafy vegetables, such as spinach, kale, broccoli, and lettuce
- Vegetable oils
- Some fruits, such as blueberries and figs
- Meat, cheese, eggs, and soybeans

WHAT KINDS OF VITAMIN K DIETARY SUPPLEMENTS ARE AVAILABLE?

Vitamin K is found in multivitamin/multimineral supplements. Vitamin K is also available in supplements of vitamin K alone or of vitamin K with a few other nutrients such as calcium, magnesium, and/or vitamin D. Common forms of vitamin K in dietary supplements are phylloquinone and phytonadione (also called "vitamin K1"), menaquinone-4, and menaquinone-7 (also called "vitamin K2").

ARE YOU GETTING ENOUGH VITAMIN K?

Vitamin K deficiency is very rare. Most people in the U.S. get enough vitamin K from the foods they eat. Also, bacteria in the colon make some vitamin K that the body can absorb. However, certain groups of people may have trouble getting enough vitamin K:

- Newborns who do not receive an injection of vitamin K at birth

- People with conditions (such as cystic fibrosis (CF), celiac disease, ulcerative colitis, and short bowel syndrome) that decrease the amount of vitamin K their body absorbs
- People who have had bariatric (weight loss) surgery

WHAT HAPPENS IF YOU DO NOT GET ENOUGH VITAMIN K

Severe vitamin K deficiency can cause bruising and bleeding problems because the blood will take longer to clot. Vitamin K deficiency might reduce bone strength and increase the risk of getting osteoporosis because the body needs vitamin K for healthy bones.

WHAT ARE SOME EFFECTS OF VITAMIN K ON HEALTH?

Scientists are studying vitamin K to understand how it affects our health. Here are some examples of what this research has shown.

Osteoporosis

Vitamin K is important for healthy bones. Some research shows that people who eat more vitamin K-rich foods have stronger bones and are less likely to break a hip than those who eat less of these foods. A few studies have found that taking vitamin K supplements improves bone strength and the chances of breaking a bone, but other studies have not. More research is needed to better understand if vitamin K supplements can help improve bone health and reduce osteoporosis risk.

Coronary Heart Disease

Scientists are studying whether low blood levels of vitamin K increase the risk of coronary heart disease (CHD), perhaps by making blood vessels that feed the heart stiffer and narrower. More research is needed to understand whether vitamin K supplements might help prevent heart disease.

CAN VITAMIN K BE HARMFUL?

Vitamin K has not been shown to cause any harm. However, it can interact with some medications, particularly warfarin (Coumadin®).

ARE THERE ANY INTERACTIONS WITH VITAMIN K THAT YOU SHOULD KNOW ABOUT?

Yes, some medications may interact with vitamin K. Here are a few examples:

Warfarin (Coumadin®)

Vitamin K can have a serious interaction with the blood thinner warfarin (Coumadin®). If you take warfarin, make sure that the amount of vitamin K you consume from food and supplements is about the same every day. A sudden change in the amount of vitamin K you get can cause dangerous bleeding (if you consume less) or blood clots (if you consume more).

Antibiotics

Antibiotics can destroy the good bacteria in your gut. Some of these bacteria make vitamin K. Using antibiotics for more than a few weeks may reduce the amount of vitamin K made in your gut and therefore, the amount available for your body to use.

Bile Acid Sequestrants

Some people take bile acid sequestrants (such as cholestyramine [Questran®] and colestipol [Colestid®]) to lower blood cholesterol levels. These medications can reduce the amount of vitamin K your body absorbs, especially if you take them for many years.

Orlistat

Orlistat (Alli® and Xenical®) is a weight-loss drug. It reduces the amount of fat your body absorbs and can decrease the absorption of vitamin K.

Tell your doctor, pharmacist, and other healthcare providers about any dietary supplements and prescription or over-the-counter (OTC) medicines you take. They can tell you if the dietary supplements might interact with your medicines or if the medicines might interfere with how your body absorbs, uses, or breaks down nutrients such as vitamin K.

Chapter 11 | Minerals

Chapter Contents

Section 11.1 | Calcium

This section includes text excerpted from "Calcium," Office of Dietary Supplements (ODS), National Institutes of Health (NIH), March 22, 2021.

WHAT IS CALCIUM AND WHAT DOES IT DO?

Calcium is a mineral found in many foods. The body needs calcium to maintain strong bones and to carry out many important functions. Almost all calcium is stored in bones and teeth, where it supports their structure and hardness.

The body also needs calcium for muscles to move and for nerves to carry messages between the brain and every body part. In addition, calcium is used to help blood vessels move blood throughout the body and to help release hormones and enzymes that affect almost every function in the human body.

HOW MUCH CALCIUM DO YOU NEED?

The amount of calcium you need each day depends on your age. Average daily recommended amounts are listed below in milligrams (mg):

Table 11.1. Amount of Calcium Recommended

Life Stage	Recommended Amount
Birth to 6 months	200 mg
Infants 7–12 months	260 mg
Children 1–3 years	700 mg
Children 4–8 years	1,000 mg
Children 9–13 years	1,300 mg
Teens 14–18 years	1,300 mg
Adults 19–50 years	1,000 mg
Adult men 51–70 years	1,000 mg

Table 11.1. Continued

Life Stage	Recommended Amount
Adult women 51–70 years	1,200 mg
Adults 71 years and older	1,200 mg
Pregnant and breastfeeding teens	1,300 mg
Pregnant and breastfeeding adults	1,000 mg

WHAT FOODS PROVIDE CALCIUM

Calcium is found in many foods. You can get recommended amounts of calcium by eating a variety of foods, including the following:

- Milk, yogurt, and cheese are the main food sources of calcium for the majority of people in the United States.
- Kale, broccoli, and Chinese cabbage are fine vegetable sources of calcium.
- Fish with soft bones that you eat, such as canned sardines and salmon, are fine animal sources of calcium.
- Most grains (such as breads, pastas, and unfortified cereals), while not rich in calcium, add significant amounts of calcium to the diet because people eat them often or in large amounts.
- Calcium is added to some breakfast cereals, fruit juices, soy and rice beverages, and tofu. To find out whether these foods have calcium, check the product labels.

WHAT KINDS OF CALCIUM DIETARY SUPPLEMENTS ARE AVAILABLE?

Calcium is found in many multivitamin-mineral supplements, though the amount varies by product. Dietary supplements that contain only calcium or calcium with other nutrients such as vitamin D are also available. Check the Supplement Facts label to determine the amount of calcium provided.

The two main forms of calcium dietary supplements are carbonate and citrate. Calcium carbonate is inexpensive, but is absorbed best when taken with food. Some over-the-counter antacid products, such as Tums® and Rolaids®, contain calcium carbonate. Each pill or chew provides 200–400 mg of calcium. Calcium citrate, a more expensive form of the supplement, is absorbed well on an empty or a full stomach. In addition, people with low levels of stomach acid (a condition more common in people older than 50) absorb calcium citrate more easily than calcium carbonate. Other forms of calcium in supplements and fortified foods include gluconate, lactate, and phosphate.

Calcium absorption is best when a person consumes no more than 500 mg at one time. So a person who takes 1,000 mg/day of calcium from supplements, for example, should split the dose rather than take it all at once.

Calcium supplements may cause gas, bloating, and constipation in some people. If any of these symptoms occur, try spreading out the calcium dose throughout the day, taking the supplement with meals, or changing the supplement brand or calcium form you take.

ARE YOU GETTING ENOUGH CALCIUM?

Many people do not get recommended amounts of calcium from the foods they eat, including:

- Boys aged 9 to 13 years
- Girls aged 9 to 18 years
- Women older than 50 years
- Men older than 70 years

When total intakes from both food and supplements are considered, many people – particularly adolescent girls – still fall short of getting enough calcium, while some older women likely get more than the upper limit.

Certain groups of people are more likely than others to have trouble getting enough calcium:

- Postmenopausal women because they experience greater bone loss and do not absorb calcium as well.

Sufficient calcium intake from food, and supplements if needed, can slow the rate of bone loss.

- Women of childbearing age whose menstrual periods stop (amenorrhea) because they exercise heavily, eat too little, or both. They need sufficient calcium to cope with the resulting decreased calcium absorption, increased calcium losses in the urine, and slowdown in the formation of new bone.
- People with lactose intolerance cannot digest this natural sugar found in milk and experience symptoms like bloating, gas, and diarrhea when they drink more than small amounts at a time. They usually can eat other calcium-rich dairy products that are low in lactose, such as yogurt and many cheeses, and drink lactose-reduced or lactose-free milk.
- Vegans (vegetarians who eat no animal products) and ovo-vegetarians (vegetarians who eat eggs, but no dairy products), because they avoid the dairy products that are a major source of calcium in other people's diets.

Many factors can affect the amount of calcium absorbed from the digestive tract, including:

- **Age.** The efficiency of calcium absorption decreases as people age. Recommended calcium intakes are higher for people over age 70.
- **Vitamin D intake.** This vitamin, present in some foods and produced in the body when skin is exposed to sunlight, increases calcium absorption.
- **Other components in food.** Both oxalic acid (in some vegetables and beans) and phytic acid (in whole grains) can reduce calcium absorption. People who eat a variety of foods do not have to consider these factors. They are accounted for in the calcium recommended intakes, which take absorption into account.
- **Many factors can also affect how much calcium the body eliminates in urine, feces, and sweat.** These include consumption of alcohol- and caffeine-containing beverages as well as intake of other nutrients

(protein, sodium, potassium, and phosphorus). In most people, these factors have little effect on calcium status.

WHAT HAPPENS IF YOU DO NOT GET ENOUGH CALCIUM

Insufficient intakes of calcium do not produce obvious symptoms in the short term because the body maintains calcium levels in the blood by taking it from the bone. Over the long term, intakes of calcium below recommended levels have health consequences, such as causing low bone mass (osteopenia) and increasing the risks of osteoporosis and bone fractures.

Symptoms of serious calcium deficiency include numbness and tingling in the fingers, convulsions, and abnormal heart rhythms that can lead to death if not corrected. These symptoms occur almost always in people with serious health problems or who are undergoing certain medical treatments.

WHAT ARE SOME EFFECTS OF CALCIUM ON HEALTH?

Scientists are studying calcium to understand how it affects health. Here are several examples of what this research has shown:

Bone Health and Osteoporosis

Bones need plenty of calcium and vitamin D throughout childhood and adolescence to reach their peak strength and calcium content by about age 30. After that, bones slowly lose calcium, but people can help reduce these losses by getting recommended amounts of calcium throughout adulthood and by having a healthy, active lifestyle that includes weight-bearing physical activity (such as walking and running).

Osteoporosis is a disease of the bones in older adults (especially women) in which the bones become porous, fragile, and more prone to fracture. Osteoporosis is a serious public-health problem for more than 10 million adults over the age of 50 in the United States. Adequate calcium and vitamin D intakes, as well as regular exercise, are essential to keep bones healthy throughout life.

Taking calcium and vitamin D supplements reduces the risk of breaking a bone and the risk of falling in frail, elderly adults who live in nursing homes and similar facilities. But, it is not clear if the supplements help prevent bone fractures and falls in older people who live at home.

Cancer

Studies have examined whether calcium supplements or diets high in calcium might lower the risks of developing cancer of the colon or rectum or increase the risk of prostate cancer. The research to date provides no clear answers. Given that cancer develops over many years, longer term studies are needed.

Cardiovascular Disease

Some studies show that getting enough calcium might decrease the risk of cardiovascular disease and stroke. Other studies find that high amounts of calcium, particularly from supplements, might increase the risk of heart disease. But, when all the studies are considered together, scientists have concluded that as long as intakes are not above the upper limit, calcium from food or supplements will not increase or decrease the risk of having a heart attack or stroke.

High Blood Pressure

Some studies have found that getting recommended intakes of calcium can reduce the risk of developing high blood pressure (hypertension). One large study, in particular, found that eating a diet high in fat-free and low-fat dairy products, vegetables, and fruits lowered blood pressure.

Preeclampsia

Preeclampsia is a serious medical condition in which a pregnant woman develops high blood pressure and kidney problems that cause protein to spill into the urine. It is a leading cause of sickness and death in pregnant women and their newborn babies. For women who get less than about 900 mg of calcium a day, taking calcium supplements during pregnancy (1,000 mg a day or more) reduces the risk of preeclampsia. But, most women in the United States who become pregnant get enough calcium from their diets.

Kidney Stones

Most kidney stones are rich in calcium oxalate. Some studies have found that higher intakes of calcium from dietary supplements are linked to a greater risk of kidney stones, especially among older adults. But, calcium from foods does not appear to cause kidney stones. For most people, other factors (such as not drinking enough fluids) probably have a larger effect on the risk of kidney stones than calcium intake.

Weight Loss

Although several studies have shown that getting more calcium helps lower body weight or reduce weight gain over time, most studies have found that calcium – from foods or dietary supplements – has little if any effect on body weight and amount of body fat.

CAN CALCIUM BE HARMFUL?

Getting too much calcium can cause constipation. It might also interfere with the body's ability to absorb iron and zinc, but this effect is not well established. In adults, too much calcium (from dietary supplements, but not food) might increase the risk of kidney stones. Some studies show that people who consume high amounts of calcium might have increased risks of prostate cancer and heart disease, but more research is needed to understand these possible links.

Most people do not get amounts above the upper limits from food alone; excess intakes usually come from the use of calcium supplements. Surveys show that some older women in the United States probably get amounts somewhat above the upper limit since the use of calcium supplements is common among these women.

The daily upper limits for calcium are listed below in milligrams (mg).

Table 11.2. Daily Upper Limits for Calcium

Life Stage	Upper Limit
Birth to 6 months	1,000 mg
Infants 7–12 months	1,500 mg
Children 1–8 years	2,500 mg
Children 9–18 years	3,000 mg
Adults 19–50 years	2,500 mg
Adults 51 years and older	2,000 mg
Pregnant and breastfeeding teens	3,000 mg
Pregnant and breastfeeding adults	2,500 mg

ARE THERE ANY INTERACTIONS WITH CALCIUM THAT YOU SHOULD KNOW ABOUT?

Calcium dietary supplements can interact or interfere with certain medicines that you take, and some medicines can lower or raise calcium levels in the body. Here are some examples:

- Calcium can reduce the absorption of these drugs when taken together:
  - Bisphosphonates (to treat osteoporosis)
  - Antibiotics of the fluoroquinolone and tetracycline families
  - Levothyroxine (to treat low thyroid activity)
  - Phenytoin (an anticonvulsant)
  - Tiludronate disodium (to treat Paget disease)
- Diuretics differ in their effects. Thiazide-type diuretics (such as Diuril® and Lozol®) reduce calcium excretion by the kidneys which in turn can raise blood calcium levels too high. But, loop diuretics (such as Lasix® and Bumex®) increase calcium excretion and thereby lower blood calcium levels.
- Antacids containing aluminum or magnesium increase calcium loss in the urine.

- Mineral oil and stimulant laxatives reduce calcium absorption.
- Glucocorticoids (such as prednisone) can cause calcium depletion and eventually osteoporosis when people use them for months at a time.

Tell your doctor, pharmacist, and other healthcare providers about any dietary supplements and medicines you take. They can tell you if those dietary supplements might interact or interfere with your prescription or over-the-counter medicines or if the medicines might interfere with how your body absorbs, uses, or breaks down nutrients.

CALCIUM AND HEALTHFUL EATING

People should get most of their nutrients from food and beverages, according to the federal government's *Dietary Guidelines for Americans 2020-2025*. Foods contain vitamins, minerals, dietary fiber, and other components that benefit health. In some cases, fortified foods and dietary supplements are useful when it is not possible to meet needs for one or more nutrients (e.g., during specific life stages such as pregnancy).

Section 11.2 | **Iron**

This section includes text excerpted from "Iron," Office of Dietary Supplements (ODS), National Institutes of Health (NIH), March 22, 2021.

WHAT IS IRON AND WHAT DOES IT DO?

Iron is a mineral that the body needs for growth and development. Your body uses iron to make hemoglobin, a protein in red blood cells that carries oxygen from the lungs to all parts of the body, and myoglobin, a protein that provides oxygen to muscles. Your body also needs iron to make some hormones.

HOW MUCH IRON DO YOU NEED?

The amount of iron you need each day depends on your age, your sex, and whether you consume a mostly plant-based diet. Average daily recommended amounts are listed below in milligrams (mg). Vegetarians who do not eat meat, poultry, or seafood need almost twice as much iron as listed in the table because the body does not absorb nonheme iron in plant foods as well as heme iron in animal foods.

Table 11.3. Amount of Iron Recommended

Life Stage	Recommended Amount
Birth to 6 months	0.27 mg
Infants 7–12 months	11 mg
Children 1–3 years	7 mg
Children 4–8 years	10 mg
Children 9–13 years	8 mg
Teens boys 14–18 years	11 mg
Teens girls 14–18 years	15 mg
Adult men 19–50 years	8 mg
Adult women 19–50 years	18 mg
Adults 51 years and older	8 mg
Pregnant teens	27 mg
Pregnant women	27 mg
Breastfeeding teens	10 mg
Breastfeeding women	9 mg

WHAT FOODS PROVIDE IRON

Iron is found naturally in many foods and is added to some fortified food products. You can get recommended amounts of iron by eating a variety of foods, including the following:

- Lean meat, seafood, and poultry
- Iron-fortified breakfast cereals and breads

- White beans, lentils, spinach, kidney beans, and peas
- Nuts and some dried fruits, such as raisins
- Iron in food comes in two forms: heme iron and nonheme iron. Nonheme iron is found in plant foods and iron-fortified food products. Meat, seafood, and poultry have both heme and nonheme iron.

Your body absorbs iron from plant sources better when you eat it with meat, poultry, seafood, and foods that contain vitamin C, such as citrus fruits, strawberries, sweet peppers, tomatoes, and broccoli.

WHAT KINDS OF IRON DIETARY SUPPLEMENTS ARE AVAILABLE?

Iron is available in many multivitamin-mineral supplements and in supplements that contain only iron. Iron in supplements is often in the form of ferrous sulfate, ferrous gluconate, ferric citrate, or ferric sulfate. Dietary supplements that contain iron have a statement on the label warning that they should be kept out of the reach of children. Accidental overdose of iron-containing products is a leading cause of fatal poisoning in children under six.

ARE YOU GETTING ENOUGH IRON?

Most people in the United States get enough iron. However, certain groups of people are more likely than others to have trouble getting enough iron:

- Teen girls and women with heavy periods
- Pregnant women and teens
- Infants (especially if they are premature or low birth weight)
- Frequent blood donors
- People with cancer, gastrointestinal (GI) disorders, or heart failure.

WHAT HAPPENS IF YOU DO NOT GET ENOUGH IRON

In the short term, getting too little iron does not cause obvious symptoms. The body uses its stored iron in the muscles, liver, spleen, and bone marrow. But, when levels of iron stored in the body become low, iron deficiency anemia sets in. Red blood cells become smaller and contain less hemoglobin. As a result, blood carries less oxygen from the lungs throughout the body.

Symptoms of iron deficiency anemia include GI upset, weakness, tiredness, lack of energy, and problems with concentration and memory. In addition, people with iron deficiency anemia are less able to fight off germs and infections, to work and exercise, and to control their body temperature. Infants and children with iron deficiency anemia might develop learning difficulties.

Iron deficiency is not uncommon in the United States, especially among young children, women under 50, and pregnant women. It can also occur in people who do not eat meat, poultry, or seafood; lose blood; have GI diseases that interfere with nutrient absorption; or eat poor diets.

WHAT ARE SOME EFFECTS OF IRON ON HEALTH?

Scientists are studying iron to understand how it affects health. Iron's most important contribution to health is preventing iron deficiency anemia and resulting problems.

Pregnant Women

During pregnancy, the amount of blood in a woman's body increases, so she needs more iron for herself and her growing baby. Getting too little iron during pregnancy increases a woman's risk of iron deficiency anemia and her infant's risk of low birth weight, premature birth, and low levels of iron. Getting too little iron might also harm her infant's brain development.

Women who are pregnant or breastfeeding should take an iron supplement as recommended by an obstetrician or other healthcare provider.

Infants and Toddlers

Iron deficiency anemia in infancy can lead to delayed psychological development, social withdrawal, and less ability to pay attention. By age 6 to 9 months, full-term infants could become iron deficient unless they eat iron-enriched solid foods or drink iron-fortified formula.

Anemia of Chronic Disease

Some chronic diseases – such as rheumatoid arthritis, inflammatory bowel disease, and some types of cancer – can interfere with the body's ability to use its stored iron. Taking more iron from foods or supplements usually does not reduce the resulting anemia of chronic disease because iron is diverted from the blood circulation to storage sites. The main therapy for anemia of chronic disease is the treatment of the underlying disease.

CAN IRON BE HARMFUL?

Yes, iron can be harmful if you get too much. In healthy people, taking high doses of iron supplements (especially on an empty stomach) can cause an upset stomach, constipation, nausea, abdominal pain, vomiting, and fainting. High doses of iron can also decrease zinc absorption. Extremely high doses of iron (in the hundreds or thousands of mg) can cause organ failure, coma, convulsions, and death. Child-proof packaging and warning labels on iron supplements have greatly reduced the number of accidental iron poisonings in children.

Some people have an inherited condition called "hemochromatosis" that causes toxic levels of iron to build up in their bodies. Without medical treatment, people with hereditary hemochromatosis can develop serious problems such as liver cirrhosis, liver cancer, and heart disease. People with this disorder should avoid using iron supplements and vitamin C supplements.

Table 11.4. Daily Upper Limits for Iron

Ages	**Upper Limit**
Birth to 12 months	40 mg
Children 1–13 years	40 mg
Teens 14–18 years	45 mg
Adults 19+ years	45 mg

The daily upper limits for iron from foods and dietary supplements are listed below. A doctor might prescribe more than the upper limit of iron to people who need higher doses for a while to treat iron deficiency.

ARE THERE ANY INTERACTIONS WITH IRON THAT YOU SHOULD KNOW ABOUT?

Yes, iron supplements can interact or interfere with medicines and other supplements you take. Here are several examples:

- Iron supplements can reduce the amount of levodopa that the body absorbs, making it less effective. Levodopa, found in Sinemet® and Stalevo®, is used to treat Parkinson disease and restless legs syndrome.
- Taking iron with levothyroxine can reduce this medication's effectiveness. Levothyroxine (Levothroid®, Levoxyl®, Synthroid®, Tirosint®, and Unithroid®) is used to treat hypothyroidism, goiter, and thyroid cancer.
- The proton pump inhibitors lansoprazole (Prevacid®) and omeprazole (Prilosec®) decrease stomach acid, so they might reduce the amount of nonheme iron that the body absorbs from food.
- Calcium might interfere with iron absorption. Taking calcium and iron supplements at different times of the day might prevent this problem.

Tell your doctor, pharmacist, and other healthcare providers about any dietary supplements and prescription or over-the-counter (OTC) medicines you take. They can tell you if the dietary supplements might interact with your medicines or if the medicines might interfere with how your body absorbs, uses, or breaks down nutrients.

Section 11.3 | **Magnesium**

This section includes text excerpted from "Magnesium," Office of Dietary Supplements (ODS), National Institutes of Health (NIH), March 22, 2021.

WHAT IS MAGNESIUM AND WHAT DOES IT DO?

Magnesium is a nutrient that the body needs to stay healthy. Magnesium is important for many processes in the body, including regulating muscle and nerve function, blood sugar levels, and blood pressure, and making protein, bone, and DNA.

HOW MUCH MAGNESIUM DO YOU NEED?

The amount of magnesium you need depends on your age and sex. Average daily recommended amounts are listed below in milligrams (mg):

Table 11.5. Amount of Magnesium Recommended

Life Stage	Recommended Amount
Birth to 6 months	30 mg
Infants 7–12 months	75 mg
Children 1–3 years	80 mg
Children 4–8 years	130 mg
Children 9–13 years	240 mg
Teen boys 14–18 years	410 mg
Teen girls 14–18 years	360 mg
Men	400–420 mg
Women	310–320 mg
Pregnant teens	400 mg
Pregnant women	350–360 mg
Breastfeeding teens	360 mg
Breastfeeding women	310–320 mg

WHAT FOODS PROVIDE MAGNESIUM

Magnesium is found naturally in many foods and is added to some fortified foods. You can get recommended amounts of magnesium by eating a variety of foods, including the following:

- Legumes, nuts, seeds, whole grains, and green leafy vegetables (such as spinach)
- Fortified breakfast cereals and other fortified foods
- Milk, yogurt, and some other milk products

WHAT KINDS OF MAGNESIUM DIETARY SUPPLEMENTS ARE AVAILABLE?

Magnesium is available in multivitamin-mineral supplements and other dietary supplements. Forms of magnesium in dietary supplements that are more easily absorbed by the body are magnesium aspartate, magnesium citrate, magnesium lactate, and magnesium chloride.

Magnesium is also included in some laxatives and some products for treating heartburn and indigestion.

ARE YOU GETTING ENOUGH MAGNESIUM?

The diets of many people in the United States provide less than the recommended amounts of magnesium. Men older than 70 and teenage girls and boys are most likely to have low intakes of magnesium. When the amount of magnesium people get from food and dietary supplements is combined, however, total intakes of magnesium are generally above recommended amounts.

WHAT HAPPENS IF YOU DO NOT GET ENOUGH MAGNESIUM

In the short term, getting too little magnesium does not produce obvious symptoms. When healthy people have low intakes, the kidneys help retain magnesium by limiting the amount lost in the urine. Low magnesium intake for a long period of time, however, can lead to magnesium deficiency. In addition, some medical conditions and medications interfere with the body's ability to absorb magnesium or increase the amount of magnesium that the body excretes, which can also lead to magnesium deficiency. Symptoms of magnesium deficiency include loss of appetite, nausea, vomiting, fatigue, and weakness. Extreme magnesium deficiency can cause numbness, tingling, muscle cramps, seizures, personality changes, and an abnormal heart rhythm.

The following groups of people are more likely than others to get too little magnesium:

- People with gastrointestinal diseases (such as Crohn disease and celiac disease)
- People with type 2 diabetes
- People with long-term alcoholism
- Older people

WHAT ARE SOME EFFECTS OF MAGNESIUM ON HEALTH?

Scientists are studying magnesium to understand how it affects health. Here are some examples of what this research has shown.

High Blood Pressure and Heart Disease

High blood pressure is a major risk factor for cardiovascular disease and stroke. Magnesium supplements might decrease blood pressure, but only by a small amount. Some studies show that people who have more magnesium in their diets have a lower risk of some types of heart disease and stroke. But, in many of these studies, it is hard to know how much of the effect was due to magnesium as opposed to other nutrients.

Type 2 Diabetes

People with higher amounts of magnesium in their diets tend to have a lower risk of developing type 2 diabetes. Magnesium helps the body break down sugars and might help reduce the risk of insulin resistance (a condition that leads to diabetes). Scientists are studying whether magnesium supplements might help people who already have type 2 diabetes control their disease. More research is needed to better understand whether magnesium can help treat diabetes.

Osteoporosis

Magnesium is important for healthy bones. People with higher intakes of magnesium have a higher bone mineral density, which is important in reducing the risk of bone fractures and osteoporosis. Getting more magnesium from foods or dietary supplements might help older women improve their bone mineral density. More research is needed to better understand whether magnesium supplements can help reduce the risk of osteoporosis or treat this condition.

Migraine Headaches

People who have migraine headaches sometimes have low levels of magnesium in their blood and other tissues. Several small studies found that magnesium supplements can modestly reduce the frequency of migraines. However, people should only take magnesium for this purpose under the care of a healthcare provider. More research is needed to determine whether magnesium supplements can help reduce the risk of migraines or ease migraine symptoms.

CAN MAGNESIUM BE HARMFUL?

Magnesium that is naturally present in food is not harmful and does not need to be limited. In healthy people, the kidneys can get rid of any excess in the urine. But, magnesium in dietary supplements and medications should not be consumed in amounts above the upper limit, unless recommended by a healthcare provider.

The daily upper limits for magnesium from dietary supplements and/or medications are listed below. For many age groups, the upper limit appears to be lower than the recommended amount. This occurs because the recommended amounts include magnesium from all sources – food, dietary supplements, and medications. The upper limits include magnesium from only dietary supplements and medications; they do not include magnesium found naturally in food.

Table 11.6. Daily Upper Limits for Magnesium

Ages	Upper Limit for Magnesium in Dietary Supplements and Medications
Birth to 12 months	Not established
Children 1–3 years	65 mg
Children 4–8 years	110 mg
Children 9–18 years	350 mg
Adults	350 mg

High intakes of magnesium from dietary supplements and medications can cause diarrhea, nausea, and abdominal cramping. Extremely high intakes of magnesium can lead to irregular heartbeat and cardiac arrest.

ARE THERE ANY INTERACTIONS WITH MAGNESIUM THAT YOU SHOULD KNOW ABOUT

Yes. Magnesium supplements can interact or interfere with some medicines. Here are several examples:

- Bisphosphonates, used to treat osteoporosis, are not well absorbed when taken too soon before or after taking dietary supplements or medications with high amounts of magnesium.
- Antibiotics might not be absorbed if taken too soon before or after taking a dietary supplement that contains magnesium.
- Diuretics can either increase or decrease the loss of magnesium through urine, depending on the type of diuretic.
- Prescription drugs used to ease symptoms of acid reflux or treat peptic ulcers can cause low blood levels of magnesium when taken over a long period of time.
- Very high doses of zinc supplements can interfere with the body's ability to absorb and regulate magnesium.

- Tell your doctor, pharmacist, and other healthcare providers about any dietary supplements and prescription or over-the-counter medicines you take. They can tell you if the dietary supplements might interact with your medicines or if the medicines might interfere with how your body absorbs, uses, or breaks down nutrients.

Section 11.4 | Potassium

This section includes text excerpted from "Potassium," Office of Dietary Supplements (ODS), National Institutes of Health (NIH), March 22, 2021.

WHAT IS POTASSIUM AND WHAT DOES IT DO?

Potassium is a mineral found in many foods. Your body needs potassium for almost everything it does, including proper kidney and heart function, muscle contraction, and nerve transmission.

HOW MUCH POTASSIUM DO YOU NEED?

The amount of potassium you need each day depends on your age and sex. Average daily recommended amounts are listed below in milligrams (mg).

Table 11.7. Amount of Potassium Recommended

Life Stage	Recommended Amount
Birth to 6 months	400 mg
Infants 7–12 months	860 mg
Children 1–3 years	2,000 mg
Children 4–8 years	2,300 mg
Children 9–13 years (boys)	2,500 mg
Children 9–13 years (girls)	2,300 mg

Table 11.7. Continued

Life Stage	Recommended Amount
Teens 14–18 years (boys)	3,000 mg
Teens 14–18 years (girls)	2,300 mg
Adults 19+ years (men)	3,400 mg
Adults 19+ years (women)	2,600 mg
Pregnant teens	2,600 mg
Pregnant women	2,900 mg
Breastfeeding teens	2,500 mg
Breastfeeding women	2,800 mg

WHAT FOODS PROVIDE POTASSIUM

Potassium is found in many foods. You can get recommended amounts of potassium by eating a variety of foods, including the following:

- Fruits, such as dried apricots, prunes, raisins, orange juice, and bananas
- Vegetables, such as acorn, squash, potatoes, spinach, tomatoes, and broccoli
- Lentils, kidney beans, soybeans, and nuts
- Milk and yogurt
- Meats, poultry, and fish

Salt substitutes. Potassium is an ingredient in many salt substitutes that people use to replace table salt. If you have kidney disease or if you take certain medications, these products could make your potassium levels too high. Talk to your healthcare provider before using salt substitutes.

WHAT KINDS OF POTASSIUM DIETARY SUPPLEMENTS ARE AVAILABLE?

Potassium is found in many multivitamin/multimineral supplements and in supplements that contain only potassium. Potassium in supplements comes in many different forms – a common form is potassium chloride, but other forms used in supplements are potassium citrate, potassium phosphate, potassium aspartate, potassium bicarbonate, and potassium gluconate. Research has not shown that any form of potassium is better than the others. Most dietary supplements provide only small amounts of potassium, no more than 99 mg per serving.

ARE YOU GETTING ENOUGH POTASSIUM?

The diets of many people in the United States provide less than recommended amounts of potassium. Even when food and dietary supplements are combined, total potassium intakes for most people are below recommended amounts.

Certain groups of people are more likely than others to have trouble getting enough potassium:

- People with inflammatory bowel disease (such as Crohn disease or ulcerative colitis)
- People who use certain medications (such as laxatives or some diuretics)
- People with pica (meaning that they eat things that are not food, such as clay)

WHAT HAPPENS IF YOU DO NOT GET ENOUGH POTASSIUM

Getting too little potassium can increase blood pressure, deplete calcium in bones, and increase the risk of kidney stones.

Prolonged diarrhea or vomiting, laxative abuse, diuretic use, eating clay, heavy sweating, dialysis, or using certain medications can cause severe potassium deficiency. In this condition, called "hypokalemia," blood levels of potassium are very low. Symptoms of hypokalemia include constipation, tiredness, muscle weakness, and not feeling well. More severe hypokalemia can cause increased urination, decreased brain function, high blood sugar levels, muscle paralysis, difficulty breathing, and irregular heartbeat. Severe hypokalemia can be life-threatening.

WHAT ARE SOME EFFECTS OF POTASSIUM ON HEALTH?

Scientists are studying potassium to understand how it affects health. Here are some examples of what this research has shown.

High blood pressure and stroke. High blood pressure is a major risk factor for coronary heart disease and stroke. People with low intakes of potassium have an increased risk of developing high blood pressure, especially if their diet is high in salt (sodium). Increasing the amount of potassium in your diet and decreasing the amount of sodium might help lower your blood pressure and reduce your risk of stroke.

Kidney stones. Getting too little potassium can deplete calcium from bones and increase the amount of calcium in urine. This calcium can form hard deposits (stones) in your kidneys, which can be very painful. Increasing the amount of potassium in your diet might reduce your risk of developing kidney stones.

Bone health. People who have high intakes of potassium from fruits and vegetables seem to have stronger bones. Eating more of these foods might improve your bone health by increasing bone mineral density (a measure of bone strength).

Blood sugar control and type 2 diabetes. Low intakes of potassium might increase blood sugar levels. Over time, this can increase the risk of developing insulin resistance and lead to type 2 diabetes. But, more research is needed to fully understand whether potassium intakes affect blood sugar levels and the risk of type 2 diabetes.

CAN POTASSIUM BE HARMFUL?

Potassium from food has not been shown to cause any harm in healthy people who have normal kidney function. Excess potassium is eliminated in the urine.

However, people who have chronic kidney disease and those who use certain medications can develop abnormally high levels of potassium in their blood (a condition called "hyperkalemia"). Examples of these medications are angiotensin-converting enzyme inhibitors, also known as "ACE inhibitors," and "potassium-sparing diuretics." Hyperkalemia can occur in these people even when they consume typical amounts of potassium from food.

Hyperkalemia can also develop in people with type 1 diabetes, congestive heart failure, liver disease, or adrenal insufficiency. Adrenal insufficiency is a condition in which the adrenal glands, located just above the kidneys, do not produce enough of certain hormones.

Even in healthy people, getting too much potassium from supplements or salt substitutes can cause hyperkalemia if they consume so much potassium that their bodies cannot eliminate the excess.

People at risk of hyperkalemia should talk to their healthcare providers about how much potassium they can safely get from food and supplements. The National Kidney Disease Education Program (NKDEP) has information about food choices that can help lower potassium levels.

ARE THERE ANY INTERACTIONS WITH POTASSIUM THAT YOU SHOULD KNOW ABOUT?

Yes, some medications may interact with potassium. Here are a few examples:

ACE inhibitors and angiotensin receptor blockers (ARBs). ACE inhibitors, such as benazepril (Lotensin®), and ARBs, such as losartan (Cozaar®), are used to treat high blood pressure, heart disease, and kidney disease. They decrease the amount of potassium lost in the urine and can make potassium levels too high, especially in people who have kidney problems.

Potassium-sparing diuretics. Potassium-sparing diuretics, such as amiloride (Midamor®) and spironolactone (Aldactone®), are used to treat high blood pressure and congestive heart failure. These medications decrease the amount of potassium lost in the urine and can make potassium levels too high, especially in people who have kidney problems.

Loop and thiazide diuretics. Loop diuretics, such as furosemide (Lasix®) and bumetanide (Bumex®), and thiazide diuretics, such as chlorothiazide (Diuril®) and metolazone (Zaroxolyn®), are used to treat high blood pressure and edema. These medications increase the amount of potassium lost in the urine and can cause abnormally low levels of potassium.

Tell your doctor, pharmacist, and other healthcare providers about any dietary supplements and prescription or over-the-counter (OTC) medicines you take. They can tell you if the dietary supplements might interact with your medicines or if the medicines might interfere with how your body absorbs, uses, or breaks down nutrients, such as potassium.

Section 11.5 | Zinc

This section includes text excerpted from "Zinc," Office of Dietary Supplements (ODS), National Institutes of Health (NIH), March 22, 2021.

WHAT IS ZINC AND WHAT DOES IT DO?

Zinc is a nutrient that people need to stay healthy. Zinc is found in cells throughout the body. It helps the immune system fight off invading bacteria and viruses. The body also needs zinc to make proteins and DNA, the genetic material in all cells. During pregnancy, infancy, and childhood, the body needs zinc to grow and develop properly. Zinc also helps wounds heal and is important for proper senses of taste and smell.

HOW MUCH ZINC DO YOU NEED?

The amount of zinc you need each day depends on your age. Average daily recommended amounts for different ages are listed below in milligrams (mg):

Table 11.8. Amount of Zinc Recommended

Life Stage	Recommended Amount
Birth to 6 months	2 mg
Infants 7–12 months	3 mg
Children 1–3 years	3 mg
Children 4–8 years	5 mg

Table 11.8. Continued

Life Stage	Recommended Amount
Children 9–13 years	8 mg
Teens 14–18 years (boys)	11 mg
Teens 14–18 years (girls)	9 mg
Adults (men)	11 mg
Adults (women)	8 mg
Pregnant teens	12 mg
Pregnant women	11 mg
Breastfeeding teens	13 mg
Breastfeeding women	12 mg

WHAT FOODS PROVIDE ZINC

Zinc is found in a wide variety of foods. You can get recommended amounts of zinc by eating a variety of foods including the following:

- Oysters, which are the best source of zinc
- Red meat, poultry, seafood such as crab and lobsters, and fortified breakfast cereals, which are also good sources of zinc
- Beans, nuts, whole grains, and dairy products, which provide some zinc

WHAT KINDS OF ZINC DIETARY SUPPLEMENTS ARE AVAILABLE?

Zinc is present in almost all multivitamin/mineral dietary supplements. It is also available alone or combined with calcium, magnesium or other ingredients in dietary supplements. Dietary supplements can have several different forms of zinc including zinc gluconate, zinc sulfate, and zinc acetate. It is not clear whether one form is better than the others.

Zinc is also found in some oral over-the-counter products, including those labeled as homeopathic medications for colds.

Use of nasal sprays and gels that contain zinc has been associated with the loss of the sense of smell, in some cases long-lasting or permanent. Currently, these safety concerns have not been found to be associated with oral products containing zinc, such as cold lozenges.

Zinc is also present in some denture adhesive creams. Using large amounts of these products, well beyond recommended levels, could lead to excessive zinc intake and copper deficiency. This can cause neurological problems, including numbness and weakness in the arms and legs.

ARE YOU GETTING ENOUGH ZINC?

Most people in the United States get enough zinc from the foods they eat.

However, certain groups of people are more likely than others to have trouble getting enough zinc:

- People who have had gastrointestinal surgery, such as weight loss surgery, or who have digestive disorders, such as ulcerative colitis or Crohn disease. These conditions can both decrease the amount of zinc that the body absorbs and increase the amount lost in the urine.
- Vegetarians because they do not eat meat, which is a good source of zinc. Also, the beans and grains they typically eat have compounds that keep zinc from being fully absorbed by the body. For this reason, vegetarians might need to eat as much as 50 percent more zinc than the recommended amounts.
- Older infants who are breastfed because breast milk does not have enough zinc for infants over 6 months of age. Older infants who do not take formula should be given foods that have zinc such as pureed meats. Formula-fed infants get enough zinc from infant formula.
- Alcoholics because alcoholic beverages decrease the amount of zinc that the body absorbs and increase the amount lost in the urine. Also, many alcoholics eat a

limited amount and variety of food, so they may not get enough zinc.
- People with sickle cell disease (SCD) because they might need more zinc.

WHAT HAPPENS IF YOU DO NOT GET ENOUGH ZINC

Zinc deficiency is rare in North America. It causes slow growth in infants and children, delayed sexual development in adolescents and impotence in men. Zinc deficiency also causes hair loss, diarrhea, eye, and skin sores, and loss of appetite. Weight loss, problems with wound healing, decreased ability to taste food, and lower alertness levels can also occur.

Many of these symptoms can be signs of problems other than zinc deficiency. If you have these symptoms, your doctor can help determine whether you might have a zinc deficiency.

WHAT ARE SOME EFFECTS OF ZINC ON HEALTH?

Scientists are studying zinc to learn about its effects on the immune system (the body's defense system against bacteria, viruses, and other foreign invaders). Scientists are also researching possible connections between zinc and the health problems discussed below.

Immune System and Wound Healing

The body's immune system needs zinc to do its job. Older people and children in developing countries who have low levels of zinc might have a higher risk of getting pneumonia and other infections. Zinc also helps the skin stay healthy. Some people who have skin ulcers might benefit from zinc dietary supplements, but only if they have low levels of zinc.

Diarrhea

Children in developing countries often die from diarrhea. Studies show that zinc dietary supplements help reduce the symptoms and duration of diarrhea in these children, many of whom are zinc deficient or otherwise malnourished. The World Health Organization and UNICEF recommend that children with diarrhea take zinc for 10–14 days (20 mg/day, or 10 mg/day for infants under 6 months). It is not clear whether zinc dietary supplements can help treat diarrhea in children who get enough zinc, such as most children in the United States.

The Common Cold

Some studies suggest that zinc lozenges or syrup (but not zinc dietary supplements in pill form) help speed recovery from the common cold and reduce its symptoms if taken within 24 hours of coming down with a cold. However, more study is needed to determine the best dose and form of zinc, as well as how long it should be taken before zinc can be recommended as a treatment for the common cold.

Age-Related Macular Degeneration

Age-related macular degeneration (AMD) is an eye disease that gradually causes vision loss. Research suggests that zinc might help slow AMD progression. In a large study among older people with AMD who were at high risk of developing advanced AMD, those who took a daily dietary supplement with 80 mg zinc, 500 mg vitamin C, 400 IU vitamin E, 15 mg beta-carotene, and 2 mg copper for about 6 years had a lower chance of developing advanced AMD and less vision loss than those who did not take the dietary supplement. In the same study, people at high risk of the disease who took dietary supplements containing only zinc also had a lower risk of getting advanced AMD than those who did not take zinc dietary supplements. People who have or are developing the disease might want to talk with their doctor about taking dietary supplements.

CAN ZINC BE HARMFUL?

Yes, if you get too much. Signs of too much zinc include nausea, vomiting, loss of appetite, stomach cramps, diarrhea, and headaches. When people take too much zinc for a long time, they sometimes have problems such as low copper levels, lower immunity, and low levels of HDL cholesterol (the "good" cholesterol).

The daily upper limits for zinc are listed below. These levels do not apply to people who are taking zinc for medical reasons under the care of a doctor:

Table 11.9. Daily Upper Limits for Zinc

Life Stage	Upper Limit
Birth to 6 months	4 mg
Infants 7–12 months	5 mg
Children 1–3 years	7 mg
Children 4–8 years	12 mg
Children 9–13 years	23 mg
Teens 14–18 years	34 mg
Adults	40 mg

ARE THERE ANY INTERACTIONS WITH ZINC THAT YOU SHOULD KNOW ABOUT?

Yes. Zinc dietary supplements can interact or interfere with medicines that you take and, in some cases, medicines can lower zinc levels in the body. Here are several examples:

- Taking a zinc dietary supplement along with quinolone or tetracycline antibiotics (such as Cipro®, Achromycin®, and Sumycin®) reduces the amount of both zinc and the antibiotic that the body absorbs. Taking the antibiotic at least 2 hours before or 4–6 hours after taking a zinc dietary supplement helps minimize this effect.
- Zinc dietary supplements can reduce the amount of penicillamine (a drug used to treat rheumatoid arthritis) that the body absorbs. They also make penicillamine work less well. Taking zinc dietary supplements at least 2 hours before or after taking penicillamine helps minimize this effect.

- Thiazide diuretics, such as chlorthalidone (brand name Hygroton®) and hydrochlorothiazide (brand names Esidrix® and HydroDIURIL®) increase the amount of zinc lost in the urine. Taking thiazide diuretics for a long time could decrease the amount of zinc in the body.

Tell your doctor, pharmacist, and other healthcare providers about any dietary supplements and medicines you take. They can tell you if those dietary supplements might interact or interfere with your prescription or over-the-counter medicines or if the medicines might interfere with how your body absorbs, uses, or breaks down nutrients.

Chapter 12 | **Antioxidants and Other Functional Foods**

Chapter Contents

Section 12.1 | **Antioxidants**

This section includes text excerpted from "Antioxidants: In Depth," National Center for Complementary and Integrative Health (NCCIH), November 2013. Reviewed May 2021.

Antioxidants are human-made or natural substances that may prevent or delay some types of cell damage. Diets high in vegetables and fruits, which are good sources of antioxidants, have been found to be healthy; however, research has not shown antioxidant supplements to be beneficial in preventing diseases. Examples of antioxidants include vitamins C and E, selenium, and carotenoids, such as beta-carotene, lycopene, lutein, and zeaxanthin.

KEY POINTS

- Vegetables and fruits are rich sources of antioxidants. There is good evidence that eating a diet that includes plenty of vegetables and fruits is healthy, and official United States government policy urges people to eat more of these foods. Research has shown that people who eat more vegetables and fruits have lower risks of several diseases; however, it is not clear whether these results are related to the amount of antioxidants in vegetables and fruits, to other components of these foods, to other factors in people's diets, or to other lifestyle choices.
- Rigorous scientific studies involving more than 100,000 people combined have tested whether antioxidant supplements can help prevent chronic diseases, such as cardiovascular diseases, cancer, and cataracts. In most instances, antioxidants did not reduce the risks of developing these diseases.
- Concerns have not been raised about the safety of antioxidants in food. However, high-dose supplements of antioxidants may be linked to health risks in some cases. Supplementing with high doses of beta-carotene may increase the risk of lung cancer in smokers. Supplementing with high doses of vitamin E may increase risks of prostate cancer and one type of stroke.

- Antioxidant supplements may interact with some medicines.
- Tell all of your healthcare providers about any complementary and integrative health approaches you use. Give them a full picture of what you do to manage your health. This will help ensure coordinated and safe care.

ABOUT FREE RADICALS, OXIDATIVE STRESS, AND ANTIOXIDANTS

Free radicals are highly unstable molecules that are naturally formed when you exercise and when your body converts food into energy. Your body can also be exposed to free radicals from a variety of environmental sources, such as cigarette smoke, air pollution, and sunlight. Free radicals can cause "oxidative stress," a process that can trigger cell damage. Oxidative stress is thought to play a role in a variety of diseases including cancer, cardiovascular diseases, diabetes, Alzheimer disease (AD), Parkinson disease (PD), and eye diseases such as cataracts, and age-related macular degeneration (AMD).

Antioxidant molecules have been shown to counteract oxidative stress in laboratory experiments (e.g., in cells or animal studies). However, there is debate as to whether consuming large amounts of antioxidants in supplement form actually benefits health. There is also some concern that consuming antioxidant supplements in excessive doses may be harmful.

Vegetables and fruits are healthy foods and rich sources of antioxidants. The Official United States government policy urges people to eat more vegetables and fruits. Concerns have not been raised about the safety of any amounts of antioxidants in food.

USE OF ANTIOXIDANT SUPPLEMENTS IN THE UNITED STATES

An analysis was conducted using data from the National Health and Nutrition Examination Survey (NHANES), (1999–2000 and 2001–2002) estimated the amounts of antioxidants adults in the United States get from foods and supplements. Supplements accounted for 54 percent of vitamin C, 64 percent of vitamin E, 14 percent of alpha- and beta-carotene, and 11 percent of selenium intake.

Safety

- High-dose antioxidant supplements may be harmful in some cases. For example, the results of some studies have linked the use of high-dose beta-carotene supplements to an increased risk of lung cancer in smokers and use of high-dose vitamin E supplements to increased risks of hemorrhagic stroke (a type of stroke caused by bleeding in the brain) and prostate cancer.
- Like some other dietary supplements, antioxidant supplements may interact with certain medications. For example, vitamin E supplements may increase the risk of bleeding in people who are taking anticoagulant drugs ("blood thinners"). There is conflicting evidence on the effects of taking antioxidant supplements during cancer treatment; some studies suggest that this may be beneficial, but others suggest that it may be harmful. The National Cancer Institute (NCI) recommends that people who are being treated for cancer must talk with their healthcare provider before taking supplements.

IF YOU ARE CONSIDERING ANTIOXIDANT SUPPLEMENTS

Do not use antioxidant supplements to replace a healthy diet or conventional medical care, or as a reason to postpone seeing a healthcare provider about a medical problem.

If you have AMD, consult your healthcare providers to determine whether supplements of the type used in the AREDS trial are appropriate for you.

If you are considering a dietary supplement, first get information on it from reliable sources. Keep in mind that dietary supplements may interact with medications or other supplements and may contain ingredients not listed on the label. Your healthcare provider can advise you. If you are pregnant or nursing a child, or if you are considering giving a child a dietary supplement, it is especially important to consult your (or your child's) healthcare provider.

Tell all of your healthcare providers about any complementary health approaches you use. Give them a full picture of what you do to manage your health. This will help ensure coordinated and safe care.

Section 12.2 | **How Good Is Soy?**

This section includes text excerpted from "Soy," National Center for Complementary and Integrative Health (NCCIH), December 2020.

- This section focuses on the use of soy by adults for health purposes.
- Soybeans have long been cultivated in Asia. Since the 1950s, they have also been produced in other parts of the world, including the Americas.
- In addition to its food uses, soy is available in dietary supplements. Soy supplements may contain soy protein, isoflavones (compounds similar in structure to the female hormone estrogen), or other components.
- Soy products are promoted for menopausal symptoms, bone health, improving memory, hypertension, and high cholesterol levels.

HOW MUCH DO WE KNOW?

Although there have been many studies on soy products, there are still uncertainties about soy's health effects.

WHAT HAVE WE LEARNED?

- Consuming soy protein in place of other proteins may lower levels of total cholesterol and LDL ("bad") cholesterol to a small extent.
- Soy isoflavone supplements or soy protein may help to reduce the frequency and severity of menopausal hot flashes, but the effect may be small.
- Observational studies indicate that among Asian women, higher dietary intakes of soy during childhood and adolescence are associated with a lower risk of breast cancer later in life. The amounts of soy in Western diets may be too low for this association to be observed. Soy products in supplement form have not been shown to reduce breast cancer risk.

- Current evidence suggests that soy isoflavone mixtures probably have a beneficial effect on bone health in postmenopausal women, but the evidence is not entirely consistent.
- Soy protein may slightly reduce blood pressure in people with hypertension.

WHAT DO WE KNOW ABOUT SAFETY?

- Except for people with soy allergies, soy is considered to be a safe food. In research studies, soy protein supplements and soy extracts rich in isoflavones have been used safely on a short-term basis; the safety of long-term use is uncertain.
- The most common side effects of soy are digestive upsets, such as constipation and diarrhea.
- Soy may alter thyroid function in people who are deficient in iodine.
- Current evidence indicates that it is safe for women who have had breast cancer or who are at risk for breast cancer to eat soy foods. However, it is uncertain whether soy isoflavone supplements are safe for these women.
- The use of soy in amounts greater than those commonly found in foods may be unsafe during pregnancy because estrogen-like substances from soy could be harmful to the fetus. Little is known about whether it is safe to use soy in amounts greater than those commonly found in foods while breastfeeding.

KEEP IN MIND

Take charge of your health – talk with your healthcare providers about any complementary health approaches you use. Together, you can make shared, well-informed decisions.

Chapter 13 | **Key Takeaways from Nutrition**

USE OILS

Oils are fats that are liquid at room temperature, like vegetable oils used in cooking. They come from many different plants and from fish. Oils are not a food group, but they provide you with important nutrients such as unsaturated fats and vitamin E. Choosing unsaturated fat in place of saturated fat can reduce your risk of heart disease and improve "good" (HDL) cholesterol levels.

A number of foods are natural sources of oils, like nuts, olives, some fish, and avocados. Most oils are high in monounsaturated or polyunsaturated fats and low in saturated fats. Foods that are mainly made of oil include mayonnaise, certain salad dressings, and soft (tub or squeeze) margarine.

The fat in some tropical plants, including coconut oil, palm oil, and palm kernel oil, are not included in the oils category because they are higher in saturated fats than other oils. For nutritional purposes, they should be considered to be solid fats. Solid fats are fats that are solid at room temperature, like butter, lard, and shortening. Solid fats come from many animal foods and can be made from vegetable oils through a process called "hydrogenation."

Common Oils Used in Cooking

- Canola oil
- Safflower oil
- Corn oil

This chapter includes text excerpted from "More Key Topics," MyPlate, U.S. Department of Agriculture (USDA), December 29, 2020.

- Cottonseed oil
- Grapeseed oil
- Olive oil
- Peanut oil
- Sesame oil*
- Soybean oil
- Sunflower oil
- Walnut oil*

Note: (*mainly used as flavoring)

LIMIT ADDED SUGARS

To build healthy eating habits and stay within calorie needs, individuals over age 2 should choose foods and beverages with little to no added sugars, and those under age 2 should avoid them altogether. Added sugars are sugars and syrups that are added to foods or beverages when they are processed or prepared. This does not include sugars found in milk and fruits.

Common Foods Containing Added Sugars

- Beverages, such as regular soft drinks, energy or sports drinks, fruit drinks, sweetened coffee and tea
- Breakfast cereals and bars
- Cakes
- Candy
- Cookies and brownies
- Ice cream and dairy desserts
- Pies and cobblers
- Sugars, jams, syrups, and sweet toppings
- Sweet rolls, pastries, and donuts

Reading the ingredient label on packaged foods can help you identify added sugars.

Names for Added Sugars*

- Anhydrous dextrose

- Fructose
- Molasses
- Brown rice syrup
- Fruit nectar
- Pancake syrup
- Brown sugar
- Glucose
- Raw sugarcane juice
- High-fructose corn syrup (HFCS)
- Sucrose
- Confectioners powdered sugar
- Honey sugar
- Corn syrup
- Invert sugar
- Sugar cane juice
- Crystal dextrose
- Liquid fructose
- White granulated sugar
- Dextrose
- Malt syrup
- Evaporated corn sweetener
- Maple syrup

LIMIT SATURATED FAT

Saturated fat is often found in forms that are solid at room temperature – examples include milk fat, butter, or the fat inside or around meat. A few food products such as coconut oil, palm oils, or whole milk remain as liquids at room temperature but are high in saturated fat.

Cut back on saturated fat by replacing foods high in saturated fat (such as butter, whole milk, cheese, and baked goods) with foods higher in unsaturated fat (found in plants and fish, such as vegetable oils, peanuts, avocado, and salmon).

Common Foods Containing Saturated Fat

- Beef fat (tallow, suet)

- Butter
- Chicken fat
- Coconut oil
- Cream
- Hydrogenated oils**
- Milk fat
- Palm and palm kernel oils
- Partially hydrogenated oils**
- Pork fat (lard) shortening
- Stick margarine

Cut back on foods containing saturated fat including:

- Desserts and baked goods, such as cakes, cookies, donuts, pastries, and croissants
- Many kinds of cheese and foods containing cheese, such as pizza, burgers, and sandwiches
- Sausages, hot dogs, bacon, and ribs
- Fried potatoes (French fries) – if fried in saturated fat or hydrogenated oil
- Regular ground beef (85 percent lean) and cuts of meat with visible fat
- Fried chicken and other chicken dishes with the skin
- Whole milk and full-fat dairy foods and dairy desserts

LIMIT SODIUM

For most people ages 14 years and older, sodium should not exceed 2,300 mg per day. Consuming less than this level is recommended for children younger than 13 years old.

The relationship between sodium intake and blood pressure is well-documented. As one goes up, so does the other. Evidence has shown that limiting sodium intake provides benefits and may reduce one's risk for heart disease and hypertension.

Common Foods Usually High in Sodium

- Mixed dishes, such as pizzas, burgers, casseroles, tacos, and sandwiches

- Processed meats, poultry, and seafood like deli meats, sausages, pepperoni, and sardines
- Sauces, dressings, and condiments
- Instant products such as flavored rice, instant noodles, ready-made pasta, and frozen entrees

Sodium is found in many of the foods we commonly eat and most of us get more than we need. Adding salt to food is a source of sodium, but it is often not the main reason for high sodium intake. Sodium is already added to a lot of the foods we buy and dishes we order. You can lower the amount of sodium you eat and drink with these tips:

- Use the Nutrition Facts label to compare the sodium in packaged foods and beverages. Choose products with less sodium.
- Buy low-sodium, reduced-sodium, or no-salt-added products.
- Look for fresh, frozen, or canned vegetables without added sauces or seasonings.
- Choose fresh or frozen poultry, seafood, and lean meats instead of prepared or ready-to-eat products so that you can control the amount of salt you add yourself.
- Cook more often at home to control the sodium in your food.
- Add herbs and spices instead of salt to recipes and dishes.

ABOUT ALCOHOL

Individuals who do not drink alcohol should not start drinking for any reason. There are some people who should not drink alcohol at all, such as women who are or who might be pregnant; under the legal drinking age; or who have certain health conditions.

Adults of legal drinking age who choose to drink should do so in moderation by limiting intake to 2 drinks or less in a day for men and 1 drink or less in a day for women, on days when alcohol is consumed. For adults who choose to drink alcoholic beverages, drinking less is better for health than drinking more.

The following count as one alcoholic drink equivalent: 12 fluid ounces of regular beer (5 percent alcohol), 5 fluid ounces of wine (12 percent alcohol), or 1.5 fluid ounces of 80 proof distilled spirits (40 percent alcohol).

Alcoholic beverages provide calories but few nutrients and should be accounted for to stay within your calorie allowance. These calories come from both alcohol and other ingredients, such as soda, juice, and added sugars. Keep additional ingredients and portion size in mind as total calories range widely, especially in cocktails and other mixed drinks.

Examples of Calories in Alcoholic Beverages

Table 13.1. Alcohol Percentage and the Amount of Calories

12 fluid ounces of regular beer (5% alcohol)	About 150 calories
5 fluid ounces of wine (12% alcohol)	About 120 calories
1.5 fluid ounces of 80 proof distilled spirits (40% alcohol)	About 100 calories
7 fluid ounces of a rum (40% alcohol) and cola	About 155 calories

Part 3 | Nutrition through the Life Span

Chapter 14 | **Infant and Toddler Nutrition**

Chapter Contents

Section 14.1 | Importance of Breast Milk for the First Six Months

This section includes text excerpted from "*Dietary Guidelines for Americans, 2020-2025*," *Dietary Guidelines for Americans* (*DGA*), U.S. Department of Agriculture (USDA), December 2020.

The time from birth until a child's second birthday is a critically important period for proper growth and development. It also is key for establishing healthy dietary patterns that may influence the trajectory of eating behaviors and health throughout the life course. During this period, nutrients critical for brain development and growth must be provided in adequate amounts. Children in this age group consume small quantities of foods, so it is important to make every bite count!

KEY RECOMMENDATIONS

- For about the first 6 months of life, exclusively feed infants human milk. Continue to feed infants human milk through at least the first year of life, and longer if desired. Feed infants iron-fortified infant formula during the first year of life when human milk is unavailable.
- Provide infants with supplemental vitamin D beginning soon after birth.
- At about 6 months, introduce infants to nutrient-dense complementary foods.
- Introduce infants to potentially allergenic foods along with other complementary foods.
- Encourage infants and toddlers to consume a variety of foods from all food groups. Include foods rich in iron and zinc, particularly for infants fed human milk.
- Avoid foods and beverages with added sugars.
- Limit foods and beverages higher in sodium.
- As infants wean from human milk or infant formula, transition to a healthy dietary pattern after 6 months is necessary.

PUTTING THE KEY RECOMMENDATIONS INTO ACTION

Feed Infants Human Milk for the First Six Months, If Possible

Exclusive human milk feeding is one of the best ways to start an infant off on the path of lifelong healthy nutrition. Exclusive human milk feeding, commonly known as "exclusive breastfeeding," refers to an infant consuming only human milk, and not in combination with infant formula and/or complementary foods or beverages (including water), except for medications or vitamin and mineral supplementation. Human milk can support an infant's nutrient needs for about the first 6 months of life, with the exception of vitamin D and potentially iron. In addition to nutrients, human milk includes bioactive substances and immunologic properties that support infant health and growth and development.

The United States data show that about 84 percent of infants born in 2017 were never breastfed with only 25 percent breastfed exclusively through age 6 months, and 35 percent continuing to be breastfed at age 12 months. Nearly one-quarter of infants were fed some human milk beyond age 12 months, with about 15 percent of toddlers being breastfed at age 18 months. Families may have a number of reasons for not having human milk for their infant. For example, a family may choose not to breastfeed, a child may be adopted, or the mother may be unable to produce a full milk supply or may be unable to pump and store milk safely due to family or workplace pressures. If human milk is unavailable, infants should be fed an iron-fortified commercial infant formula (i.e., labeled with iron) regulated by the U.S. Food and Drug Administration (FDA), which is based on standards that ensure nutrient content and safety. Infant formulas are designed to meet the nutritional needs of infants and are not needed beyond age 12 months. It is important to take precautions to ensure that expressed human milk and prepared infant formula are handled and stored safely.

Donor Human Milk

If families do not have sufficient human milk for their infant but want to feed their infant human milk, they may look for alternative ways to obtain it. It is important for the family to obtain pasteurized donor human milk from a source, such as an accredited human milk bank, that has screened its donors and taken appropriate safety precautions. When human milk is obtained directly from individuals or through the Internet, the donor is unlikely to have been screened for infectious diseases, and it is unknown whether the human milk has been collected or stored in a way to reduce possible safety risks to the baby.

Proper Handling and Storage of Human Milk and Infant Formula

- Wash hands thoroughly before expressing human milk or preparing to feed human milk or infant formula.
- If expressing human milk, ensure pump parts are thoroughly cleaned before use.
- If preparing powdered infant formula, use a safe water source and follow instructions on the label.
- Refrigerate freshly expressed human milk within 4 hours for up to 4 days. Previously frozen and thawed human milk should be used within 24 hours. Thawed human milk should never be refrozen. Refrigerate prepared infant formula for up to 24 hours.
- Do not use a microwave to warm human milk or infant formula. Warm safely by placing the sealed container of human milk or infant formula in a bowl of warm water or under warm, running tap water.
- Once it has been offered to the infant, use or discard leftovers quickly (within 2 hours for human milk or 1 hour for infant formula).
- Thoroughly wash all infant feeding items, such as bottles and nipples. Consider sanitizing feeding items for infants younger than 3 months of age, infants born prematurely, or infants with a compromised immune system.

Homemade infant formulas and those that are improperly and illegally imported into the United States without the mandated FDA review and supervision should not be used. Toddler milk or toddler formulas should not be fed to infants, as they are not designed to meet the nutritional needs of infants.

Provide Infants Supplemental Vitamin D Beginning Soon after Birth

All infants who are fed human milk exclusively or who receive both human milk and infant formula (mixed fed) will need a vitamin D supplement of 400 IU per day beginning soon after birth. Infant formula is fortified with vitamin D, thus, when an infant is receiving full feeds of infant formula, vitamin D supplementation is not needed. Families who do not wish to provide a supplement directly to their infant should discuss with a healthcare provider the risks and benefits of maternal high-dose supplementation options. Even when consuming a varied diet, achieving adequate vitamin D from foods and beverages (natural sources) alone is challenging, suggesting that young children may need to continue taking a vitamin D supplement after age 12 months. Parents, caregivers, and guardians should consult with a healthcare provider to determine how long supplementation is necessary.

Supplemental Vitamin B_{12}

Human milk has sufficient vitamin B_{12} to meet infant needs unless the mother's vitamin B_{12} status is inadequate. This can occur for different reasons, including when the mother eats a strictly vegan diet without any animal source foods. When the mother is at risk of vitamin B_{12} deficiency, human milk may not provide sufficient vitamin B_{12}. In these cases, the mother and/or infant-fed human milk may require a vitamin B_{12} supplement. Parents, caregivers, and guardians should consult with a healthcare provider to determine whether supplementation is necessary.

Section 14.2 | **Introducing Six Months Infants to Nutrient-Dense Complimentary Food**

This section includes text excerpted from "*Dietary Guidelines for Americans, 2020-2025*" *Dietary Guidelines for Americans* (*DGA*), U.S. Department of Agriculture (USDA), December 2020.

At about age 6 months, infants should be introduced to nutrient-dense, developmentally appropriate foods to complement human milk or infant formula feedings. Some infants may show developmental signs of readiness before age 6 months, but introducing complementary foods before age 4 months is not recommended. Waiting until after age 6 months to introduce foods also is not recommended. Starting around that time, complementary foods are necessary to ensure adequate nutrition and exposure to flavors, textures, and different types of foods. Infants should be given age- and developmentally-appropriate foods to help prevent choking. It is important to introduce potentially allergenic foods along with other complementary foods. For infants fed human milk, it is particularly important to include complementary foods that are rich in iron and zinc when starting complementary foods. About one-third (32 percent) of infants in the United States are introduced to complementary foods and beverages before age 4 months, highlighting the importance of providing guidance and support to parents, guardians, and caregivers on the timing of introduction to complementary foods. Early introduction of complementary foods and beverages is higher among infants receiving infant formula (42 percent) or a combination of infant formula and human milk (32 percent) than among infants exclusively fed human milk (19 percent).

DEVELOPMENTAL READINESS FOR BEGINNING TO EAT SOLID FOODS

The age at which infants reach different developmental stages will vary. Typically between age 4 and 6 months, infants develop the gross motor, oral, and fine motor skills necessary to begin to eat complementary foods. As an infant's oral skills develop, the thickness and texture of foods can gradually be varied. Signs that an infant is ready for complementary foods include:

- Being able to control head and neck
- Sitting up alone or with support
- Bringing objects to the mouth
- Trying to grasp small objects, such as toys or food
- Swallowing food rather than pushing it back out onto the chin

Infants and young children should be given age- and developmentally-appropriate foods to help prevent choking. Foods, such as hot dogs, candy, nuts and seeds, raw carrots, grapes, popcorn, and chunks of peanut butter are some of the foods that can be a choking risk for young children. Parents, guardians, and caregivers are encouraged to take steps to decrease choking risks, including:

- Offering foods in the appropriate size, consistency, and shape that will allow an infant or young child to eat and swallow easily
- Making sure the infant or young child is sitting up in a high chair or other safe, supervised place
- Ensuring an adult is supervising feeding during mealtimes
- Not putting infant cereal or other solid foods in an infant's bottle. This could increase the risk of choking and will not make the infant sleep longer.

INTRODUCE INFANTS TO POTENTIALLY ALLERGENIC FOODS ALONG WITH OTHER COMPLEMENTARY FOODS

Potentially allergenic foods (e.g., peanuts, egg, cow milk products, tree nuts, wheat, crustacean shellfish, fish, and soy) should be introduced when other complementary foods are introduced to an infant's diet. Introducing peanut-containing foods in the first year reduces the risk that an infant will develop a food allergy to peanuts. Cow milk, as a beverage, should be introduced at age 12 months or later. There is no evidence that delaying the introduction of allergenic foods, beyond when other complementary foods are introduced, helps to prevent food allergy.

For Infants at High Risk of Peanut Allergy, Introduce Peanut-Containing Foods at Age 4 to 6 Months

If an infant has severe eczema, egg allergy, or both (conditions that increase the risk of peanut allergy), age-appropriate, peanut-containing foods should be introduced into the diet as early as age 4 to 6 months. This will reduce the risk of developing peanuts allergy. Caregivers should check with the infant's healthcare provider before feeding the infant peanut-containing foods. A blood test or skin prick may be recommended to determine whether peanuts should be introduced to the infant. More information is available in the Addendum Guidelines for the Prevention of Peanut Allergy in the United States at (www.niaid.nih.gov/sites/default/files/addendum-peanut-allergy-prevention-guidelines.pdf).

ENCOURAGE INFANTS AND TODDLERS TO CONSUME A VARIETY OF COMPLEMENTARY FOODS AND BEVERAGES TO MEET ENERGY AND NUTRIENT NEEDS

Parents, caregivers, and guardians are encouraged to introduce foods across all the food groups that fit within a family's preferences, cultural traditions, and budget. Complementary foods and beverages should be rich in nutrients, meet calorie and nutrient requirements during this critical period of growth and development, and stay within the limits of dietary components, such as added sugars and sodium. Although the *Dietary Guidelines* does not provide a recommended dietary pattern for infants ages 6 through 11 months, infants should be on the path to a healthy dietary pattern that is recommended for those ages 12 through 23 months. In the United States, some dietary components are of public-health concern for infants and toddlers. Iron is a dietary component of public-health concern for underconsumption among older infants ages 6 through 11 months who are fed primarily human milk and consume inadequate iron from complementary foods. Older infants who are fed primarily human milk also underconsume zinc and protein from complementary foods, and vitamin D, choline, and potassium are notably under-consumed by all older infants. During the second year of life, the dietary components of public-health concern for underconsumption are vitamin D, calcium, dietary fiber, and potassium and for overconsumption are added sugars and sodium.

Introduce Iron-Rich Foods to Infants Starting at about 6 Months Old

Iron-rich foods (e.g., meats and seafood rich in heme iron and iron-fortified infant cereals) are important components of the infant's diet from age 6 through 11 months to maintain adequate iron status, which supports neurologic development and immune function. Infants are typically born with body stores of iron adequate for about the first 6 months of life, depending on gestational age, maternal iron status, and timing of umbilical cord clamping. By age 6 months, however, infants require an external source of iron apart from human milk. Caregivers of infants exclusively fed human milk should talk with their pediatric care provider about whether there may be a need for infants supplementation with iron before age 6 months. A complementary food source of iron beginning at about 6 months is particularly important for infants fed human milk because the iron content of human milk is low and maternal iron intake during lactation does not increase its content. In the United States, an estimated 77 percent of infants fed human milk have inadequate iron intake during the second half of infancy, highlighting the importance of introducing iron-rich foods starting at age 6 months. Infants receiving most of their milk feeds as iron-fortified infant formula are likely to need less iron from complementary foods beginning at 6 months of age. After age 12 months, children have a lower iron requirement, but good food sources of iron are still needed to maintain adequate iron status and prevent deficiency.

Introduce Zinc-Rich Foods to Infants Starting at about 6 Months Old

Zinc-rich complementary foods (e.g., meats, beans, zinc-fortified infant cereals) are important from age 6 months onwards to support adequate zinc status, which supports growth and immune function. Although the zinc content of human milk is initially high and efficiently absorbed, the concentration declines over the first 6 months of lactation and is not affected by maternal zinc intake. During the second half of infancy, approximately half (54 percent) of United States infants fed human milk have inadequate zinc intake. Prioritizing zinc-rich foods starting at 6 months of age to complement human milk feedings will help infants meet their requirement for zinc.

Encourage a Variety of Foods from All Food Groups to Infants Starting at about Six Months Old

To support nutrient adequacy, foster acceptance of healthy foods, and set intakes on a path toward a healthy pattern, it is important to encourage foods from all food groups. Because very young children are being exposed to new textures and flavors for the first time, it may take up to 8 to 10 exposures for an infant to accept a new type of food. Repeated offering of foods, such as fruits and vegetables increases the likelihood of an infant accepting them. A nutrient-dense, diverse diet from age 6 through 23 months of life includes a variety of food sources from each food group.

- Protein foods, including meats, poultry, eggs, seafood, nuts, seeds, and soy products, are important sources of iron, zinc, protein, choline, and long-chain polyunsaturated fatty acids. The long-chain polyunsaturated fatty acids, specifically the essential omega-3 and omega-6 fatty acids supplied through seafood, nuts, seeds, and oils, influence the infant's fatty acid status and are among the key nutrients needed for the rapid brain development that occurs through the infant's first 2 years of life. Some types of fish, such as salmon and trout are also natural sources of vitamin D. To limit exposure to methyl mercury from seafood, the U.S. Food and Drug Administration (FDA) and the U.S. Environmental Protection Agency (EPA) issued joint guidance regarding the types of seafood to choose.
- Vegetables and fruits, especially those rich in potassium, vitamin A, and vitamin C, should be offered to infants and toddlers age 6 through 23 months. The

vegetable subgroup of beans, peas, and lentils also provides a good source of protein and dietary fiber.
- For dairy, families can introduce yogurt and cheese, including soy-based yogurt, before 12 months. However, infants should not consume cow milk, as a beverage, or fortified soy beverage, before age 12 months as a replacement for human milk or infant formula. In the second year of life, when calcium requirements increase, dairy products, including milk, yogurt, cheese, and fortified soy beverages and soy yogurt provide a good source of calcium. Vitamin D-fortified milk and soy beverages also provide a good source of vitamin D. For those younger than the age of 2, offer dairy products without added sugar.
- Grains, including iron-fortified infant cereal, play an important role in meeting nutrient needs during this life stage. Infant cereals fortified with iron include oat, barley, multigrain, and rice cereals. Rice cereal fortified with iron is a good source of nutrients for infants, but rice cereal should not be the only type of cereal given to infants. Offering young children whole grains more often than refined grains will increase dietary fiber as well as potassium intake during the second year of life and help young children establish healthy dietary practices.

Section 14.3 | **Healthy Dietary Pattern during a Toddler's Second Year of Life**

This section includes text excerpted from "*Dietary Guidelines for Americans, 2020-2025*," *Dietary Guidelines for Americans* (*DGA*), U.S. Department of Agriculture (USDA), December 2020.

In the second year of life, toddlers consume less human milk, and infant formula is not recommended. Calories and nutrients should predominantly be met from a healthy dietary pattern of age-appropriate foods and beverages. The Healthy U.S.-Style Dietary Pattern presented here is intended for toddlers ages 12 through 23 months who no longer consume human milk or infant formula. The pattern represents the types and amounts of foods needed to meet energy and nutrition requirements for this period. For toddlers who are still consuming human milk (approximately one-third at 12 months and 15 percent at 18 months), a healthy dietary pattern should include a similar combination of nutrient-dense complementary foods and beverages.

Table 14.1 displays the Healthy U.S.-style Dietary Pattern to illustrate the specific amounts and limits for food groups and other dietary components that make up healthy dietary patterns. The pattern is provided at calorie levels ranging from 700 to 1,000 calories per day, which are appropriate for most toddlers ages 12 through 23 months. A healthy dietary pattern includes a variety of nutrient-dense fruits, vegetables, grains, protein foods (including lean meats, poultry, eggs, seafood, nuts, and seeds), dairy (including milk, yogurt, and cheese), and oils. Based on the FDA and the EPA's joint "advice about eating fish," young children should eat seafood lowest in methyl mercury, and certain species of seafood should be avoided. If young children are lower in body weight, they should eat less seafood than the amounts in the Healthy U.S.-Style Dietary Pattern.

After food group and subgroup recommendations are met, a small number of calories are allocated to oils. The recommendation to limit saturated fat to less than 10 percent of calories per day does not apply to those younger than age 2, and the inclusion of higher-fat versions of dairy is a notable difference in the pattern for toddlers ages 12 through 23 months compared to patterns for ages 2 and older. However, no calories remain in the pattern for additional saturated fat or for added sugars. To illustrate the concept of nutrient density, this dietary pattern requires careful choices of foods and beverages but does not require the inclusion of fortified products specifically formulated for infants or toddlers to meet nutrient recommendations.

Make Healthy Shifts to Empower Toddlers to Eat Nutrient-Dense Foods in Dietary Patterns

Science shows that early food preferences influence later food choices. Make the first choice the healthiest choices that set the toddlers on a path of making nutrient-dense choices in the years to come. Examples of shifts in common choices to healthier, more nutrient-dense food choices include:

- Cereal with added sugars to cereals with minimal added sugars
- Fruit product with added sugars to fruit (e.g., canned in 100 percent juice)
- Fried vegetables to roasted vegetables
- High sodium snacks to vegetables
- High sodium meats to ground lean meats
- Beverages with added sugars
- Unsweetened beverages

Table 14.1. Healthy U.S.-Style Dietary Pattern for Toddlers Ages 12 through 23 Months Who Are No Longer Receiving Human Milk or Infant Formula

Calorie Level of Pattern[a]	**700**	**800**	**900**	**1,000**
Food Group or Subgroup[b,c]	Daily Amount of Food from Each Group[d] (Vegetable and protein foods subgroup amounts are per week.)			
Vegetables (cup eq/day)	2/3	¾	1	1
	Vegetable Subgroups in Weekly Amounts			
Dark-Green Vegetables (cup eq/wk)	1	1/3	½	½
Red and Orange Vegetables (cup eq/wk)	1	1 ¾	2 ½	2 ½
Beans, Peas, Lentils (cup eq/wk)	¾	1/3	½	½
Starchy Vegetables (cup eq/wk)	1	1 ½	2	2
Other Vegetables (cup eq/wk)	¾	1 ¼	1 ½	1 ½
Fruits (cup eq/day)	**½**	**¾**	**1**	**1**
Grains (ounce eq/day)	**1 ¾**	**2 ¼**	**2 ½**	**3**

Table 14.1. Continued

Calorie Level of Pattern[a]	**700**	**800**	**900**	**1,000**
Whole Grains (ounce eq/day)	1 ½	2	2	2
Refined Grains (ounce eq/day)	¼	¼	½	1
Dairy (cup eq/day)	**1**	**1 ¾**	**2**	**2**
Protein Foods (ounce eq/day)	**2**	**2**	**2**	**2**
	Protein Foods Subgroups in Weekly Amounts			
Meats, Poultry (ounce eq/wk)	8 ¾	7	7	7 ¾
Eggs (ounce eq/wk)	2	2 ¾	2 ½	2 ½
Seafood (ounce eq/wk)e	2-3	2-3	2-3	2-3
Nuts, Seeds, Soy Products (ounce eq/wk)	1	1	1 ¼	1 ¼
Oils (grams/day)	**9**	**9**	**8**	**13**

[a]***Calorie level ranges:*** *Energy levels are calculated based on median length and body weight reference individuals. Calorie needs vary based on many factors. The DRI calculator for healthcare professionals, available at (www.nal.usda.gov/fnic/dri-calculator), can be used to estimate calorie needs based on age, sex, and weight.*

[b]*Definitions for each food group and subgroup and quantity (i.e., cup or ounce equivalents)*

[c]*All foods are assumed to be in nutrient-dense forms and prepared with minimal added sugars, refined starches, or sodium. Foods are also lean or in low-fat forms with the exception of dairy, which includes whole-fat fluid milk, reduced-fat plain yogurts, and reduced-fat cheese. There are no calories available for additional added sugars, saturated fat, or to eat more than the recommended amount of food in a food group.*

[d]*In some cases, food subgroup amounts are greatest at the lower calorie levels to help achieve nutrient adequacy when a relatively small number of calories are required.*

[e]*If consuming up to 2 ounces of seafood per week, children should only be fed cooked varieties from the "best choices" list in the FDA/EPA joint "Advice About Eating Fish," available at (www.fda.gov/food/consumers/advice-about-eating-fish) and (www.epa.gov/choose-fish-and-shellfish-wisely). If consuming up to 3 ounces of seafood per week, children should only be fed cooked varieties from the "Best Choices" list that contain even lower methylmercury: flatfish (e.g., flounder), salmon, tilapia, shrimp, catfish, crab, trout, haddock, oysters, sardines, squid, pollock, anchovies, crawfish, mullet, scallops, whiting, clams, shad, and Atlantic mackerel. If consuming up to 3 ounces of seafood per week, many commonly consumed varieties of seafood should be avoided because they cannot be consumed at 3 ounces per week by children without the potential of exceeding safe methylmercury limits; examples that should not be consumed include canned light tuna or white (albacore) tuna, cod, perch, black sea bass.*

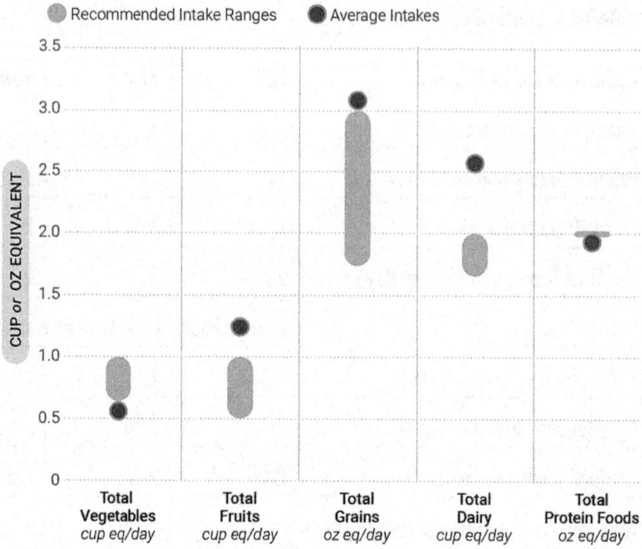

Figure 14.1. Average Daily Food Group Intakes Compared to Recommended Intake Ranges *(Source: Average Intakes: Analysis of What We Eat in America, NHANES 2007–2016, day 1 dietary intake data, weighted. Recommended Intake Ranges: Healthy U.S.-Style Dietary Patterns.)*

DIETARY INTAKES OF TODDLERS DURING THE SECOND YEAR OF LIFE

Current Intakes: Ages 12 to 23 Months

Average intakes of the food groups are compared to the range of recommended intakes at the calorie levels most relevant to males and females in this age group. Additionally, the average intake and range of intakes of added sugars, saturated fats, and sodium are displayed. Average intakes compared to recommended intake ranges of the subgroups for grains are represented in daily amounts; subgroups for vegetables and protein foods are represented in weekly amounts.

Average Intakes of Added Sugars, Saturated Fat, and Sodium

ADDED SUGARS

- Limit: Avoid
- Average intakes: 104 kcals

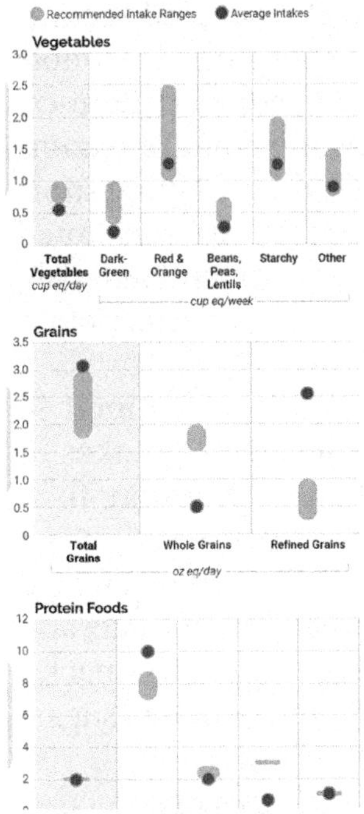

Figure 14.2. Average Intakes of Subgroups Compared to Recommended Intake Ranges: Ages 12 through 23 Months *(Source: Average Intakes: Analysis of What We Eat in America, NHANES 2007–2016, day 1 dietary intake data, weighted. Recommended Intake Ranges: Healthy U.S.-Style Dietary Patterns.)*

SATURATED FAT

- Limit: N/A
- Average intakes: 167 kcals

SODIUM

- Limit: 1,200 mg
- Average intakes: 1,586 mg

Approximately 60 percent of toddlers meet or exceed recommended intakes for fruit. A majority of fruit is consumed as whole fruit (fresh, canned, puréed, frozen) or as 100 percent fruit juice. The average intake of total vegetables is below the range of recommended amounts, with nearly 90 percent of toddlers falling short of recommendations. About one-half of vegetables are consumed on their own, one-quarter are consumed as part of a mixed dish, and nearly 5 percent are consumed as savory snacks (e.g., potato chips).

Total grains, particularly refined grains, are consumed in amounts that exceed recommendations. Conversely, intakes of whole grains fall short of recommended amounts for more than 95 percent of toddlers. A majority of grains are consumed through breads, rolls, tortillas, or other bread products or as part of a mixed dish. Ten percent of grains come from sweet bakery products and approximately 15 percent come from crackers and savory snacks. Many of these categories are top sources of sodium or added sugars in this age group.

Average intakes of dairy foods, most of which are consumed as milk, generally exceed recommended amounts in this age group. Intakes of yogurt and cheese account for about 10 percent of dairy intakes. Plant-based beverages and flavored milk each makeup about 2 percent of dairy intakes among toddlers.

Protein food intakes fall within the recommended range, on average. Intakes of meats, poultry, and eggs make up a majority of protein foods intakes, however, seafood intakes in this age group is low. Children in this age group can reduce sodium intake by eating less cured or processed meats including hot dogs, deli meats, and sausages.

Due to the relatively high nutrient needs of toddlers, a healthy dietary pattern has virtually no room for added sugars. Toddlers consume an average of more than 100 calories from added sugars each day, ranging from 40 to 250 calories a day (about 2.5 to 16 teaspoons). Sugar-sweetened beverages, particularly fruit drinks, contribute more than 25 percent of total added sugars intakes and sweet bakery products contribute about 15 percent. Other food category sources contribute a smaller proportion of total added

Table 14.2. Signs a Child Is Hungry or Full

Birth through Age 5 Months	
A child may be hungry if she or he:	**A child may be full if she or he:**
Puts hands to mouth	Closes mouth
Turns head toward breast or bottle	Turns head away from breast or bottle
Puckers, smacks, or licks lips	Relaxes hands
Has clenched hands	
Age 6 through 23 Months	
A child may be hungry if she or he:	**A child may be full if she or he:**
Reaches for or points to food	Pushes food away
Opens her or his mouth when offered a spoon or food	Closes her or his mouth when food is offered
Gets excited when she or he sees food	Turns her or his head away from food
Uses hand motions or makes sounds to let you know she or he is still hungry	Uses hand motions or makes sounds to let you know she or he is still full

sugars on their own, but the wide variety of sources, which include yogurts, ready-to-eat cereals, candy, fruits, flavored milk, milk substitutes, baby food products, and bread, points to the need to make careful choices across all foods.

SUPPORTING HEALTHY EATING

Parents, guardians, and caregivers play an important role in nutrition during this life stage because infants and toddlers are fully reliant on them for their needs. In addition to "what" to feed children, "how" to feed young children also is critical. As noted above, repeated exposure to foods can increase the acceptance of new foods. Another important concept is responsive feeding, a feeding style that emphasizes recognizing and responding to the hunger or fullness cues of an infant or young child.

Responsive Feeding

Responsive feeding is a term used to describe a feeding style that emphasizes recognizing and responding to the hunger or fullness cues of an infant or young child. Responsive feeding helps young children learn how to self-regulate their intake. See Table 14.2 for some examples of signs a child may show for hunger and fullness when she or he is a newborn through age 5 months and signs a child may start to show between age 6 through 23 months. It is important to listen to the child's hunger and fullness cues to build healthy eating habits during this critical age. If parents, guardians, or caregivers have questions or concerns, a conversation with a healthcare provider will be helpful.

Chapter 15 | **Children and Food**

Chapter Contents

Section 15.1 | **Childhood Nutrition Facts**

This section contains text excerpted from the following sources: Text in this section begins with excerpts from "Childhood Nutrition Facts," Centers for Disease Control and Prevention (CDC), February 15, 2021; Text under the heading "Healthy U.S.-Style Dietary Pattern for Children Ages Two through Eight" is excerpted from "*Dietary Guidelines for Americans, 2020-2025,*" *Dietary Guidelines for Americans* (*DGA*), U.S. Department of Agriculture (USDA), December 2020.

Healthy eating in childhood and adolescence is important for proper growth and development and to prevent various health conditions. The *Dietary Guidelines for Americans, 2020–2025* recommend that people aged two years or older follow a healthy eating pattern that includes the following:

- A variety of fruits and vegetables
- Whole grains
- Fat-free and low-fat dairy products
- A variety of protein foods
- Oils

These guidelines also recommend that individuals limit calories from solid fats (major sources of saturated and *trans* fatty acids) and added sugars, and reduce sodium intake. Unfortunately, most children and adolescents do not follow the recommendations set forth in the *Dietary Guidelines for Americans.*

BENEFITS OF HEALTHY EATING

Healthy eating can help individuals achieve and maintain a healthy body weight, consume important nutrients, and reduce the risk of developing health conditions such as:

- High blood pressure (HBP)
- Heart disease
- Type 2 diabetes
- Cancer
- Osteoporosis
- Iron deficiency
- Dental caries (cavities)

DIET AND ACADEMIC PERFORMANCE

- Schools are in a unique position to provide students with opportunities to learn about and practice healthy eating behaviors.
- Eating a healthy breakfast is associated with improved cognitive function (especially memory), reduced absenteeism, and improved mood.
- Adequate hydration may also improve cognitive function in children and adolescents, which is important for learning.

EATING BEHAVIORS OF YOUNG PEOPLE

- Between 2001 and 2010, consumption of sugar-sweetened beverages among children and adolescents decreased but still accounts for 10 percent of total caloric intake.
- Between 2003 and 2010, total fruit intake and whole fruit intake among children and adolescents increased. However, most youth still do not meet fruit and vegetable recommendations.
- Empty calories from added sugars and solid fats contribute to 40 percent of daily calories for children and adolescents age 2–18 years – affecting the overall quality of their diets. Approximately half of these empty calories come from six sources: soda, fruit drinks, dairy desserts, grain desserts, pizza, and whole milk. Most youths do not consume the recommended amount of total water.

HEALTHY U.S.-STYLE DIETARY PATTERN FOR CHILDREN AGES TWO THROUGH EIGHT

In early childhood (ages 2 through 4), females require about 1,000 to 1,400 calories per day and males require about 1,000 to 1,600 calories per day. With the transition to school-age (ages 5 through 8), females require about 1,200 to 1,800 calories per day and males require about 1,200 to 2,000 calories per day.

Table 15.1. Healthy U.S.-Style Dietary Pattern for Children Ages 2 through 8, with Daily or Weekly Amounts from Food Groups, Subgroups, and Components

CALORIE LEVEL OF PATTERN [a]	1,000	1,200	1,400	1,600	1,800	2,000
FOOD GROUP OR SUBGROUP	**Daily Amount of Food from Each Group** (Vegetable and protein foods subgroup amounts are per week.)					
Vegetables (cup eq/day)	**1**	**1 1/2**	**1 1/2**	**2**	**2 1/2**	**2 1/2**
	Vegetable Subgroups in Weekly Amounts					
Dark-Green Vegetables (cup eq/wk)	1/2	1	1	1 1/2	1 1/2	1 1/2
Red & Orange Vegetables (cup eq/wk)	2 1/2	3	3	4	5 1/2	5 1/2
Beans, Peas, Lentils (cup eq/wk)	1/2	1/2	1/2	1	1 1/2	1 1/2
Starchy Vegetables (cup eq/wk)	2	3 1/2	3 1/2	4	5	5
Other Vegetables (cup eq/wk)	1 1/2	2 1/2	2 1/2	3 1/2	4	4
Fruits (cup eq/day)	**1**	**1**	**1 1/2**	**1 1/2**	**1 1/2**	**2**
Grains (ounce eq/day)	**3**	**4**	**5**	**5**	**6**	**6**
Whole Grains (ounce eq/day)	1 1/2	2	2 1/2	3	3	3
Refined Grains (ounce eq/day)	1 1/2	2	2 1/2	2	3	3
Dairy (cup eq/day)	**2**	**2 1/2**	**2 1/2**	**2 1/2**	**2 1/2**	**2 1/2**
Protein Foods (ounce eq/day)	**2**	**3**	**4**	**5**	**5**	**5 1/2**
	Protein Foods Subgroups in Weekly Amounts					
Meats, Poultry, Eggs (ounce eq/wk)	10	14	19	23	23	26
Seafood (ounce eq/wk)[b]	2-3 [c]	4	6	8	8	8
Nuts, Seeds, Soy Products (ounce eq/wk)	2	2	3	4	4	5
Oils (grams/day)	**15**	**17**	**17**	**22**	**22**	**24**

Table 15.1. Continued

CALORIE LEVEL OF PATTERN[a]	**1,000**	**1,200**	**1,400**	**1,600**	**1,800**	**2,000**
Limit on Calories for Other Uses (kcal/day)	**130**	**80**	**90**	**150**	**190**	**280**
Limit on Calories for Other Uses (%/day)[d]	13%	7%	6%	9%	10%	14%

[a]Calorie level ranges: Ages 2 through 4, Females: 1,000-1,400 calories; Males: 1,000-1,600 calories. Ages 5 through 8, Females: 1,200-1,800 calories; Males: 1,200-2,000 calories.
[b]The U.S. Food and Drug Administration (FDA) and the U.S. Environmental Protection Agency (EPA) provide joint advice regarding seafood consumption to limit methylmercury exposure for children. Depending on body weight, some children should choose seafood lowest in methylmercury or eat less seafood.
[c]If consuming up to 3 ounces of seafood per week, children should only be fed cooked varieties from the "Best Choices" list that contain even lower methylmercury. If consuming up to 3 ounces of seafood per week, many commonly consumed varieties of seafood should be avoided because they cannot be consumed at 3 ounces per week by children without the potential of exceeding safe methylmercury limits.
[d]Foods are assumed to be in nutrient-dense forms; lean or low-fat; and prepared with minimal added sugars, refined starches, saturated fat, or sodium. If all food choices to meet food group recommendations are in nutrient-dense forms, a small number of calories remain within the overall limit of the pattern (i.e., limit on calories for other uses). The number of calories depends on the total calorie level of the pattern and the amounts of food from each food group required to meet nutritional goals.

Section 15.2 | **Helping Your Child in Developing Healthy Food Habits**

This section includes text excerpted from "Helping Your Child: Tips for Parents and Other Caregivers," National Institute of Diabetes and Digestive and Kidney Diseases (NIDDK), October 2019.

WHAT SHOULD YOUR CHILD EAT AND DRINK?

Just like adults, children need to consume foods and beverages that are packed with nutrients. Also, like adults, children should consume just enough calories to fuel their daily living and activities. The *2015–2020 Dietary Guidelines for Americans* suggest balancing calories you consume with physical activity. The guidelines also recommend improving eating habits to promote health, reduce the risk of disease, and reduce overweight and obesity. Americans ages 2 years and older are encouraged to consume a variety of healthy foods and beverages. Suggested items include:

- Fruits, vegetables, unsalted nuts, and seeds, and whole grains*

- Fat-free or low-fat dairy products, including milk, yogurt, cheese, and/or fortified nondairy beverages
- A variety of protein foods, including seafood, lean meats and poultry, eggs, legumes (beans and peas), nuts, seeds, and soy products

**Please make sure your child can tolerate these foods and is not allergic to them*

WHAT FOODS AND BEVERAGES SHOULD BE LIMITED?

Youth and adults are also encouraged to get less:

- Refined grains
- Added sugars
- Saturated fats, such as lard, butter, and margarine, which are often solid at room temperature
- Salt (sodium)

Added sugars, solid fats, and salt often occur in pizzas, chips, crackers, sodas, sugar-sweetened drinks, desserts, such as cookies or cake, and fast foods. If children and teens consume these foods and beverages, these items should be limited to a healthy eating plan.

Another step is to make sure your children have breakfast to spark the energy they need to focus in school. Some studies suggest that eating breakfast regularly may decrease children's chances of developing obesity.

HOW CAN YOU HELP YOUR CHILD EAT BETTER?

Use less fat, salt, and sugar. Here are some ideas to help you and your child follow a healthy eating plan:

- Cook with fewer solid fats. Use olive or canola oil instead of butter or margarine. Bake or roast foods instead of frying. You can get a crunchy texture with "oven-frying" recipes that involve little or no oil.
- Choose and prepare foods with less salt. Keep the salt shaker off the table. Have cut-up fruits and vegetables on hand for snacks instead of salty snacks such as chips or crackers.

- Limit the amount of sugar your child eats. Choose hot or cold cereals with no added sugar or low sugar.
- Fill half of your child's plate with fruits and vegetables.
- Learn about age-appropriate portion sizes and how to avoid oversized portions.

Serve nutrient-rich foods and beverages. Many foods and beverages are particularly rich in key nutrients and vitamins – such as potassium, calcium, vitamin D, and dietary fiber – that are important to your children's health and development. Here are some ideas for boosting your children's intake of these nutrients:

- Offer more fruit for breakfast, snacks, and desserts. Add dark green, red, and orange vegetables to stews and soups. Add beans (black, kidney, pinto), peas, and lentils to casseroles and salads. For meal planning ideas and healthy recipes, see Nutrition.gov (www.nutrition.gov).
- Serve more low-fat milk and milk products. If your child cannot digest much lactose, called "lactose intolerance," serve lactose-free milk, cheese, or yogurt. (Lactose is the sugar in milk that may cause some people stomach pain and bloating when they drink milk or eat milk products.) Your child can also try nondairy drinks, such as soy, almond, or rice drinks enriched with calcium or vitamin D.
- Serve fresh, frozen, or canned salmon, shrimp, and light tuna (not albacore). For young children, you may serve safe types of seafood (www.fda.gov/media/102331/download) 1–2 times a week in child-sized portions, starting with 1-ounce portions at age 2.
- Replace the refined grains (breads, pasta, rice) your child eats with whole grains. Eat more bran. Check Nutrition Facts labels to find products high in dietary fiber. Look at the ingredients list to be sure that whole grains are one of the first items.

Think about the drink:

- Serve more water.

- Offer low-fat or fat-free milk instead of whole milk.
- Avoid serving sugar-sweetened beverages and fruit-flavored drinks.
- Offer fresh fruit, which has more fiber than juice. If serving juice, offer small portions of 100 percent fruit juice.
- Offer healthy snacks. Along with their meals, snacks can help children get enough nutrients to help them stay healthy. Buy or prepare single-serving snacks for younger children to help them get just enough to satisfy their hunger. Visit the children's section of ChooseMyPlate (www.myplate.gov/children) to help you and your kids select a satisfying snack (www.myplate.gov/ten-tips-snack-tips-for-parents).

Try to keep healthy food in the house for snacks and meals for the whole family. Offer snacks such as:

- Sliced apples, oranges, pears, and carrots
- Whole-grain bread served with low-fat cheese, favorite spread, or roasted veggies
- Fresh, frozen, or canned vegetables

Keep two more things in mind when choosing healthy snacks.

- Read Nutrition Facts labels to choose the appropriate serving size. Remember that the serving size on nutrition labels applies to adults' dietary needs and is based on a 2,000-calorie diet. So, the right serving size for most children will probably be smaller than what is on the package, depending on the child's age, size, and activity level. Visit the parents' section of Nutrition Facts label: Read the label youth Outreach Materials (www.fda.gov/food/nutrition-education-resources-materials/nutrition-facts-label-read-label-youth-outreach-materials) to find tools for helping your children make healthful food choices and understand how to read the Nutrition Facts label on food packages.

- Children of preschool age and younger can easily choke on foods. Be careful with foods that may be hard to chew, small and round, or sticky. Examples are hard vegetables, whole grapes, hard chunks of cheese, raisins, nuts and seeds, and popcorn. Select snacks with care for children in this age group.

Share food time together:

- Plan to have sit-down meals with your children, and serve everyone the same thing.
- Involve your children in planning and preparing meals. Children may be more willing to eat the dishes they help prepare.
- Try to limit how much food or beverages your child consumes on the go and away from home. That will help you control the calories, sugar, and fat your children consume. To serve more homemade meals, cook large batches of soup, stew, or casseroles and freeze them as a time saver. For handy tips on quick and easy homemade meals, visit (www.choosemyplate.gov).
- Limit eating at home to specific areas such as the kitchen or dining room – not in front of a TV or while using another electronic screen.

Section 15.3 | **Food Allergies in Children**

This section contains text excerpted from the following sources: Text in this section begins with excerpts from "Food Allergies," Centers for Disease Control and Prevention (CDC), June 8, 2020; Text beginning with the heading "Food Allergy Symptoms in Children" is excerpted from "Voluntary Guidelines for Managing Food Allergies in Schools and Early Care and Education Programs," Centers for Disease Control and Prevention (CDC), May 21, 2021.

Food allergies are a growing food safety and public-health concern that affect an estimated 8 percent of children in the United States. That is 1 in 13 children or about 2 students per classroom. A food allergy occurs when the body has a specific and reproducible immune response to certain foods. The body's immune response can be severe and life-threatening, such as anaphylaxis. Although the immune system normally protects people from germs, in people with food allergies, the immune system mistakenly responds to food as if it were harmful.

There is no cure for food allergies. Strict avoidance of the food allergen is the only way to prevent a reaction. However, because it is not always easy or possible to avoid certain foods, staff in schools, out-of-school time, and Early Care and Education Programs (ECE) should develop plans for preventing an allergic reaction and responding to a food allergy emergency, including anaphylaxis. Early and quick recognition and treatment can prevent serious health problems or death.

Eight foods or food groups account for most serious allergic reactions in the United States:

- Milk, eggs, fish, crustacean shellfish, wheat, soy, peanuts, and tree nuts.

The symptoms and severity of allergic reactions to food can be different between individuals and can also be different for one person over time. Anaphylaxis is a sudden and severe allergic reaction that may cause death. Not all allergic reactions will develop into anaphylaxis and more than 40 percent (2 in 5) of children with food allergies in the United States have been treated in the emergency department.

MANAGING FOOD ALLERGIES AT SCHOOL

The Centers for Disease Control and Prevention (CDC) in consultation with the U.S. Department of Education (ED), several federal agencies, and many stakeholders, developed *Voluntary Guidelines for Managing Food Allergies In Schools* and early care and education programs (www.cdc.gov/healthyschools/foodallergies/pdf/20_316712-A_FA_guide_508tag.pdf) to provide practical information and recommendations for each of the five priority areas that should be addressed in each school's or ECE program's Food Allergy Management Prevention Plan:

- Ensure the daily management of food allergies in individual children.
- Prepare for food allergy emergencies.
- Provide professional development on food allergies for staff members.
- Educate children and family members about food allergies.
- Create and maintain a healthy and safe educational environment.

FOOD ALLERGY SYMPTOMS IN CHILDREN

Children with food allergies might communicate their symptoms in the following ways:

- It feels like something is poking my tongue
- My tongue (or mouth) is tingling (or burning)
- My tongue (or mouth) itches
- My tongue feels like there is hair on it
- My mouth feels funny
- There is a frog in my throat; there is something stuck in my throat
- My tongue feels full (or heavy)
- My lips feel tight
- It feels like there are bugs in there (to describe itchy ears)
- It (my throat) feels thick
- It feels like a bump is on the back of my tongue (throat)

FOOD ALLERGIES AND ASTHMA

One-third of children with food allergies also have asthma, which increases their risk of experiencing a severe or fatal reaction. Data also suggest that children with asthma and food allergies have more visits to hospitals and emergency departments (EDs) than children who do not have asthma.

Because asthma can pose serious risks to the health of children with food allergies, schools, and ECE programs must consider these risks when they develop plans for managing food allergies.

FATAL FOOD ALLERGY REACTIONS

Risk factors:

- Delayed administration of epinephrine
- Reliance on oral antihistamines alone to treat symptoms
- Consuming alcohol and food allergen at the same time

Groups at higher risk:

- Adolescents and young adults
- Children with a known food allergy
- Children with a prior history of anaphylaxis
- Children with asthma, particularly those with poorly controlled asthma

EMOTIONAL IMPACT ON CHILDREN WITH FOOD ALLERGIES AND THEIR PARENTS

The health of a child with a food allergy can be compromised at any time by an allergic reaction to food that is severe or life-threatening. Many studies have shown that food allergies have a significant effect on the psychosocial well-being of children with food allergies and their families.

Parents of a child with a food allergy may have constant fear about the possibility of a life-threatening reaction and stress from constant vigilance needed to prevent a reaction. They also have to trust their child to the care of others, make sure their child is safe outside the home, and help their child have a normal sense of identity.

Children with food allergies may also have constant fear and stress about the possibility of a life-threatening reaction. The fear of ingesting a food allergen without knowing it can lead to coping strategies that limit social and other daily activities. Children can carry emotional burdens because they are not accepted by other people, they are socially isolated, or they believe they are a burden to others. They also may have anxiety and distress that is caused by teasing, taunting, harassment, or bullying by peers, teachers, or other adults. School and ECE program staff must consider these factors as they develop plans for managing the risk of food allergy for children with food allergies.

Section 15.4 | **School Meal Programs**

This section includes text excerpted from "School Meals," Centers for Disease Control and Prevention (CDC), April 27, 2021.

WHAT ARE SCHOOL MEAL PROGRAMS?

Many schools provide students with access to meals through federal school meal programs including the National School Lunch Program (NSLP) (www.fns.usda.gov/nslp) and the School Breakfast Program (SBP) (www.fns.usda.gov/sbp/school-breakfast-program). These programs are administered by the U.S. Department of Agriculture (USDA) and state agencies by reimbursing schools for providing healthy meals to students.

WHO CAN PARTICIPATE IN SCHOOL MEAL PROGRAMS?

All students can participate in school meal programs, and some students are eligible to receive free or reduced-price meals. The USDA has extended flexibilities to allow free meals to be available to all children, regardless of household income, through June 30, 2022.

BENEFITS OF SCHOOL MEALS

Research shows that students who participate in the school meal programs consume more whole grains, milk, fruits, and vegetables during meal times and have better overall diet quality, than nonparticipants. And, eating breakfast at school is associated with better attendance rates, fewer missed school days, and better test scores. Meals served through these programs must meet specific nutrition requirements (www.fns.usda.gov/cn/nutrition-standards-school-meals). These requirements were revised in 2012 to include more fruits, vegetables, whole grains, and decrease the amount of sodium and trans fat. Research shows that these changes have helped make school meals more nutritious.

Schools can encourage students to participate in the school meal programs by:

- Providing meals that are nutritious and appealing

- Obtaining input from students and parents about items they would like to see served in the meals
- Ensuring that students have adequate time to eat their meal (at least 10 minutes for breakfast and 20 minutes for lunch)
- Preventing the overt identification of students who are eligible to receive free or reduced-price meals

Section 15.5 | **Smart Snacks**

This section contains text excerpted from the following sources: Text under the heading "What Are Smart Snacks in School?" is excerpted from "Smart Snacks," Centers for Disease Control and Prevention (CDC), May 29, 2019; Text beginning with the heading "Why Are Smart Snacks Important?" is excerpted from "Guide to Smart Snacks in School for School Year 2019-2020," Food and Nutrition Service (FNS), U.S. Department of Agriculture (USDA), March 23, 2021.

WHAT ARE SMART SNACKS IN SCHOOL?

Smart Snacks in School refer to the national nutrition standards for foods and beverages sold outside of the federal reimbursable school meal programs during the school day. These items are called "competitive foods" because they can compete with participation in school meal programs.

As of the 2014–2015 school year, all competitive foods and beverages sold during the school day must meet or exceed Smart Snacks in School nutrition standards, which include limits on fat, sugar, sodium, and calorie content. These standards are the minimum requirement for schools, but states and local education agencies can continue to implement stronger nutrition standards for all competitive foods in schools.

WHY ARE SMART SNACKS IMPORTANT?

- More than a quarter of kids' daily calories may come from snacks.
- Kids who have healthy eating patterns are more likely to perform better academically.

- Kids consume more healthy foods and beverages during the school day. When there are Smart Snacks available, the healthy choice is the easy choice.
- Smart Snacks Standards are a federal requirement for all foods sold outside the National School Lunch Program (NSLP) and School Breakfast Program (SBP).

WHICH FOOD AND BEVERAGES SOLD AT SCHOOL NEED TO MEET THE SMART SNACKS STANDARDS?

- Any food and beverage sold to students at schools during the school day,* other than those foods provided as part of the school meal programs.
- Examples include à la carte items sold in the cafeteria and foods sold in school stores, snack bars, and vending machines.
- Food and beverages sold during fundraisers, unless these items are not intended for consumption at school or are otherwise exempt by your state agency.

* The school day is defined as midnight before to 30 minutes after the end of the school day.

HOW CAN YOU TELL IF YOUR SNACK MEETS THE SMART SNACKS STANDARDS?

- See if your snack is listed in the products section of the Alliance for a Healthier Generation's Smart Foods Planner (foodplanner.healthiergeneration.org/products). These products were determined to meet the Smart Snacks Standards based on the product's ingredient statement and Nutrition Facts panel.
- Enter information from the food or beverage's Nutrition Facts panel and ingredients list into the Alliance for a Healthier Generation's Smart Snacks Product Calculator (foodplanner.healthiergeneration.org/calculator). It is important to note that the standards are for the food items as packaged and sold. Therefore, if the item is labeled as

Table 15.2. The Nutrient Standards for Calories, Sodium, Sugar, and Fats

Nutrient	**Snack**	**Entrée**
Calories	200 calories or less	350 calories or less
Sodium	200 mg or less	480 mg or less
Total Fat	35% of calories or less	35% of calories or less
Saturated Fat	Less than 10% of calories	Less than 10% of calories
Trans Fat	0 g	0 g
Sugar	35% by weight or less	35% by weight or less

having two servings per package, then the information in the Nutrition Facts panel must be multiplied by two. The Smart Snacks Product Calculator does this math for you.

- If your snack does not have a nutrition label because it is made from scratch, then you may need to calculate the nutrition information. Your school nutrition program may have nutrient analysis software approved by the United States Department of Agriculture (USDA); (www.fns.usda.gov/tn/usdaapproved-nutrient-analysis-software) which can be used to evaluate recipes.

WHAT ARE THE SMART SNACKS STANDARDS FOR FOOD?

To qualify as a Smart Snack, a snack or entrée must first meet the general nutrition standards:

- Be a grain product that contains 50 percent or more whole grains by weight (have whole grain as the first ingredient)
- Have as the first ingredient a fruit, a vegetable, a dairy product, or a protein food
- Be a combination food that contains at least ¼ cup of fruit and/or vegetable

Chapter 16 | **Nutrition Information for Teens and Young Adults**

Chapter Contents

Section 16.1 | **Teens and Healthy Eating**

This section includes text excerpted from "Take Charge of Your Health: A Guide for Teenagers," National Institute of Diabetes and Digestive and Kidney Diseases (NIDDK), December 2016. Reviewed May 2021.

TAKING CHARGE OF YOUR HEALTH

As you get older, you are able to start making your own decisions about a lot of things that matter most to you. You may choose your own clothes, music, and friends. You also may be ready to make decisions about your body and health.

Making healthy decisions about what you eat and drink, how active you are, and how much sleep you get is a great place to start. Here you will learn:

- How your body works – how your body uses the food and drinks you consume and how being active may help your body "burn" calories?
- How to choose healthy food and drinks?
- How to get moving and stay active?
- How getting enough sleep is important to staying healthy?
- How to ease into healthy habits and keep them up?
- How to plan healthy meals and physical activities that fit your lifestyle?

How Does the Body Use Energy?

Your body needs the energy to function and grow. Calories from food and drinks give you that energy. Think of food as energy to charge up your battery for the day. Throughout the day, you use energy from the battery to think and move, so you need to eat and drink to stay powered up. Balancing the energy you take in through food and beverages with the energy you use for growth, activity, and daily living is called "energy balance." Energy balance may help you stay a healthy weight.

How Many Calories Does Your Body Need?

Different people need different amounts of calories to be active or stay a healthy weight. The number of calories you need depends on whether you are female or male, your genes, how old you are, your height and weight, whether you are still growing, and how active you are, which may not be the same every day.

How Should You Manage or Control Your Weight?

Some teens try to lose weight by eating very little; cutting out whole groups of foods such as foods with carbohydrates, or carbs skipping meals, or fasting. These approaches to losing weight could be unhealthy because they may leave out important nutrients your body needs. In fact, unhealthy dieting could get in the way of trying to manage your weight because it may lead to a cycle of eating very little and then overeating because you get too hungry. Unhealthy dieting could also affect your mood and how you grow.

Smoking, making yourself vomit, or using diet pills or laxatives to lose weight may also lead to health problems. If you make yourself vomit, or use diet pills or laxatives to control your weight, you could have signs of a serious eating disorder and should talk with your healthcare professional or another trusted adult right away. If you smoke, which increases your risk of heart disease, cancer, and other health problems, quit smoking as soon as possible.

If you think you need to lose weight, talk with a healthcare professional first. A doctor or dietitian may be able to tell you if you need to lose weight and how to do so in a healthy way.

CHOOSE HEALTHY FOODS AND DRINKS

Healthy eating involves taking control of how much and what types of food you eat, as well as the beverages you drink. Try to replace foods high in sugar, salt, and unhealthy fats with fruits, vegetables, whole grains, low-fat protein foods, and fat-free or low-fat dairy foods.

Fruits and Vegetables

Make half of your plate fruits and vegetables. Dark green, red, and orange vegetables have high levels of the nutrients you need, such as vitamin C, calcium, and fiber. Adding tomato and spinach – or any other available greens that you like – to your sandwich is an easy way to get more veggies in your meal.

Grains

Choose whole grains such as whole-wheat bread, brown rice, oatmeal, and whole-grain cereal, instead of refined-grain cereals, white bread, and white rice.

Protein

Power up with low-fat or lean meats such as turkey or chicken, and other protein-rich foods, such as seafood, egg whites, beans, nuts, and tofu.

Dairy

Build strong bones with fat-free or low-fat milk products. If you cannot digest lactose – the sugar in milk that can cause stomach pain or gas – choose lactose-free milk or soy milk with added calcium. Fat-free or low-fat yogurt is also a good source of dairy food.

Fats

Fat is an important part of your diet. Fat helps your body grow and develop, and may even keep your skin and hair healthy. But, fats have more calories per gram than protein or carbs, and some are not healthy.

Some fats, such as oils that come from plants and are liquid at room temperature, are better for you than other fats. Foods that contain healthy oils include avocados, olives, nuts, seeds, and seafood such as salmon and tuna fish.

Solid fats such as butter, stick margarine, and lard, are solid at room temperature. These fats often contain saturated and *trans* fats, which are not healthy for you. Other foods with saturated fats include fatty meats, and cheese and other dairy products made from whole milk. Take it easy on foods such as fried chicken, cheeseburgers, and fries, which often have a lot of saturated and *trans* fats. Options to consider include a turkey sandwich with mustard or a lean-meat, turkey, or veggie burger.

Your body needs a small amount of sodium, which is mostly found in salt. But, getting too much sodium from your foods and drinks can raise your blood pressure, which is unhealthy for your heart and your body in general. Even though you are a teen, it is important to pay attention to your blood pressure and heart health now to prevent health problems as you get older.

Try to consume less than 2,300 mg, or no more than one teaspoon, of sodium a day. This amount includes the salt in already prepared food, as well as the salt you add when cooking or eating your food.

Processed foods, such as those that are canned or packaged, often have more sodium than unprocessed foods, such as fresh fruits and vegetables. When you can choose fresh or frozen fruits and veggies over processed foods, try adding herbs and spices instead of salt to season your food if you make your own meals. Remember to rinse canned vegetables with water to remove extra salt. If you use packaged foods, check the amount of sodium listed on the Nutrition Facts label.

Limit Added Sugars

Some foods, such as fruit, are naturally sweet. Other foods, such as ice cream and baked desserts, as well as some beverages, have added sugars to make them taste sweet. These sugars add calories but not vitamins or fiber. Try to consume less than 10 percent of your daily calories from added sugars in food and beverages. Reach for an apple or banana instead of a candy bar.

Control Your Food Portions

A portion is how much food or beverage you choose to consume at one time, whether in a restaurant, from a package, at school or a friend's, or at home. Many people consume larger portions than they need, especially when away from home. Ready-to-eat meals – from a restaurant, grocery store, or at school – may give you larger portions than your body needs to stay charged up.

Just one super-sized, fast food meal may have more calories than you need in a whole day. And, when people are served more food, they may eat or drink more – even if they do not need it. This habit may lead to weight gain. When consuming fast food, choose small portions or healthier options, such as a veggie wrap or salad instead of fries or fried chicken.

Be Media Smart

Advertisements, TV shows, the internet, and social media may affect your food and beverage choices and how you choose to spend your time. Many ads try to get you to consume high-fat foods and sugary drinks. Be aware of some of the tricks ads use to influence you:

- An ad may show a group of teens consuming a food or drink, or using a product to make you think all teens are or should be doing the same. The ad may even use phrases such as "all teens need" or "all teens are."
- Advertisers sometimes show famous people using or recommending a product because they think you will want to buy products that your favorite celebrities use.
- Ads often use cartoon figures to make a food, beverage, or activity look exciting and appealing to young people.

Do Not Skip Meals

Skipping meals might seem like an easy way to lose weight, but it actually may lead to weight gain if you eat more later to make up for it. Even if you are really busy with school and activities, it is important to try not to skip meals. Follow these tips to keep your body charged up all day and to stay healthy:

- **Eat breakfast every day.** Breakfast helps your body get going. If you are short on time in the morning, grab something to go, such as an apple or banana.
- **Pack your lunch on school days.** Packing your lunch may help you control your food and beverage portions and increases the chances that you will eat it because you made it.

- **Eat dinner with your family.** When you eat home-cooked meals with your family, you are more likely to consume healthy foods. Having meals together also gives you a chance to reconnect with each other and share news about your day.
- **Get involved in grocery shopping and meal planning at home.** Going food shopping and planning and preparing meals with family members or friends can be fun. Not only can you choose a favorite grocery store, and healthy foods and recipes, you also have a chance to help others in your family eat healthy too.

Healthy Eating Tips

- Try to limit foods such as cookies, candy, frozen desserts, chips, and fries, which often have a lot of sugar, unhealthy fat, and salt.
- For a quick snack, try recharging with a pear, apple, or banana; a small bag of baby carrots; or hummus with sliced veggies.
- Do not add sugar to your food and drinks.
- Drink fat-free or low-fat milk and avoid sugary drinks. Soda, energy drinks, sweet tea, and some juices have added sugars, a source of extra calories. The *2015-2020 Dietary Guidelines* call for getting less than 10 percent of your daily calories from added sugars.

Section 16.2 | The Importance of Calcium for Tweens and Teens

This section includes text excerpted from "Building Strong Bones: Calcium Information for Health Care Providers," *Eunice Kennedy Shriver* National Institute of Child Health and Human Development (NICHD), January 2006. Reviewed May 2021.

You can play a critical role in making sure tweens* and teens get 1,300 mg of calcium every day – at least 3 cups of low-fat or fat-free milk, plus other calcium-rich foods – to build strong bones for life.

Calcium is essential to overall health and bone development, but most children and teenagers are not getting enough. In fact, fewer than one in 10 girls and just more than one in four boys 9 to 13 years of age are at or above their adequate intake of calcium.

You can help children achieve lifelong bone health by talking to parents and young people about the importance of calcium consumption, especially during 11 to 15 years of age, a time of critical bone growth. Children and teenagers can get most of their daily calcium from three cups of low-fat or fat-free milk (900 mg), but they also need additional servings of calcium-rich foods to get the 1,300 mg of calcium necessary for optimal bone development.

Research suggests many parents do not know that children and teenagers need almost twice as much calcium as children younger than 9 years of age.

**Note: Tweens are kids ages 9 to 12.*

HOW DOES PEDIATRIC BONE DEVELOPMENT INFLUENCE OSTEOPOROSIS LATER IN LIFE?

The tween and teen years are critical for bone development because most bone mass accumulates during this time. In the years of peak skeletal growth, teenagers accumulate more than 25 percent of adult bone, and by the time teens finish their growth spurts around 17 years of age, 90 percent of their adult bone mass is established. Calcium is critical to building bone mass for supporting physical activity throughout life, and for reducing the risk of bone fractures, especially those due to osteoporosis. The onset of osteoporosis later in life is influenced by two important factors:

- Peak bone mass attained in the first two to three decades of life
- The rate at which bone is lost in the later years

Although the consequences of low-calcium consumption may not be visible in childhood, the *Eunice Kennedy Shriver* National Institute of Child Health and Human Development (NICHD) recognizes lack of calcium intake as a serious and growing threat to the health of young people later in life. At a time when they require more nutrients to feed their rapidly growing and developing bodies, tweens, and teens who do not get enough calcium are at increased risk for osteoporosis later in life.

ARE THERE ANY SPECIAL CALCIUM RECOMMENDATIONS FOR LACTATING OR PREGNANT TEENS?

Increasing dietary calcium does not prevent the loss of calcium that occurs during lactation, and the calcium lost seems to be regained after weaning. Therefore, the Dietary Reference Intakes do not recommend increasing calcium intake for lactating adolescents above normal levels for that age group. However, the 1994 *NIH Consensus Statement on Optimal Calcium Intake* recommends that lactating teenagers and young adults increase their calcium intake to up to 1,500 mg per day.

Section 16.3 | **Healthy Eating Tips for Teen Girls**

This section includes text excerpted from "Healthy Eating for Girls," girlshealth.gov, Office on Women's Health (OWH), January 20, 2016. Reviewed May 2021.

There are low-fat diets, heart-healthy diets, high-protein diets, and low-carb diets. No wonder girls sometimes are confused about what they should and should not eat. Understanding nutrition really is not so hard, though. Check out this helpful menu:

- Foods to eat
- Foods to limit
- How much food do you need to eat?

FOODS TO EAT

Some foods can help protect your health. Try to focus more on these foods.

- Fruits and vegetables are packed with vitamins and minerals. They also have fiber, which helps you feel full and is great for you. Try to fill half your plate with a variety of different fruits and veggies. And, instead of

drinking juice, try to munch on whole fruits, whether frozen, canned, or dried.
- Whole grains have lots of health benefits, including possibly helping prevent heart disease. At least half your grains should be whole grains. This includes whole wheat, oatmeal, and brown rice. (It even includes popcorn – just watch out for added butter and salt.)
- Fat-free and low-fat milk products are great. They are especially good for a girl during her childhood and teen years because she needs them to build strong bones. Look for fat-free or low-fat cheese, yogurt, and other dairy products. If you cannot drink milk, try soy drinks fortified with calcium and vitamin D.
- Protein helps your body heal, gives you energy, and more. Choose a mix of different protein foods. Good options include fish and other seafood, poultry (without the skin), lean meats, beans and peas, eggs, soy products, and unsalted nuts and seeds. Try to pick fish and shellfish in place of some meat and poultry.

You can get great tips on ways to fill your plate with healthy foods (www.myplate.gov/ten-tips).

FOODS TO LIMIT

Some foods are not good for your health if you eat too much of them. Try to have less of these.
- Solid fats, which are fats that are solid at room temperature. Solid fats usually are high in saturated fat and *trans* fat, and eating too much of them can cause problems such as heart disease. Oils that have unsaturated fat are a much healthier choice.
- Sodium is found in table salt and lots of prepared foods. Eating too much sodium can cause health problems such as high blood pressure.
- Added sugars mean you are getting extra calories without any extra nutrients. Added sugars are often hiding out in your soda, cookies, candy, and sugary cereals.

- Refined grains are grains that have had some of the nutrients removed. Choose whole grains because they have all the nutrients.
- Cholesterol can increase your risk of heart disease. Check the Nutrition Facts label (www.girlshealth.gov/nutrition/healthy_eating/food_labels.html) on foods you eat to see how much cholesterol they have. Try to eat as little cholesterol as possible. Cholesterol usually comes from foods such as ice cream, steak, and other animal products.

HOW MUCH FOOD DO YOU NEED TO EAT?

Eating a healthy amount of food helps your body do all the important jobs it needs to do. Eating a lot more than you need or not eating enough can prevent your body from working well.

Eating too much or too little also can stop you from being at a healthy weight. How much you need to eat depends on things such as your age, sex, and how active you are.

Your body also needs a healthy mix of foods. For example, your body cannot work well if you eat piles of protein and little else. The MyPlate food guide (www.girlshealth.gov/nutrition/healthy_eating/pyramid.html) can help you figure out how much of each type of food you need.

The Hungry Hiker game lets you load a hiker's plate with different foods. If you give her the right mix, she can make it to her mountaintop!

Section 16.4 | **Female Athlete Triad**

This section includes text excerpted from "Do You Exercise a Lot?" girlshealth.gov, Office on Women's Health (OWH), May 7, 2018.

Being active is great. In fact, girls should be active at least an hour each day. Sometimes, though, a girl will be very active (such as running every day or playing a competitive sport), but not eat enough to fuel her activity. This can lead to health problems. Following are the problems that can happen if girls do not eat enough to fuel their activity:

- A problem called "low energy availability"
- Period (menstrual) problems
- Bone problems

These three sometimes are called the "female athlete triad." ("triad" means a group of three). They sometimes also are called "athletic performance and energy deficit." (This means you have a "deficit," or lack, of the energy your body needs to stay healthy.)

A PROBLEM CALLED "LOW ENERGY AVAILABILITY"

Your body needs healthy food to fuel the things it does, like fight infections, heal wounds, and grow. If you exercise, your body needs extra food for your workout. You can learn how much food to eat based on your activity level. "Energy availability" means the fuel from food that is not burned up by exercise and so is available for growing, healing, and more. If you exercise a lot and do not get enough nutrition, you may have low energy availability. That means your body will not be as healthy and strong as it should be. Some female athletes diet to lose weight. They may do this to qualify for their sport or because they think losing weight will help them perform better. But, eating enough healthy food is key to having the strength you need to succeed. Also, your body needs good nutrition to make hormones that help with things like healthy periods and strong bones. Sometimes, girls may exercise too much and eat too little because they have an eating disorder. Eating disorders are serious and can even lead to death, but they are treatable.

PERIOD (MENSTRUAL) PROBLEMS

If you are very active, or if you just recently started getting your period (menstruating), you may skip a few periods. But, if you work out really hard and do not eat enough, you may skip a lot of periods (or not get your period to begin with) because your body cannot make enough of the hormone estrogen. You may think you would not mind missing your period, but not getting your period should be taken seriously. Not having your period can mean your body is not building enough bone, and the teenage years are the main time for building strong bones. If you have been getting your period regularly and then miss three periods in a row, see your doctor. Not having your period could be a sign of a serious health problem or of being pregnant. Also, consult your doctor if you are 15 years old and still have not gotten your period.

BONE PROBLEMS

Being physically active helps build strong bones. But, you can hurt your bones if you do not eat enough healthy food to fuel all your activity. That is because your body will not be able to make the hormones needed to build strong bones. Learn about how much food active girls need to eat. One sign that your bones are weak is getting stress fractures, which are tiny cracks in bones. Some places you could get these cracks are your feet, legs, ribs, and spine. Even if you do not have problems with your bones when you are young, not taking good care of them now can be a problem later in life. Your skeleton is almost completely formed by age 18, so it is important to build strong bones early in life. If you do not, then later on you could wind up with osteoporosis, which is a disease that makes it easier for bones to break.

Chapter 17 | Nutrition Needs for Women

Chapter Contents

Section 17.1 | Healthy Eating and Women

This section includes text excerpted from "Healthy Eating and Women," Office on Women's Health (OWH), U.S. Department of Health and Human Services (HHS), March 14, 2019.

The food and drink choices you make every day affect your health now and later in life. Choosing healthy foods and drinks more often can help prevent or manage many health problems that affect women. And, studies show that when a woman eats healthy, everyone in her household is more likely to eat healthy.

WHAT IS HEALTHY EATING?

Healthy eating is a way of eating that improves your health and helps prevent disease. It means choosing different types of healthy food from all of the food groups (fruits, vegetables, grains, dairy, and proteins), most of the time, in the correct amounts for you. Healthy eating also means not eating a lot of foods with added sugar, sodium (salt), and saturated and *trans* fats.

Healthy eating also means getting nutrients primarily from food rather than from vitamins or other supplements. Some women might need vitamins, minerals, or other supplements at certain times in life such as before or during pregnancy. But, most women, most of the time, should get their essential nutrients from what they eat and drink.

What you eat and drink is influenced by where you live, the types of foods available in your community and in your budget, your culture and background, and your personal preferences. Often, healthy eating is affected by things that are not directly under your control, such as how close the grocery store is to your house or job. Focusing on the choices you can control will help you make small changes in your daily life to eat healthier.

HOW MANY CALORIES DO YOU NEED?

The amount of calories you need is based on your physical activity level, age, height, weight, and other unique health considerations, such as whether you are pregnant or breastfeeding.

WHAT DOES HEALTHY EATING LOOK LIKE?

Think about filling your plate with foods from the five food groups – fruits, vegetables, grains, proteins, and dairy – at each meal. Snacks can be a good way to fill in fruits and whole grains you might have missed at meals. Most of us do not need complicated calorie counting programs or special recipes for healthy eating.

Some simple tips to improve your eating habits are to eat more vegetables, snack on fruit more often, and cook at home more each week.

- **Fruits and vegetables.** Everyone needs to eat fruits and vegetables every day. Try to fill about half of your plate with fruits or vegetables at meals. Most women do not get enough fruits and vegetables. Eat whole fruit (not juice) and try different types of vegetables during the week.
- **Protein.** Eat different types of foods with protein, including seafood, lean meats, poultry, eggs, legumes (beans and peas), nuts, seeds, and soy products. Most women do not eat enough seafood to meet weekly recommendations of 8 to 10 ounces (or about two servings a week).
- **Grains.** Make at least half your grains whole grains, such as brown rice, whole-wheat pasta, or whole-wheat bread. Most women do not eat enough whole grains.
- **Dairy.** Women should get three cups of dairy each day, but most women get only half that amount. If you cannot drink milk, try to eat low-fat plain yogurt or low-fat cheese. Dairy products are among the best food sources of mineral calcium, but some vegetables such as kale and broccoli also have calcium, as do some fortified foods such as fortified soymilk, fortified cereals, and many fruit juices. Most girls 9 to 18 years of age and women older than 50 years of age need more calcium for good bone health.
- **Oils.** When cooking, try to use oils from plants instead of solid fats such as butter, margarine, or coconut oil. Most women eat too much solid fat through packaged

foods such as chips or salad dressing, and not enough healthy fats such as olive oil or the type of fat in seafood.

Healthy eating means not eating a lot of food with added sugars, saturated and *trans* fat, and sodium (salt). Healthy eating means eating fruits, vegetables, whole grains, healthy types of protein and dairy, and not eating or drinking too many calories for your body type.

DOES HEALTHY EATING INCLUDE A SPECIFIC DIET OR TYPE OF FOOD?

No. There is no one special ingredient or vitamin that will make you healthy and cure illness. One of the keys to healthy eating is your overall pattern of eating.

You do not have to spend a lot of money, follow a very strict diet, or eat only specific types of food to eat healthily. Healthy eating is not about skipping meals or certain nutrients. Healthy eating is not limited to certain types of food, such as organic, gluten free, or enriched food. It is not limited to certain patterns of eating, such as high protein.

You also do not have to stop eating all of your favorite foods. You can eat a variety of foods, including less healthy favorites, as long as you do not eat them all the time and keep the amount small.

Some diets have been shown by researchers to prevent disease and help people reach and maintain a healthy weight. Get started with one of these:

- Healthy U.S.-style eating plan
- Mediterranean-style eating plan
- Vegetarian eating plan
- DASH diet (Dietary Approaches to Stop Hypertension)

WHY IS HEALTHY EATING IMPORTANT FOR EVERYONE?

Healthy eating helps:

- Your body and brain get the energy you need to think and be physically active

- Your body gets the essential vitamins and minerals you need to stay alive and healthy. For example, your body needs iron to help deliver oxygen to all of your muscles and organs. Vitamin C helps your body make new skin cells and collagen. Vitamin A helps you see better at night.
- You reach and maintain a healthy weight
- Lower your risk of diseases, such as heart disease and diabetes

The old saying "you are what you eat" is true. What you eat and drink becomes the building blocks for all of the cells in your body. Over time, your food and drink choices make a difference in your health.

HOW DO YOUR NUTRITIONAL NEEDS CHANGE THROUGHOUT LIFE?

Women's nutritional needs change as their bodies change during different stages of their lives.

- **During the teen years.** Girls 9 to 18 years of age need more calcium and vitamin D to build strong bones and help prevent osteoporosis later in life. Girls need 1,300 milligrams (mg) of calcium and 600 international units (IUs) of vitamin D every day. Girls 14 to 18 years of age also need more iron than boys (15 mg compared to 11 mg).
- **Young adults.** Teen girls and young women usually need more calories than when they were younger, to support their growing and developing bodies. After about 25 years of age, a woman's resting metabolism (the number of calories her body needs to sustain itself at rest) goes down. To maintain a healthy weight after 25 years of age, women need to gradually reduce their calories and increase their physical activity.
- **Before and during pregnancy.** You need more of certain nutrients than usual to support your health and your baby's development. These nutrients include protein, calcium, iron, and folic acid. Many

doctors recommend prenatal vitamins or a folic acid supplement during this time. Many health insurance plans also cover folic acid supplements prescribed by your doctor during pregnancy. You also need to avoid some foods, such as certain kinds of fish.

- **During breastfeeding.** Continue eating healthy foods while breastfeeding. You may also need to drink more water. Nursing mothers may need about 13 cups of water a day. Try drinking a glass of water every time you nurse and with each meal.
- **After menopause.** Lower levels of estrogen after menopause raise your risk for chronic diseases such as heart disease, stroke, and diabetes, and osteoporosis, a condition that causes your bones to become weak and break easily. What you eat also affects these chronic diseases. Talk to your doctor about healthy eating plans and whether you need more calcium and vitamin D to protect your bones. Most women also need fewer calories as they age, because of less muscle and less physical activity.

HOW MUCH FIBER SHOULD YOU EAT?

Fiber is an important part of an overall healthy eating plan. Good sources of fiber include fortified cereal, many whole-grain breads, beans, fruits (especially berries), dark green leafy vegetables, all types of squash, and nuts. Look on the Nutrition Facts label for fiber content in processed foods such as cereals and breads. Use the search tool on the USDA page (fdc.nal.usda.gov/ndb/search/list) to find the amount of fiber in whole foods such as fruits and vegetables.

Most women do not get enough fiber.

- Women 19 to 30 years of age need 28 grams of fiber every day.
- Women 31 to 50 years of age need 25 grams of fiber every day.
- Women 51 years of age or older need 22 grams of fiber every day.

WHY IS FIBER GOOD FOR WOMEN'S HEALTH?

Not getting enough fiber can lead to constipation and can raise your risk for other health problems. Part of healthy eating is choosing fiber-rich foods, including beans, berries, and dark green leafy vegetables, every day. Fiber helps lower your risk for diseases that affect many women, such as heart disease, diabetes, irritable bowel syndrome (IBS), and colon cancer. Fiber also helps you feel full, so it can help you reach and maintain a healthy weight.

WHY IS SEAFOOD GOOD FOR WOMEN'S HEALTH?

In addition to other nutrients, seafood has two important omega-3 fatty acids: eicosapentaenoic acid and docosahexaenoic acid, more commonly called "EPA" and "DHA." These fatty acids may affect:

- Risk for heart disease
- Risk for preterm birth (also called "premature birth")
- Growth and development in unborn babies and breastfed infants

HOW CAN YOU GET ENOUGH OMEGA-3 FATTY ACIDS?

Here are some ways to get omega-3 fatty acids:

- **Eat seafood.** Salmon, tuna, trout, anchovies, and sardines have high amounts of omega-3 fatty acids. One way to get more seafood is to make it your main protein choice a couple of times a week.
- **Eat nuts, seeds, and oils with omega-3 fatty acids.** Foods high in omega-3 fatty acids include walnuts, flaxseeds, flaxseed oil, soybean oil and canola oil.
- **Eat foods with added omega-3 fatty acids.** Some foods may have added omega-3 fatty acids (called "fortified" on the label), including some types of eggs, yogurt, juices, milk, or soy beverages.
- **Take a fish oil supplement.** If it is difficult to get enough omega-3 fatty acids from food, your doctor or nurse may recommend a supplement (an over-the-counter (OTC) pill). Vegetarian women who do not eat seafood especially may benefit from vegetarian omega-3 supplements.

ARE LOW-FAT OR LOW-CARB DIETS SAFE FOR WOMEN?

Yes, low-fat and low-carbohydrate (carb) diets can be safe, but you should always talk to your doctor or nurse before limiting the amount of any specific nutrient such as fat or carbs. Fats and carbs are essential, which means your body needs them to work correctly and for good health.

- Low-carb diets can help you lose weight, but they can also limit the amount of fiber you get each day. Most women do not get enough fiber. Low-carb diets can also be difficult to continue in the long term. Carbohydrates are a type of essential nutrient, meaning that your body has to have carbs to work correctly.
- Low-fat diets also can help you lose weight. But, the amount of weight loss is usually small. You can lose weight and lower your risk for heart disease and stroke if you follow an overall healthy pattern of eating that includes more fruits, vegetables, whole grains, and beans that are high in fiber, nuts, low-fat dairy, and fish, in addition to staying away from *trans* fat and saturated fat.

For weight loss what is more important is eating healthy carbs and unsaturated fats and limiting the amount of calories you take in. It helps to cut out or eat less of foods that do not have essential vitamins, minerals, or nutrients. Make sure you read the Nutrition Facts label carefully.

Section 17.2 | Menopause and Diet

This section contains text excerpted from the following sources: Text in this section begins with excerpts from "Menopause Basics," Office on Women's Health (OWH), U.S. Department of Health and Human Services (HHS), March 18, 2019; Text under the heading "What Unique Nutritional Needs Do Women Have?" is excerpted from "Healthy Eating and Women," Office on Women's Health (OWH), U.S. Department of Health and Human Services (HHS), March 14, 2019; Text under the heading "What Are Some Natural Remedies for Menopause Symptoms?" is excerpted from "Menopause Treatment," Office on Women's Health (OWH), U.S. Department of Health and Human Services (HHS), May 23, 2019.

Menopause is when your period stops permanently. Menopause is a normal part of a woman's life. It is sometimes called "the change of life." Menopause does not happen all at once. As your body transitions to menopause over several years, you may have menopause symptoms and irregular periods. The average age for menopause in the United States is 52 years of age.

Menopause is when your periods stop permanently and you can no longer get pregnant. You have reached menopause only after it has been a full year since your last period. This means you have not had any bleeding, including spotting, for 12 months in a row.

After menopause your ovaries make very low levels of the hormones estrogen and progesterone. These low hormone levels can raise your risk for certain health problems.

WHAT UNIQUE NUTRITIONAL NEEDS DO WOMEN HAVE?

Women have some unique nutritional needs, including needing more of certain vitamins and minerals during pregnancy or after menopause.

- **Calories.** Most times, women need fewer calories. That is because women naturally have less muscle, more body fat, and are usually smaller. On average, adult women need between 1,600 and 2,400 calories a day. Women who are more physically active may need more calories. Find out how many calories you need each day, based on your age, height, weight, and activity level.
- **Vitamins and minerals.** Calcium, iron, and folic acid are particularly important for women.

- **Reproductive health.** Women have different nutritional needs during different stages of life, such as during pregnancy and breastfeeding or after menopause.
- **Health problems.** Women are more likely to have some health problems related to nutrition, such as celiac disease and lactose intolerance, and vitamin and mineral deficiencies, such as iron-deficiency anemia.
- **Metabolism.** Women process some substances differently and burn fewer calories at rest and during exercise than men do.

WHAT ARE SOME NATURAL REMEDIES FOR MENOPAUSE SYMPTOMS?

Some women report relief for hot flashes and other menopause symptoms with complementary or alternative therapies. Talk to your doctor or nurse before taking any herbal or vitamin supplement. The U.S. Food and Drug Administration (FDA) does not regulate supplements in the same way they regulate medicines. Many supplements can interfere with medicines and make them work incorrectly or not at all.

Some research studies show relief from premenstrual syndrome (PMS) symptoms with these herbal supplements, but other studies do not. Many herbal supplements should not be used with other medicines. Some herbal supplements women use for menopause symptoms are:

- **Black cohosh.** The underground stems and roots of black cohosh are used fresh or dried to make tea, capsules, pills, or liquid extracts. Black cohosh is used to help treat menopausal symptoms, such as hot flashes.
- **Red clover.** It has phytoestrogens, which are similar to estrogen. Phytoestrogens are also found in some cereals, vegetables, legumes (peas, beans, soy). You can take red clover in tea or as a pill. Red clover may not be safe for women who should not take menopausal hormone therapy with estrogen.

- **Soy.** It is a plant in the pea family. The seeds of soy are soybeans. Soybeans make isoflavones, a type of phytoestrogen. Soy can be found in dietary supplements or added to foods such as cheese and pasta. Soybeans can be cooked and eaten or used to make foods such as tofu and soy milk. Soy may not be safe for women who should not take menopausal hormone therapy with estrogen.
- **Mind and body practices.** Yoga, tai chi, and acupuncture may help reduce menopause symptoms, including sleep and mood problems, stress, and muscle and joint pain. One study also found that hypnosis (a trance-like state during which your mind is relaxed) helped decrease hot flashes by 74 percent.

Research continues on these and other alternative ways of relieving menopause. Talk to your doctor or nurse before trying natural remedies.

Section 17.3 | **The Importance of Folic Acid for Women of Childbearing Age**

This section includes text excerpted from "Folic Acid," National Center on Birth Defects and Developmental Disabilities (NCBDDD), Centers for Disease Control and Prevention (CDC), April 19, 2021.

The Centers for Disease Control and Prevention (CDC) urges all women of reproductive age to take 400 micrograms (mcg) of folic acid each day, in addition to consuming food with folate from a varied diet.

ABOUT FOLIC ACID

Folic acid is a B vitamin. Our bodies use it to make new cells. Think about the skin, hair, and nails. These – and other parts of the body – make new cells each day. Folic acid is the synthetic (i.e., not generally occurring naturally) form of folate that is used in supplements and in fortified foods such as rice, pasta, bread, and some breakfast cereals.

WHY FOLIC ACID IS IMPORTANT BEFORE AND DURING PREGNANCY

During early development, folic acid helps form the neural tube. Folic acid is very important because it can help prevent some major birth defects of the baby's brain (anencephaly) and spine (spina bifida).

WOMEN OF REPRODUCTIVE AGE NEED 400 MCG OF FOLIC ACID EVERY DAY

- All women of reproductive age should get 400 mcg of folic acid each day to get enough folic acid to help prevent some birth defects because:
  - About half of U.S. pregnancies are unplanned.
  - Major birth defects of the baby's brain or spine occur very early in pregnancy (3–4 weeks after conception), before most women know they are pregnant.
- When taking folic acid, a higher dose than 400 mcg of folic acid each day is not necessarily better to prevent neural tube defects (NTDs), unless a doctor recommends taking more due to other health conditions.
  - When planning to become pregnant, women who have already had a pregnancy affected by a neural tube defect should consult with their health-care provider. The CDC recommends that these women consume 4,000 mcg of folic acid each day one month before becoming pregnant and through the first three months of pregnancy.

WHEN TO START TAKING FOLIC ACID

Every woman of reproductive age needs to get folic acid every day, whether she is planning to get pregnant or not, to help make new cells.

ARE FOLATE AND FOLIC ACID THE SAME THING?

The terms "folate" and "folic acid" are often used interchangeably, even though they are different. Folate is a general term to describe many different types of vitamin B_9.

Types of folate can include:

- Dihydrofolate (DHF)
- Tetrahydrofolate (THF)
- 5, 10-methylenetetrahydrofolate (5, 10-Methylene-THF)
- 5-methyltetrahydrofolate (5-Methyl-THF or 5-MTHF)

Food fortification is a way to add vitamins or minerals, or both, to foods. Some rice, pasta, bread, and breakfast cereals are fortified with folic acid. These foods are labeled "enriched." Folic acid is a specific type of folate that does not generally occur naturally.

Folic acid is ideal to use for food fortification. It is more stable than types of natural food folate. Heat and light can easily break down types of natural food folate. Folic acid is better suited for food fortification because many fortified products, such as bread and pasta, are cooked.6

The CDC recommends that women of reproductive age who could become pregnant consume at least 400 micrograms (mcg) of folate every day. However, it's difficult to get 400 mcg of folate through diet alone. You can get 400 mcg of folic acid each day by taking a vitamin with folic acid in it, eating fortified foods, or a combination of the two, in addition to consuming a balanced diet rich in natural food folate.

HOW TO GET ENOUGH FOLIC ACID

In addition to eating foods with folate from a varied diet, women can get folic acid from:

- **Taking a vitamin that has folic acid in it.**
    - Most vitamins sold in the United States have the recommended daily amount of folic acid (400 mcg) that women need.
    - Vitamins can be found at the most local pharmacy, grocery, or discount stores. Check the label on the

  bottle to be sure it contains 100 percent of the daily value of folic acid, which is 400 mcg.
- **Eating fortified foods.**
  - You can find folic acid in some breads, breakfast cereals, and corn masa flour.
  - Be sure to check the Nutrient Facts label, and look for a product that has "100 percent" next to folate.
- **Getting a combination of the two.** Take a vitamin that has folic acid in it and eat fortified foods.

Section 17.4 | Nutrition: Tips for Pregnant Moms

This section includes text excerpted from "Tips for Pregnant Moms," Food and Nutrition Service (FNS), U.S. Department of Agriculture (USDA), December 2016. Reviewed May 2021.

Making healthy food choices along with regular physical activity will help fuel your baby's growth and keep you healthy during pregnancy.

FIND YOUR HEALTHY EATING STYLE

Choose a variety of foods and beverages to build your own healthy eating style. Include foods from all food groups: fruits, vegetables, grains, dairy, and protein foods.

The amount and types of food you eat is an important part of a healthy eating style. Before you eat, think about what and how much food goes on your plate or in your cup, bowl, or glass.

MAKING HEALTHY FOOD CHOICES

- Make half your plate fruits and vegetables. Choose fresh, frozen, canned, dried, and 100 percent juice. Make sure to include dark green, red, and orange vegetables; beans and peas; and starchy vegetables.
- Make at least half your grains whole grains. Try oatmeal, popcorn, whole-grain bread, and brown rice.

- Move to low-fat or fat-free milk, yogurt, or cheese. Fortified soy beverages also count.
- Vary your protein routine. Choose seafood, lean meats and poultry, eggs, beans and peas, soy products, and unsalted nuts and seeds.
- Use the Nutrition Facts label and ingredients list to limit items higher in sodium, saturated fat, and added sugars. Drink water instead of sugary drinks. Choose vegetable oils instead of butter.
- Enriched grains, beans, peas, oranges, spinach, or other dark green leafy vegetables can help you get the folate-rich food you need.

DAILY FOOD CHECKLIST

The Checklist shows slightly more amounts of food during the 2nd and 3rd trimesters because you have changing nutritional needs. This is a general checklist. You may need more or less amounts of food.*

Table 17.1. Daily Food Checklist for Pregnant Moms

Food Group	1st Trimester	2nd and 3rd Trimesters	What Counts As 1 Cup or 1 Ounce?
Eat this amount from each group daily.*			
Fruits	2 cups	2 cups	1 cup fruit or 100% juice and ½ cup dried fruit
Vegetables	2½ cups	3 cups	1 cup raw or cooked vegetables or 100% juice and 2 cups raw leafy vegetables
Grains	6 ounces	8 ounces	1 slice bread; 1 ounce ready-to-eat cereal; and ½ cup cooked pasta, rice, or cereal
Protein Foods	5½ ounces	6½ ounces	1 ounce lean meat, poultry, or seafood; ¼ cup cooked beans; ½ ounce nuts or 1 tbsp peanut butter; and 1 egg
Dairy	3 cups	3 cups	1 cup milk; 8 ounces yogurt; 1½ ounces natural cheese; and 2 ounces processed cheese

**If you are not gaining weight or gaining too slowly, you may need to eat a little more from each food group. If you are gaining weight too fast, you may need to cut back by decreasing the amount or change the types of food you are eating.*

Seafood

Seafood is part of a healthy diet. Omega-3 fats in seafood can have important health benefits for you and your developing baby. Salmon, sardines, and trout are some choices higher in omega-3 fats and lower in contaminants such as mercury.

- Eat at least 8 and up to 12 ounces of a variety of seafood each week from choices that are lower in mercury.
- Eat all types of tuna, but limit white (albacore) tuna to 6 ounces each week.
- Do not eat tilefish, shark, swordfish, and king mackerel since they are highest in mercury.

Being Physically Active

Unless your doctor advises you not to be physically active, include 2½ hours each week of physical activity such as brisk walking, dancing, gardening, or swimming. The activity can be done for at least 10 minutes at a time, and preferably spread throughout the week. Avoid activities with a high risk of falling or injury.

VISIT YOUR DOCTOR REGULARLY

Doctors' Recommendation

- Pregnant women and women who may be pregnant need to avoid alcohol and smoking. Ask for advice about caffeine, dietary supplements, and drug use.
- In addition to eating a healthy diet, take a prenatal vitamin and mineral supplement containing folic acid.
- Feed your baby only human milk (also known as "breastmilk") for the first six months.

How Much Weight Should You Gain?

- The right weight gain depends on your weight when you became pregnant. If your weight was in the healthy range, you should gain between 25 and 35 pounds. If you were overweight or underweight before becoming pregnant, the advice is different.
- Gain weight gradually. For most women, this means gaining a total of 1 to 4 pounds during the first three months. Gain 2 to 4 pounds each month from the 4th to 9th month.

Chapter 18 | Nutrition for Older Persons

Chapter Contents

Section 18.1 | **Healthy Eating after 50**

This section contains text excerpted from the following sources: Text in this section begins with excerpts from "AgePage: Healthy Eating after 50," National Institute on Aging (NIA), National Institutes of Health (NIH), October 2019; Text beginning with the heading "Healthy Dietary Patterns for Adults Aged 60" is excerpted from "*Dietary Guidelines for Americans, 2020-2025*," *Dietary Guidelines for Americans* (*DGA*), U.S. Department of Agriculture (USDA), December 2020.

Choosing healthy foods is a smart thing to do – no matter your age! Healthy habits such as eating well and being physically active can help you reduce your risk of chronic diseases such as heart disease, diabetes, and osteoporosis. Here are some tips to get you started:

- Eat many different colors and types of vegetables and fruits.
- Make sure at least half your grains are whole grains.
- Limit saturated fat (found mostly in butter, beef fat, and coconut, palm, and palm kernel oils) and *trans* fats (found in processed foods such as store-bought baked goods, pizza, and margarine).
- Eat "good" (poly and monounsaturated) fats, such as those found in seeds, nuts, avocados, and fatty fish such as salmon. Any fats added in cooking should come from plant-based oils such as olive or canola oils.
- Eat eight ounces of seafood per week. Certain fish, such as salmon, shad, and trout, contain less mercury than large fish, such as tuna. Mercury can be harmful.

HOW MUCH SHOULD YOU EAT?

How much you should eat depends on how active you are. If you eat more calories than your body uses, you gain weight.

What Are Calories?

Calories are a way to count how much energy is in food. The energy you get from food helps you do the things you need to do each day. Try to choose foods that have a lot of the nutrients you need, but not many calories.

Just counting calories is not enough for making smart choices. Think about this: a medium banana, one cup of flaked cereal, 1 1/2 cups of cooked spinach, one tablespoon of peanut butter, or one cup of one percent milk all have roughly the same number of calories. But, the foods are different in many ways. Some have more nutrients than others do. For example, milk gives you more calcium than a banana, and peanut butter gives you more protein than cereal. Some food can make you feel more full than others.

COMMON PROBLEMS OLDER ADULTS HAVE WITH EATING

Does your favorite chicken dish taste different? As you age, your sense of taste and smell may change, and foods may seem to lose flavor. Try extra spices, herbs, or lemon juice to add flavor. Also, medicines may change how food tastes. They can also make you feel less hungry. Talk to your doctor if this is a problem.

Maybe some of the foods you used to eat no longer agree with you. For example, some people become lactose intolerant. They have stomach pain, gas, or diarrhea after eating or drinking something with milk in it. Your doctor can test to see if you are lactose intolerant.

Are you finding it harder to chew your food? If you have dentures, maybe they do not fit, or your gums are sore. If so, a dentist can help you. Until then, you might want to eat softer foods that are easier to chew.

These are just a few possible problems older adults may have with eating.

How Many Calories Do People Over Age 50 Need Each Day?

A woman:

- Who is not physically active needs about 1,600 calories
- Who is somewhat active needs about 1,800 calories
- Who has an active lifestyle needs about 2,000–2,200 calories

A man:

- Who is not physically active needs about 2,000–2,200 calories

- Who is somewhat active needs about 2,200–2,400 calories
- Who has an active lifestyle needs about 2,400–2,800 calories

Here Is a Tip

Aim for at least 150 minutes (21⁄2 hours) of physical activity each week.

Try to be active throughout the day to reach this goal, and avoid sitting for a long time.

DO OLDER ADULTS NEED TO DRINK WATER?

With age, you might lose some of your sense of thirst. Do not wait until you feel thirsty to drink water or other fluids. Unless your doctor has told you to limit fluids, drink plenty of liquids such as water, milk, or broth.

Try to add liquids throughout the day. You could try low-fat soup for a snack or drink a glass of water when you take a pill. Do not forget to take sips of water, milk, or juice between bites during a meal.

WHAT ABOUT FIBER

Fiber is found in foods from plants – fruits, vegetables, beans, nuts, seeds, and whole grains. Eating more fiber can help prevent stomach or intestinal problems, such as constipation. It might also help lower cholesterol and blood sugar. It is better to get fiber from food than dietary supplements. Start adding fiber slowly. That will help avoid gas. Here are some tips for adding fiber:

- Eat cooked dry beans, peas, and lentils.
- Leave the skin on your fruit and vegetables if possible but wash them first.
- Choose whole fruit over fruit juice.
- Eat whole-grain breads and cereals.

SHOULD YOU CUT BACK ON SALT?

The usual way people get sodium is by eating salt. The body needs sodium, but too much can make blood pressure go up in some people. Many foods contain some sodium, especially those high in protein. However, most fresh fruits and vegetables do not have much sodium. Salt is added to many canned, boxed, and prepared foods.

People tend to eat more salt than they need. If you are 51 or older, about one teaspoon of table salt – 2,300 milligrams (mg) sodium – is all you need each day. That includes all the sodium in your food and drink, not just the salt you add. If you have high blood pressure or prehypertension, try to limit sodium to 1,500 mg, or about 2/3 teaspoon, per day.

Try to avoid adding salt during cooking or at the table. Eat fewer salty snacks and processed foods, such as lunch meats, potato chips, or frozen dinners.

Look for the word sodium, not salt, on the Nutrition Facts panel. Choose foods labeled "low sodium," "no salt added," "unsalted," or "salt-free." The amount of sodium in the same kind of food can vary greatly among brands, so check the label.

Here Is a Tip

Spices, herbs, and lemon juice add flavor to your food, so you will not miss the salt.

WHAT ABOUT FAT

Fat in your diet comes from two places – the fat already in food and the fat added when you cook. Fat gives you energy and helps your body function, but it is high in calories. Some types of fat, such as mono- and poly-unsaturated fats, provide your body with important nutrients and can be good for you in the right amounts. Other types of fat, such as *trans* fat and saturated fat, can be bad for your health. To lower the fat in your diet:

- Choose cuts of meat, fish, or poultry (with the skin removed) with less fat. Trim off any extra fat before cooking.
- Use low-fat or fat-free dairy products and salad dressings.
- Choose unsaturated fats, such as olive, canola, or vegetable oil, for cooking. Check the label.

- Do not fry foods. Instead, broil, roast, bake, stir-fry, steam, microwave, or boil them.

KEEP FOOD SAFE

As you grow older, you must take extra care to keep your food safe to eat. It is harder for you to fight off infections, and some foods could make you very sick.

Handle raw meat, poultry, seafood, and eggs with care. Keep them apart from foods that will not be cooked or are already cooked. Use hot, soapy water to wash your hands, tools, and work surfaces as you cook.

Do not depend on sniffing or tasting food to tell what is bad. Try putting dates on the foods in your fridge. Check the "use by" date on foods. If in doubt, toss it out.

Make sure food gets into the refrigerator no more than two hours after it is bought or cooked. Use or freeze leftovers within three to four days.

CAN YOU AFFORD TO EAT RIGHT?

If your budget is limited, it might take some planning to be able to pay for the foods you should eat. Here are some suggestions:

- Buy only the foods you need – a shopping list will help.
- Buy only as much food as you will use. If you buy in bulk, buy only as much as you can use before it goes bad.
- Choose foods with plain (generic) labels or store brands – they often cost less than name brands.
- Plan your meals around food that is on sale.
- Divide leftovers into small servings, label, and date, and freeze to use within a few months.

Federal government programs are available to help people with low incomes buy groceries.

HEALTHY DIETARY PATTERNS FOR ADULTS AGED 60

Table 18.1. Healthy U.S.-Style Dietary Pattern for Adults Ages 60 and Older

CALORIE LEVEL OF PATTERN[a]	1,600	1,800	2,000	2,200	2,400	2,600
FOOD GROUP OR SUBGROUP[b]	Daily Amount of Food from Each Group (Vegetable and protein foods subgroup amounts are per week.)					
Vegetables (cup eq/day)	2	2 1/2	2 1/2	3	3	3 1/2
	Vegetable Subgroups in Weekly Amounts					
Dark-Green Vegetables (cup eq/wk)	1 1/2	1 1/2	1 1/2	2	2	2 1/2
Red & Orange Vegetables (cup eq/wk)	4	5 1/2	5 1/2	6	6	7
Beans, Peas, Lentils (cup eq/wk)	1	1 1/2	1 1/2	2	2	2 1/2
Starchy Vegetables (cup eq/wk)	4	5	5	6	6	7
Other Vegetables (cup eq/wk)	3 1/2	4	4	5	5	5 1/2
Fruits (cup eq/day)	1 1/2	1 1/2	2	2	2	2
Grains (ounce eq/day)	5	6	6	7	8	9
Whole Grains (ounce eq/day)	3	3	3	3 1/2	4	4 1/2
Refined Grains (ounce eq/day)	2	3	3	3 1/2	4	4 1/2
Dairy (cup eq/day)	3	3	3	3	3	3
Protein Foods (ounce eq/day)	5	5	5 1/2	6	6 1/2	6 1/2
	Protein Foods Subgroups in Weekly Amounts					
Meats, Poultry, Eggs (ounce eq/wk)	23	23	26	28	31	31
Seafood (ounce eq/wk)	8	8	9	9	10	10

Table 18.1. Continued

CALORIE LEVEL OF PATTERN[a]	1,600	1,800	2,000	2,200	2,400	2,600
Nuts, Seeds, Soy Products (ounce eq/wk)	4	4	5	5	5	5
Oils (grams/day)	22	24	27	29	31	34
Limit on Calories for Other Uses (kcal/day)	100	140	240	250	320	350
Limit on Calories for Other Uses (%/day)	7%	8%	12%	12%	13%	5

[a]Calorie level ranges: Females: 1,600–2,200 calories; Males: 2,000–2,600 calories. Energy levels are calculated based on median height and body weight for healthy body mass index (BMI) reference individuals. For adults, the reference man is five feet 10 inches tall and weighs 154 pounds. The reference woman is five feet four inches tall and weighs 126 pounds. Calorie needs vary based on many factors. The DRI calculator for healthcare professionals, available at (nal.usda.gov/fnic/dri-calculator), can be used to estimate calorie needs based on age, sex, height, weight, and physical activity level.

[b]All foods are assumed to be in nutrient-dense forms; lean or low-fat and prepared with minimal added sugars; refined starches, saturated fat, or sodium. If all food choices to meet food group recommendations are in nutrient-dense forms, a small number of calories remain within the overall limit of the pattern (i.e., limit on calories for other uses). The number of calories depends on the total calorie level of the pattern and the amounts of food from each food group required to meet nutritional goals. Calories up to the specified limit can be used for added sugars, saturated fat, and/or alcohol, or to eat more than the recommended amount of food in a food group.

**NOTE: The total dietary pattern should not exceed Dietary Guidelines limits for added sugars, saturated fat, and alcohol; be within the Acceptable Macronutrient Distribution Ranges for protein, carbohydrate, and total fats; and stay within calorie limits. Values are rounded.*

CURRENT INTAKES OF ADULTS AGED 60 AND OVER

The figures highlight the dietary intakes of older adults, including the healthy eating index-2015 score, which is an overall measure of how intakes align with the *Dietary Guidelines,* as well as information on the components of a healthy diet – specifically, the food groups. Figure 18.1 displays the average intakes of the food groups compared to the range of recommended intakes at the calorie levels most relevant to males and females in this age group. Additionally, the percent of older adults exceeding the recommended limits for added sugars, saturated fat, and sodium are shown, along with average intakes of these components.

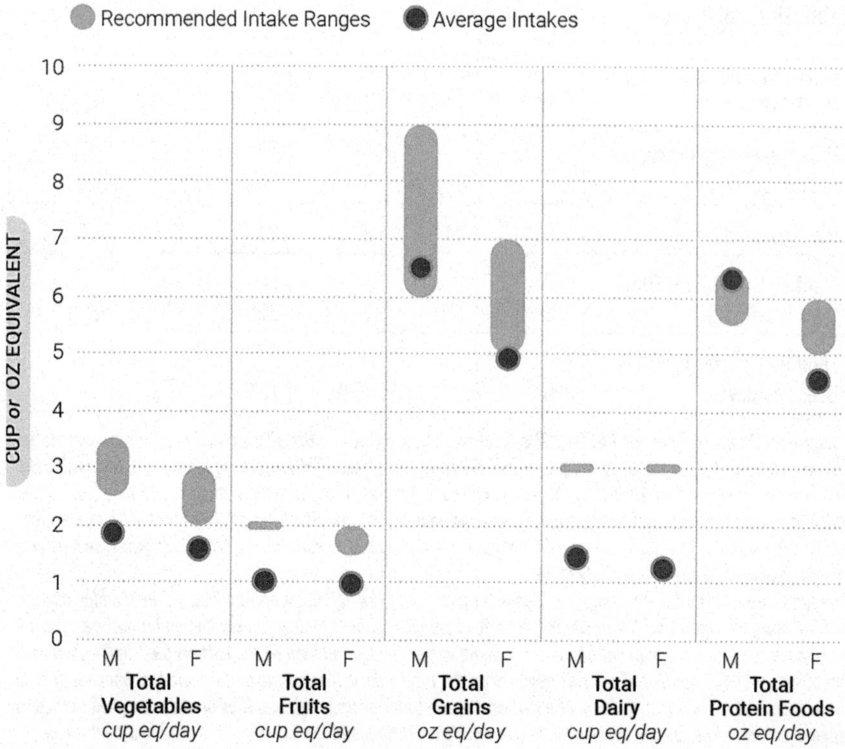

Figure 18.1. Average Intakes of Subgroups Compared to Recommended Intake Ranges: Ages 60 and Older

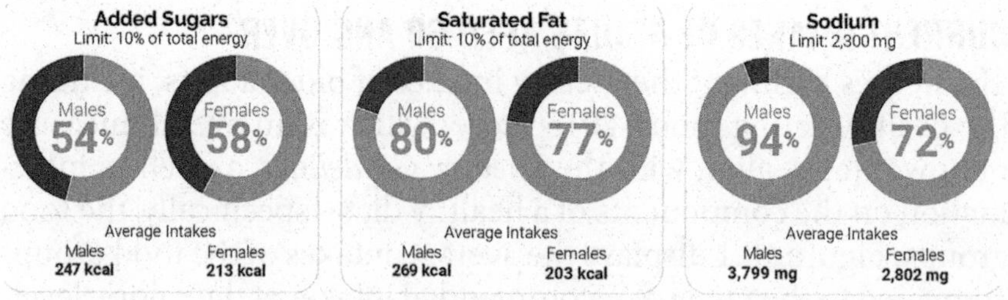

Figure 18.2. Percent Exceeding Limits and Recommended Limits of Added Sugars, Saturated Fat, and Sodium *(Source: Average Intakes and HEI-2015 Scores: Analysis of What We Eat in America, NHANES 2015–2016, day 1 dietary intake data, weighted. Recommended Intake Ranges: Healthy U.S.-Style Dietary Patterns. Percent Exceeding Limits: What We Eat in America, NHANES 2013–2016, 2 days dietary intake data, weighted.)*

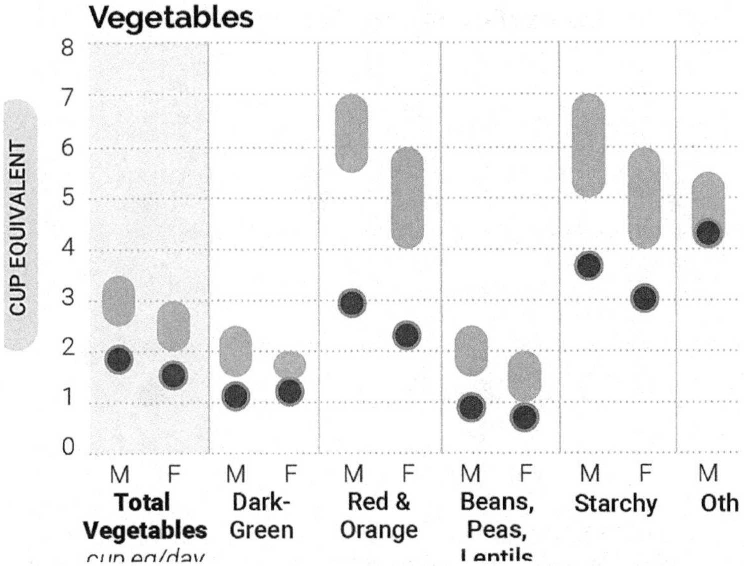

Figure 18.3. Recommended Vegetable Intake Ranges: Aged 60 and Older

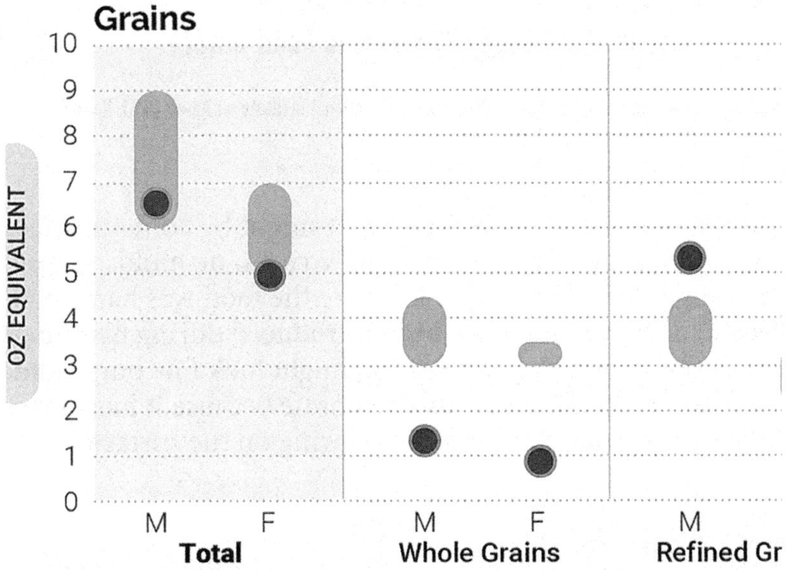

Figure 18.4. Recommended Grains Intake Ranges: Aged 60 and Older

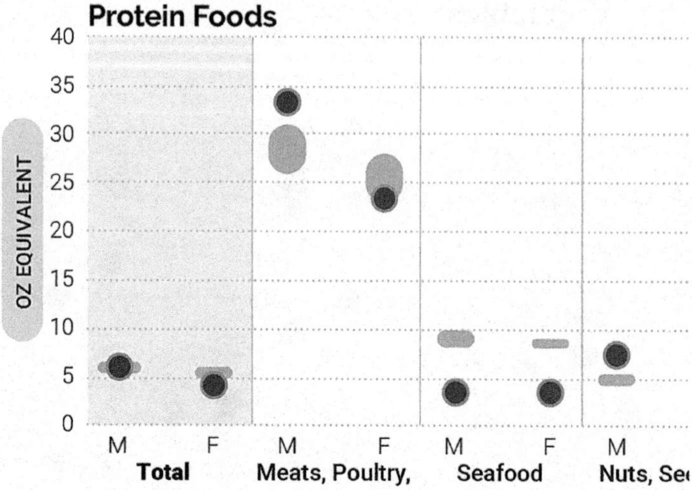

Figure 18.5. Recommended Protein Intake Ranges: Aged 60 and Older *(Source: Average Intakes: Analysis of What We Eat in America, NHANES 2015–2016, day 1 dietary intake data, weighted. Recommended Intake Ranges: Healthy U.S.-Style Dietary Patterns.)*

Section 18.2 | Older Adults and Food Safety

This section includes text excerpted from "Food Safety," National Institute on Aging (NIA), National Institutes of Health (NIH), April 30, 2019.

Food can be unsafe for many reasons. It might be contaminated by germs – microbes such as bacteria, viruses, or molds. These microbes might have been present before the food was harvested or collected, or they could have been introduced during handling or preparation. In either case, the food might look fine but, could make you very sick. Food can also be unsafe because it has "gone bad." Sometimes, you may see mold growing on the surface.

AVOID GETTING SICK FROM YOUR FOOD

For an older person, a food-related illness can be life-threatening. As you age, you have more trouble fighting off microbes. Health problems, such as diabetes or kidney disease, also make you more likely to get sick from eating foods that are unsafe. So be careful about how food is prepared and stored.

Some foods present higher risks than others. Here are some tips on selecting lower risk food options:

- Eat fish, shellfish, meat, and poultry that have been cooked to a safe minimum internal temperature, instead of eating the food raw or undercooked.
- Drink pasteurized milk and juices instead of the unpasteurized versions.
- Make sure pasteurized eggs or egg products are used in recipes that call for raw or undercooked eggs, such as homemade Caesar salad dressings, raw cookie dough, or eggnog.
- Always wash vegetables, including all salad ingredients, before eating. Cooked vegetables also are a lower-risk option than raw vegetables.
- Choose cooked sprouts instead of raw sprouts.
- Choose hard or processed cheeses, cream cheese, or mozzarella, or any cheese that is clearly labeled "Made from Pasteurized Milk" instead of soft cheese made from unpasteurized (raw) milk, such as Brie, Camembert, blue-veined, or queso fresco.
- Heat up hot dogs, deli meats, and luncheon meats to 165 °F (steaming hot), instead of eating the meat unheated.

Changing Taste and Smell

As you grow older, your senses of taste and smell might change. Some illnesses, such as COVID–19, or health conditions can change your senses of smell and taste. Certain medicines might also make things taste different. If you cannot rely on your sense of taste or smell to tell that food is spoiled, be extra careful about how you handle your food. If something does not look, smell, or taste right, throw it out – do not take a chance with your health.

Smart Storage

Food safety starts with storing your food properly. Sometimes that is as simple as following directions on the container. For example, if the label says "refrigerate after opening," do that! It is also a good idea to keep any canned and packaged items in a cool place.

When you are ready to use a packaged food, check the date on the label. That bottle of juice might have been in your cabinet so long it is now out of date.

Try to use refrigerated leftovers within three or four days to reduce your risk of food poisoning. Throw away foods older than that or those that show moldy areas.

Foods and Medicines

Some foods, and also caffeine and alcohol, are unsafe to take with certain medicines. A food-medicine interaction can prevent a medicine from working the way it should, cause a side effect from medicine to get worse, cause a new side effect, or change the way your body processes the food or medicine. For example, some statins (cholesterol medicines) act differently on the body if you consume large amounts of grapefruit juice. Every time you use a new medicine, check the label for interactions. If you have any questions, talk to your doctor or pharmacist.

FOOD SAFETY FOR OLDER ADULTS WHEN COOKING

When preparing foods, follow four basic steps – clean, separate, cook, and chill.

Clean

Wash your hands, the cutting board, and the counter with hot, soapy water, and make sure knives and other utensils are clean before you start to prepare food. Clean the lids of cans before opening. Rinse fruits and vegetables under running water, but do not use soap or detergent. Do not rinse raw meat or poultry before cooking – you might contaminate other things by splashing disease-causing microbes around.

Keep your refrigerator clean, especially the vegetable and meat bins. When there is a spill, use hot, soapy water to clean it up.

Separate

Keep raw meat, poultry, seafood, and eggs (and their juices and shells) away from foods that will not be cooked. That begins in your grocery cart – put raw vegetables and fruit in one part of the cart, maybe the top part.

Products such as meat and fish should be put in plastic bags and placed in a separate part of the cart. At checkout, make sure the raw meat and seafood are not mixed with other items in your bags.

When you get home, keep things such as raw meat separate from fresh fruit and vegetables (even in your refrigerator). Do not let the raw meat juices drip on foods that will not be cooked before they are eaten.

When you are cooking, it is also important to keep ready-to-eat foods such as fresh produce or bread apart from food that will be cooked. Use a different knife and cutting board for fresh produce than you use for raw meat, poultry, and seafood. Or, use one set, and cut all the fresh produce before handling foods that will be cooked.

Wash your utensils and cutting board in hot, soapy water or the dishwasher, and clean the counter and your hands afterwards. If you put raw meat, poultry, or seafood on a plate, wash the plate in hot, soapy water before reusing it for cooked food.

Cook

Use a food thermometer. Put it in the thickest part of the food you are cooking to check that the inside has reached the right temperature. The chart below shows what the temperature should be inside food before you stop cooking it. No more runny fried eggs or hamburgers that are pink in the middle.

Bring sauces, marinades, soups, and gravy to a boil when reheating.

No matter what temperature you set your oven at, the temperature inside your food needs to reach the level shown here to be safe.

Table 18.2. The USDA-Recommended Safe Minimum Internal Temperatures

Type of Food	Minimum Internal Temperature
All meats and seafood	145 °F (with a 3-minute rest time)
All ground meats	160 °F
Egg dishes	160 °F
All poultry	165 °F
Hot dogs and luncheon meats	165 °F

Chill

Keeping foods cold slows the growth of microbes, so your refrigerator should always be at 40 °F or below. The freezer should be at 0 °F or below. But, just because you set the thermostat for 40 °F does not mean it actually reaches that temperature. Use refrigerator/freezer thermometers to check.

Put food in the refrigerator within two hours of buying or cooking it. If the outside temperature is over 90 °F, refrigerate within one hour. Put leftovers in a clean, shallow container that is covered and dated. Use or freeze leftovers within three to four days.

FOOD SAFETY FOR OLDER ADULTS WHEN EATING OUT

It is nice to take a break from cooking or get together with others for a meal at a restaurant. But, do you think about food safety when you eat out? You should.

- Pick a tidy place with clean tables and floors.
- If your city or state requires restaurants to post a cleanliness rating near the front door, check it out.
- Do not be afraid to ask the waiter or waitress how items on the menu are prepared. For example, could you have the tuna cooked well instead of seared? Or, if you find out the Caesar salad dressing is made with raw eggs, ask for another salad dressing.
- Consider avoiding buffets. Sometimes food in buffets sits out for a while and might not be kept at the proper temperature – whether hot or cold.

- If you take leftovers home, get them into the refrigerator within two hours – sooner if the temperature outside is above 90 °F.

Section 18.3 | **Overcoming Roadblocks to Healthy Eating**

This section includes text excerpted from "Overcoming Roadblocks to Healthy Eating," National Institute on Aging (NIA), National Institutes of Health (NIH), April 30, 2019.

ARE YOU TIRED OF COOKING OR EATING ALONE?

Maybe you are tired of planning and cooking dinners every night. Have you considered potluck meals? If everyone brings one part of the meal, cooking is a lot easier, and there might be leftovers to share. Or try cooking with a friend to make a meal you can enjoy together. Also look into having some meals at a nearby senior center, community center, or religious facility. Not only will you enjoy a free or low-cost meal, but you will have some company while you eat.

DO YOU HAVE PROBLEMS CHEWING FOOD?

Do you avoid some foods because they are hard to chew? People who have problems with their teeth or dentures often avoid eating meat, fruits, or vegetables and might miss out on important nutrients. If you are having trouble chewing, see your dentist to check for problems. If you wear dentures, the dentist can check how they fit.

IS IT SOMETIMES HARD TO SWALLOW YOUR FOOD?

If the food seems to get stuck in your throat, it might be that less saliva in your mouth is making it hard for you to swallow your food. Or, there may be other reasons you are having trouble swallowing your food, including problems with the muscles or nerves in your throat, problems with your esophagus, or gastroesophageal reflux disease (GERD). Talk to your doctor about what might be causing your swallowing issues.

DOES FOOD TASTE DIFFERENT?

Are foods not as tasty as you remember? It might not be the cook's fault! Maybe your sense of taste, smell, or both have changed. Growing older, having dental problems, and medication side effects can cause your senses to change. Taste and smell are important for a healthy appetite and eating. Try adding fresh herbs, spices, or lemon juice to your plate. If you drink alcohol or smoke, cutting back can improve your sense of taste.

DO YOU FEEL SAD AND YOU DO NOT WANT TO EAT?

Feeling blue now and then is normal, but if you continue to feel sad, ask your doctor for help. Being unhappy can cause a loss of appetite. Help might be available. You might need to talk with someone trained to work with people who are depressed.

ARE YOU JUST NOT HUNGRY?

Maybe you are not sad, but just cannot eat very much. Changes to your body as you age can cause some people to feel full sooner than they did when younger. Or lack of appetite might be the side effect of a medicine you are taking – your doctor might be able to suggest a different drug.

Try being more physically active. In addition to all the other benefits of exercise and physical activity, it may make you hungrier.

If you are not hungry because food just is not appealing, there are ways to make it more interesting. Make sure your foods are seasoned well, but not with extra salt. Try using lemon juice, vinegar, or herbs to boost the flavor of your food.

Vary the shape, color, and texture of foods you eat. When you go shopping, look for a new vegetable, fruit, or seafood you have not tried before or one you have not eaten in a while. Sometimes grocery stores have recipe cards near items. Or ask the produce staff or meat or seafood department staff for suggestions about preparing the new food. You can also find recipes online.

Foods that are overcooked tend to have less flavor. Try cooking or steaming your vegetables for a shorter time, and see if that gives them a crunch that will help spark your interest.

DO YOU HAVE TROUBLE GETTING ENOUGH CALORIES?

If you are not eating enough, add snacks throughout the day to help you get more nutrients and calories. Raw vegetables with hummus, low-fat cheese and whole-grain crackers, a piece of fruit, unsalted nuts, or peanut butter are good examples. You can try putting shredded low-fat cheese on your soup or popcorn or sprinkling nuts or wheat germ on yogurt or cereal.

If you are eating so little that you are losing weight but do not need to, your doctor might suggest a protein nutrition supplement. Sometimes these supplements help undernourished people gain a little weight. If so, they should be used as snacks between meals or after dinner, not in place of a meal and not right before one. Ask your doctor how to choose a supplement.

ARE PHYSICAL PROBLEMS MAKING IT HARD TO EAT?

Sometimes illnesses such as Parkinson disease, stroke, or arthritis can make it harder for you to cook or feed yourself. Your doctor might recommend an occupational therapist. She or he might suggest rearranging things in your kitchen, make a custom splint for your hand, or give you special exercises to strengthen your muscles. Devices such as special utensils and plates might make mealtime easier or help with food preparation.

CAN FOODS AND MEDICINES INTERACT?

Medicines can change how food tastes, make your mouth dry or take away your appetite. In turn, some foods can change how certain medicines work. You might have heard that grapefruit juice is a common culprit when used with any of several drugs. Chocolate, licorice, and alcohol are some of the others. Whenever your doctor prescribes a new drug for you, be sure to ask about any food-drug interactions.

ARE YOU LACTOSE INTOLERANT?

Some older people have uncomfortable stomach and intestinal symptoms after they have dairy products. Your doctor can do tests to learn whether or not you do indeed need to limit or avoid foods with lactose when you eat. If so, talk to your healthcare provider about how to meet your calcium and vitamin D needs. Even lactose-intolerant people might be able to have small amounts of milk when taken with food. There are nondairy food sources of calcium, lactose-free milk and milk products, calcium- and vitamin D-fortified foods, and supplements.

ARE WEIGHT ISSUES ADDING TO FRAILTY?

Some older adults do not get enough of the right nutrients. These problems can put you at risk of developing weak bones and muscles, which can make you frail and unable to do daily activities. Obesity is a growing problem in the United States, and the number of older people who are overweight or obese is also increasing. But, just losing weight is not necessarily the answer. That is because sometimes when older people lose weight, they lose even more muscle than fat. That puts them at greater risk of becoming frail and falling. They also might lose bone strength and be at risk for a broken bone. Exercise helps you keep muscle and bone. Also, for some people, a few extra pounds late in life can act as a safety net should they get a serious illness that limits how much they can eat for a while.

The *Dietary Guidelines* encourage people 65 and older who are overweight to try to avoid gaining more weight. Those who are very overweight (obese) might be helped by intentional weight loss, especially if they are at risk for heart disease. So, if you think you weigh too much, check with your doctor before starting a diet. She or he can decide whether or not losing a few pounds will be good for you and how you can safely lose weight.

Section 18.4 | **Dietary Supplements**

This section contains text excerpted from the following sources: Text in this section begins with excerpts from "Dietary Supplements for Older Adults," National Institute on Aging (NIA), National Institutes of Health (NIH), April 23, 2021; Text beginning with the heading "Vitamins and Minerals for Older Adults" is excerpted from "Vitamins and Minerals for Older Adults," National Institute on Aging (NIA), National Institutes of Health (NIH), January 1, 2021.

Dietary supplements are substances you might use to add nutrients to your diet or to lower your risk of health problems, such as osteoporosis or arthritis. Dietary supplements come in the form of pills, capsules, powders, gel tabs, extracts, or liquids. They might contain vitamins, minerals, fiber, amino acids, herbs or other plants, or enzymes. Sometimes, the ingredients in dietary supplements are added to foods, including drinks. A doctor's prescription is not needed to buy dietary supplements.

SHOULD YOU TAKE A DIETARY SUPPLEMENT?

Eating a variety of healthy foods is the best way to get the nutrients you need. However, some people do not get enough vitamins and minerals from their daily diet, and their doctors may recommend a supplement. Dietary supplements may provide nutrients that might be missing from your daily diet. When that is the case, your doctors may recommend a dietary supplement to provide missing nutrients.

If you are thinking about using dietary supplements:

- **Learn.** Find out as much as you can about any dietary supplement you might take. Talk with your doctor, your pharmacist, or a registered dietitian. A supplement that seemed to help your neighbor might not work for you. If you are reading fact sheets or checking websites, be aware of the source of the information. Could the writer or group profit from the sale of a particular supplement?
- **Remember.** Just because something is said to be "natural" does not mean it is safe or good for you. It could have side effects. It might make the medicine

your doctor prescribed for you either weaker or stronger. It could also be harmful to you if you have certain medical conditions.
- **Tell your doctor.** She or he needs to know if you decide to use a dietary supplement. Do not diagnose or treat any health condition without first checking with your doctor.
- **Buy wisely.** Choose brands that your doctor, dietitian, or pharmacist recommends. Do not buy dietary supplements with ingredients you do not need. Do not assume that more is better. It is possible to waste money on unneeded supplements.
- **Check the science.** Make sure any claim about a dietary supplement is based on scientific proof. The company making the dietary supplement should be able to send you information on the safety and/or effectiveness of the ingredients in a product, which you can then discuss with your doctor. Remember, if something sounds too good to be true, it probably is.

WHAT IF YOU ARE OVER 50?

People over age 50 may need more of some vitamins and minerals than younger adults do. Your doctor or a dietitian can tell you whether you need to change your diet or take a vitamin or mineral supplement to get enough of these:
- **Calcium** works with vitamin D to keep bones strong at all ages. Bone loss can lead to fractures in both older women and men. Calcium is found in milk and milk products (fat-free or low fat is best), canned fish with soft bones, dark-green leafy vegetables such as kale, and foods with calcium added, such as breakfast cereals.
- **Vitamin D.** Most people's bodies make enough vitamin D if they are in the sun for 15 to 30 minutes at least twice a week. But, if you are older, you may not be able to get enough vitamin D that way. Try adding vitamin D-fortified milk and milk products, vitamin D-fortified

cereals, and fatty fish to your diet, and/or use a vitamin D supplement.

- **Vitamin B_6.** This vitamin is needed to form red blood cells. It is found in potatoes, bananas, chicken breasts, and fortified cereals.
- **Vitamin B_{12}** helps keep your red blood cells and nerves healthy. While older adults need just as much vitamin B_{12} as other adults, some have trouble absorbing the vitamin naturally found in food. If you have this problem, your doctor may recommend that you eat foods, such as fortified cereals that have this vitamin added, or use a B_{12} supplement.

ARE DIETARY SUPPLEMENTS SAFE?

Scientists are still working to answer this question. The U.S. Food and Drug Administration (FDA) checks prescription medicines, such as antibiotics or blood pressure medicines, to make sure they are safe and do what they promise. The same is true for over-the-counter (OTC) drugs, such as pain and cold medicines.

The FDA does not have authority over dietary supplements in the same way it does prescription medicines. The federal government does not regularly test what is in dietary supplements, and companies are not required to share information on the safety of a dietary supplement with the FDA before they sell it. The companies are responsible for making sure the supplement is safe, but the FDA does not evaluate the safety of the product before the supplement is sold. So, just because you see a dietary supplement on a store shelf does not mean it is safe, that it does what the label says it will, or that it contains what the label says it contains.

If the FDA receives reports of possible problems with a supplement, it will issue warnings about products that are clearly unsafe. The FDA may also take these supplements off the market. The Federal Trade Commission (FTC) looks into reports of ads that might misrepresent what dietary supplements do. A few private groups, such as the U.S. Pharmacopeia, NSF International, ConsumerLab.com, and the Natural Products Association (NPA), have their own "seals of approval" for dietary supplements. To get such a seal, products must be made by following good manufacturing procedures, must contain what is listed on the label, and must not have harmful levels of ingredients that do not belong there, like lead.

VITAMINS AND MINERALS FOR OLDER ADULTS

Vitamins and minerals are two of the main types of nutrients that your body needs to survive and stay healthy. Find information on some of the essential vitamins recommended for older adults and how to get the recommended amount within your diet.

Vitamins help your body grow and work the way it should. There are 13 essential vitamins – vitamins A, C, D, E, K, and B vitamins (thiamine, riboflavin, niacin, pantothenic acid, biotin, B_6, B_{12}, and folate).

Vitamins have different jobs to help keep the body working properly. Some vitamins help you resist infections and keep your nerves healthy, while others may help your body get energy from food or help your blood clot properly. By following the *Dietary Guidelines,* you will get enough of most of these vitamins from food.

Like vitamins, minerals also help your body function. Minerals are elements that our bodies need to function that can be found on the earth and in foods. Some minerals, such as iodine and fluoride, are only needed in very small quantities. Others, such as calcium, magnesium, and potassium, are needed in larger amounts. As with vitamins, if you eat a varied diet, you will probably get enough of most minerals.

HOW CAN YOU GET THE VITAMINS AND MINERALS YOU NEED?

It is usually better to get the nutrients you need from food, rather than a pill. That is because nutrient-dense foods contain other things that are good for you, such as fiber.

Most older people can get all the nutrients they need from foods. But if you are not sure, talk with your doctor or a registered dietitian to find out if you are missing any important vitamins or minerals. She or he may recommend a vitamin or dietary supplement.

If you do need to supplement your diet, look for a supplement that contains the vitamin or mineral you need without a lot of other unnecessary ingredients. Read the label to make sure the dose is not too large. Avoid supplements with mega-doses. Too much of some vitamins and minerals can be harmful, and you might be paying for supplements you do not need. Your doctor or pharmacist can recommend brands that fit your needs.

Here Is a Tip

Different foods in each food group have different nutrients. Picking an assortment within every food group throughout the week will help you get many nutrients. For example, choose seafood instead of meat twice a week. The variety of foods will make your meals more interesting, too.

MEASUREMENTS FOR VITAMINS AND MINERALS

Vitamins and minerals are measured in a variety of ways. The most common are:

- Milligram–mg (a milligram is one-thousandth of a gram)
- Microgram–mcg (a microgram is one-millionth of a gram. 1,000 micrograms is equal to one milligram).
- International unit–IU (the conversion of milligrams and micrograms into IU depends on the type of vitamin or drug)

RECOMMENDED SODIUM INTAKE FOR OLDER ADULTS

Sodium is another important mineral. In most Americans' diets, sodium primarily comes from salt (sodium chloride). Whenever you add salt to your food, you are adding sodium. But the *Dietary Guidelines* show that most of the sodium we eat does not come from our saltshakers – it is added to many foods during processing or preparation. We all need some sodium, but too much over time can lead to high blood pressure, which can raise your risk of having a heart attack or stroke.

Table 18.3. Key Vitamins and Minerals for People Over Age 51

Vitamin/ Mineral	Men Age 51+	Women Age 51+	Food Sources
Vitamin D	If you are age 51–70, you need at least 15 mcg (600 IU) each day, but not more than 100 mcg (4,000 IU). If you are over age 70, you need at least 20 mcg (800 IU), but not more than 100 mcg (4,000 IU).	If you are age 51–70, you need at least 15 mcg (600 IU) each day, but not more than 100 mcg (4,000 IU). If you are over age 70, you need at least 20 mcg (800 IU), but not more than 100 mcg (4,000 IU).	You can get vitamin D from fatty fish, fish liver oils, fortified milk and milk products, and fortified cereals.
Vitamin B_{12}	2.4 mcg every day	2.4 mcg every day	You can get this vitamin from meat, fish, poultry, milk, and fortified breakfast cereals. Some people over age 50 have trouble absorbing the vitamin B_{12} found naturally in foods. They may need to take vitamin B_{12} supplements and eat foods fortified with this vitamin.
Calcium	Men aged 51–70 need 1,000 mg each day. Men aged 71 need 1,200 mg each day. Do not consume more than 2,000 mg each day.	1,200 mg each day Do not consume more than 2,000 mg each day.	Calcium is a mineral that is important for strong bones and teeth, so there are special recommendations for older people who are at risk for bone loss. You can get calcium from milk and other dairy, some forms of tofu, dark-green leafy vegetables, soybeans, canned sardines and salmon with bones, and calcium-fortified foods.

Table 18.3. Continued

Vitamin/ Mineral	Men Age 51+	Women Age 51+	Food Sources
Magnesium	420 mg each day	320 mg each day	This mineral, generally, is found in foods containing dietary fiber, such as green leafy vegetables, whole grains, legumes, and nuts and seeds. Breakfast cereals and other fortified foods often have added magnesium. Magnesium is also present in tap, mineral, or bottled drinking water.
Potassium	Men need 3,400 mg each day.	Most women age 51 and older need 2,600 mg each day.	Many different fruits, vegetables, meats, and dairy foods contain potassium. Foods high in potassium include dried apricots, lentils, and potatoes. Adults get a lot of their potassium from milk, coffee, tea, and other nonalcoholic beverages.
Sodium	Men 51 and older should reduce their sodium intake to 2,300 mg each day. That is about 1 teaspoon of salt and includes sodium added during manufacturing or cooking as well as at the table when eating. If you have high blood pressure or prehypertension, limiting sodium intake to 1,500 mg per day, about 2/3 teaspoon of salt, may be helpful.	Women 51 and older should reduce their sodium intake to 2,300 mg each day. That is about 1 teaspoon of salt and includes sodium added during manufacturing or cooking as well as at the table when eating. If you have high blood pressure or prehypertension, limiting sodium intake to 1,500 mg per day, about 2/3 teaspoon of salt, may be helpful.	Preparing your own meals at home without using a lot of processed foods or salt will allow you to control how much sodium you get.

Table 18.3. Continued

Vitamin/ Mineral	Men Age 51+	Women Age 51+	Food Sources
Vitamin B_6	Most men 51 and older should aim for 1.7 mg each day.	Most women 51 and older should aim for 1.5 mg each day.	Vitamin B_6 is found in a wide variety of foods. The richest sources of vitamin B_6 include fish, beef liver, potatoes and other starchy vegetables, and fruit (other than citrus).
Vitamin A	Most men 51 and older should aim for 900 mcg RAE.	Most women 51 and older should aim for 700 mcg RAE each day.	Vitamin A can be found in products such as eggs and milk. It can also be found in vegetables and fruits, such as carrots and mangoes.
Vitamin C	Most men 51 and older should aim for 75 mg each day.	Most women 51 and older should aim for 90 mg each day.	Fruits and vegetables are some of the best sources of vitamin C. Citrus fruits, tomatoes, and potatoes can be a large source of vitamin C.
Vitamin E	Most men age 51 and older should aim for 15 mg each day.	Most women age 51 and older should aim for 15 mg each day.	Vitamin E can be found in nuts such as peanuts and almonds and can be found in vegetable oils, too. It can also be found in green vegetables, such as broccoli and spinach.
Vitamin B_1 (Thiamin)	Most men 51 and older should aim for 1.2 mg each day.	Most women 51 and older should aim for 1.1 mg each day.	You can find vitamin B1 in meat – especially pork – and fish. It is also in whole grains and some fortified breads, cereals, and pastas.
Vitamin B_2 (Riboflavin)	Most men 51 and older should aim for 1.3 mg each day.	Most women 51 and older should aim for 1.1 mg each day.	You can find vitamin B2 in eggs and organ meat, such as liver and kidneys, and lean meat. You can also find it in green vegetables, such as asparagus and broccoli.

Table 18.3. Continued

Vitamin/ Mineral	Men Age 51+	Women Age 51+	Food Sources
Vitamin B_3 (Niacin)	Most men 51 and older should aim for 16 mg each day.	Most women 51 and older should aim for 14 mg each day.	Vitamin B3 can be found in some types of nuts, legumes, and grains. It can also be found in poultry, beef, and fish.
Vitamin K	Most men 51 and older should aim for 120 mg each day.	Most women should aim for 90 mg each day.	Vitamin K can be found in many foods including green leafy vegetables, such as spinach and kale and in some fruits, such as blueberries and figs. It can also be found in cheese, eggs, and different meats.
Folate	Most men age 51 and older should aim for 400 mcg DFE each day.	Most women age 51 and older should aim for 400 mcg DFE each day.	Folate can be found in vegetables and fruit, such as broccoli, brussel sprouts, spinach, and oranges. It can also be found in nuts, beans, and peas.

How much sodium is okay? People 51 and older should reduce their sodium intake to 2,300 mg each day. That is about one teaspoon of salt and includes sodium added during manufacturing or cooking as well as at the table when eating. If you have high blood pressure or prehypertension, limiting sodium intake to 1,500 mg per day, about 2/3 teaspoon of salt, may be helpful. Preparing your own meals at home without using a lot of processed foods or salt will allow you to control how much sodium you get. Try using less salt when cooking, and do not add salt before you take the first bite. If you make this change slowly, you will get used to the difference in taste. Also look for grocery products marked "low sodium," "unsalted," "no salt added," "sodium-free," or "salt-free." Also, check the Nutrition Facts label to see how much sodium is in a serving.

Eating more fresh vegetables and fruit also helps – they are naturally low in sodium and provide more potassium. Get your sauce and dressing on the side and use only as much as you need for taste.

Part 4 | **Lifestyle and Nutrition**

Chapter 19 | **Smart Supermarket Shopping**

Chapter Contents

Section 19.1 | **Planning for Healthy Food Shopping**

This section includes text excerpted from "Shopping for Food That's Good for You," National Institute on Aging (NIA), National Institutes of Health (NIH), April 29, 2019.

Many people say a successful trip to the grocery store starts with a shopping list. Throughout the week, try to keep a list of food and supplies you need. Keeping to a list helps you follow a budget because you will be less likely to buy on impulse. A prepared grocery list will help you choose healthy types of foods.

When making your shopping list, check your staples. Staples are nice to have around if you cannot go grocery shopping. These include items, such as:

- Whole-grain cereal
- Flour
- Cans of low-sodium soup and tuna fish
- Dried fruit
- Bags of frozen vegetables or fruits
- Frozen or bottled 100 percent juice
- Powdered dry milk or ultra-pasteurized, shelf-stable milk
- Pasta or rice
- Low-sodium sauce in a jar

MAKE SHOPPING EASIER

A trip to the grocery store can be a chore for anyone, but as you get older, you might have some new reasons for not going. For example, getting around a big food store might be difficult. What can you do?

- Some stores have motorized carts, which you can use
- Ask if there is an employee who can help you reach things or push your cart
- If your store has a pharmacy department, you might find a seat there if you get tired
- Plan to shop at a time of day when you are rested and the store is not busy so you will not have to stand in a long checkout line

- Check with your local area agency on aging (www.n4a.org) to see if there are volunteers in your area who can help

Some people think a grocery delivery service is helpful. You will want to ask about fees and other charges before deciding if this service would work for you. Many require access to a computer for ordering.

Shopping for healthy foods, especially fresh fruits and vegetables, might be hard where you live. People who live in rural areas or some city neighborhoods often have trouble finding larger supermarkets. Instead, they have to shop at convenience stores and small neighborhood markets. Sometimes smaller stores have limited selections of fresh foods.

You might try talking to the managers or owners. Let them know that you and others are interested in buying more fresh fruits and vegetables, whole-grain products, and low-fat milk products.

Here is a tip. Some grocery stores have special shelf tags or food labels that help you identify healthier choices – for example, high fiber, no added sugar, low in saturated fat, or whole grain. If your grocery store features healthy choices, this can help you find them quickly when you shop, but always read the Nutrition Facts label to compare products.

COMMUNITY SUPPORTED AGRICULTURE

Try to find a community supported agriculture (CSA) group (www.nal.usda.gov/afsic/community-supported-agriculture). The CSAs are membership or subscription groups that allow you to buy in-season fruits and vegetables directly from local farmers. Each week you receive a variety of the food being harvested at that time. LocalHarvest is one organization that can help you find a CSA in your area.

Farmers' markets or vegetable stands offer fresh fruits and vegetables in season and might cost less than what you find in the grocery store. To find farmers' markets in your area, check with LocalHarvest, or your local government. Or you can search an online listing of farmers' markets.

You might also get help from the federal government to pay for vegetables and fruits from farmers' markets through the Seniors Farmers' Market Nutrition Program (SFMNP). They provide coupons you can use at farmers' markets and roadside stands.

Section 19.2 | Healthy Eating on a Budget

This section contains text excerpted from the following sources: Text in this section begins with excerpts from "Make a Plan," MyPlate, U.S. Department of Agriculture (USDA), December 30, 2020; Text under the heading "Tips for Every Aisle" is excerpted from "Shop Smart," MyPlate, U.S. Department of Agriculture (USDA), December 30, 2020.

Making a plan before heading to the store can help you get organized, save money, and choose healthy options.

PLAN YOUR WEEKLY MEAL

Here are some simple tips to get you started:

- **See what you already have.** Look in your freezer, cabinets, and refrigerator. You can save money by using these items in the upcoming week's meals.
- **Write down your meals.** It is helpful to write out your meals for the week including breakfast, lunch, dinner, and snacks.
- **List out recipes to try.** Find new ideas for healthy and low-cost meals based on what you have on hand, foods your family enjoys, and foods that are good buys.
- **Think about your schedule.** Choose meals you can easily prepare when you are short on time. Save ones that take longer for days off or when family members are free to help.
- **Plan to use leftovers.** Think about making larger recipes with enough servings for another meal. On busy days, just heat and serve.
- **Make a grocery list.** Organize your grocery list by store section or food groups to make shopping quick and easy.

- **Build your shopping list as you go.** Keep an ongoing list of foods you need on your refrigerator or on a free mobile app and add items as you run out. Some mobile apps allow you to sync grocery lists with others in your household.
- **Buy a combination of fresh, frozen, and nonperishable items.** Plan for a mix of fresh, frozen, and shelf-stable foods in your meals. Eat your fresh food first so it does not go bad. Stock your freezer and pantry with items you can eat later.

SAVE MORE AT THE STORE

- **Ask around.** Ask friends, family, or post a question on social media to see where others shop and find great bargains! Grocery stores, ethnic markets, dollar stores, retail supercenters, and wholesale clubs may offer good deals.
- **Read the sales flyer.** Sales flyers usually come out midweek and can be found at the store's entrance, in the newspaper, on their website, or on social media pages.
- **Eat before you shop.** Grocery shopping while hungry can lead to impulse buying and unhealthy food choices. This is a simple, yet effective way to keep you on task.
- **Join your store's loyalty program.** Most stores offer a free loyalty program. Get special offers, coupons, and discounts for being a member.
- **Get fresh produce to your door.** Search online for low-cost produce delivery services in your area. Or support local farms by joining a Community Supported Agriculture (CSA) program.

TIPS FOR EVERY AISLE

Fruits and Vegetables

Find fruits and vegetables in the produce section, frozen foods, and in the canned and pantry food aisles. Compare prices to find the best buys.

- Buy "in season" produce which is usually less expensive and at peak flavor. Buy only what you can use before it spoils.
- Choose fruit canned in 100 percent fruit juice and vegetables with "low sodium" or "no salt added" on the label. These products are just as nutritious as fresh and often cost less.
- If you have the freezer space, stock up on frozen vegetables without added sauces or butter. Frozen vegetables are as good for you as fresh and may cost less.
- Canned and frozen fruits and vegetables last much longer than fresh and a quick way to add fruits and vegetables to your meal.

Grains

Find grains in many areas of the store, including the bread, cereal, snack, and pasta and rice aisles.

- Make half your grains whole grains. Types of whole grains include whole wheat, brown rice, bulgur, buckwheat, oatmeal, whole-grain cornmeal, whole oats, and whole rye.
- While shopping, check ingredient lists and pick the items that have a whole grain listed first.
- Rice and pasta are budget-friendly grain options.
- Choose hot cereals, such as plain oatmeal or whole-grain dry cereal.
- Try new whole-grain snack ideas, such as switching to whole-wheat crackers or popping your own popcorn.

Protein Foods

Find protein foods throughout the entire store. They can be found in the fresh meat case, frozen foods section, dairy case, and canned and pantry food aisles.

- Some great low-cost protein foods include beans, peas, and lentils, such as kidney beans, lima beans, split peas, and garbanzo beans (chickpeas). Beans, peas, and lentils cost far less than a similar amount of other protein foods.

- To lower meat costs, buy the family-sized or value pack and freeze what you do not use. Choose lean meats, such as chicken or turkey. When choosing ground beef, make sure it is lean (at least 93 percent lean) ground beef.
- Seafood does not have to be expensive. Try buying canned tuna, salmon, or sardines – these stores well and are a low-cost option.
- Do not forget about eggs! They are a great low-cost option that is easy to prepare.

Dairy

Find dairy foods in the refrigerated and pantry aisles.

- Choose low-fat or fat-free milk. These products provide just as much calcium, but fewer calories than whole and two percent milk.
- Buy the larger size of low-fat plain yogurt instead of individual flavored yogurt. Then add your own flavors by mixing in fruits.
- When it comes to cheese, look for "reduced fat," or "low fat" on the label.
- Always check the "sell by" date to make sure you are buying the freshest dairy products.

Other

- Drink water instead of buying sodas or other sugary drinks. Water is easy on your wallet and has zero calories. A reusable water bottle is a great way to have water with you on the go.
- Save time, money, and calories by skipping the chip and cookie aisles.
- Choose the checkout lane without the candy, especially if you have kids with you.

Chapter 20 | **Healthy Vegetarianism**

BEANS, PEAS, AND LENTILS ARE UNIQUE FOODS

Beans, peas, and lentils belong to a group of vegetables called "pulses." This group includes all beans, peas, and lentils cooked from dry, canned, or frozen, such as kidney beans, pinto beans, black beans, pink beans, black-eyed peas, garbanzo beans (chickpeas), split peas, pigeon peas, mung beans, and lentils. Lentils come in varieties that are mostly identified by their colors, such as brown, black, red, and green. Green peas, green lima beans, and green (string) beans are not part of the beans, peas, and lentils subgroup because their nutrient content is more similar to other vegetable subgroups. Green peas and green lima beans are grouped with starchy vegetables. Green (string) beans are grouped with other vegetables, such as onions, avocado, beets, and cabbage.

You can choose to count beans, peas, and lentils as part of the vegetable group or the protein foods group depending on how they fit into your overall eating pattern. They are excellent sources of dietary fiber and nutrients, such as folate and potassium, similar to vegetables. They are also excellent sources of plant protein and provide other nutrients, such as iron and zinc, similar to protein foods. Because they are similar to meats, poultry, and seafood in their contribution of certain nutrients, beans, peas, and lentils are vegetarian options within the protein foods group. Due to their

This chapter contains text excerpted from the following sources: Text beginning with the heading "Beans, Peas, and Lentils Are Unique Foods" is excerpted from "Beans, Peas, and Lentils," MyPlate, U.S. Department of Agriculture (USDA), January 2, 2021; Text under the heading "Healthy Vegetarian Dietary Patterns" is excerpted from "*Dietary Guidelines for Americans, 2020-2025,*" *Dietary Guidelines for Americans* (*DGA*), U.S. Department of Agriculture (USDA), December 2020; Text under the heading "Vegetarian Diet for Women" is excerpted from "Vegetarian Eating," Office on Women's Health (OWH), U.S. Department of Health and Human Services (HHS), March 14, 2019.

high-nutrient content, consuming beans, peas, and lentils is recommended for everyone, including people who also eat meat, poultry, and seafood regularly.

HOW TO COUNT BEANS, PEAS, AND LENTILS

Generally, individuals who regularly eat meat, poultry, and seafood would count beans, peas, and lentils in the vegetable group. Vegetarians, vegans, and individuals who seldom eat meat, poultry, or seafood would count some of the beans, peas, and lentils they eat in the protein foods group. Here is an example for both ways:

Count the number of ounce-equivalents of all meat, poultry, seafood, eggs, nuts, seeds, and soy products eaten.

1. If the total is equal to or more than the suggested intake from the protein foods group (which ranges from 2 ounce-equivalents for the 1,000 calorie plan to 7 ounce-equivalents for the 2,800 calorie plan and above) then count any beans, peas, or lentils eaten as part of the beans, peas, and lentils subgroup in the vegetable group.
2. If the total is less than the suggested intake from the protein foods group, then count any beans, peas, and lentils eaten toward the suggested intake level until it is reached. (1/4 cup of cooked beans, peas, or lentils counts as 1 ounce-equivalent in the protein foods group.) After the suggested intake level in the protein foods group is reached, count any additional beans, peas, or lentils eaten as part of the beans, peas, and lentils subgroup in the vegetable group.

Example 1: (For the 2,000-calorie plan)

Foods eaten (protein foods group only – not a complete daily list):

- 3½ ounces chicken
- 2 ounces tuna fish
- ½ cup black beans

The 3½ ounces of chicken and 2 ounces of tuna fish equal 5½ ounce-equivalents in the protein foods group, which meets the recommendation at this calorie level. Therefore, the ½ cup of black beans counts as ½ cup of vegetables, towards meeting the 1½ cups per week recommendation for the beans, peas, and lentils subgroup in the 2,000-calorie plan.

Example 2: (For the 2,000-calorie plan)

Foods eaten (protein foods group only – not a complete daily list):

- 2 eggs
- 1½ tbsp. peanut butter
- ½ cup chickpeas

The 2 eggs and 1½ tbsp. peanut butter equals 3½ ounce-equivalents in the protein foods group. Two more ounces are needed to meet the 5½ ounce recommendation for this group. This ½ cup of chickpeas can help with meeting the remaining 2 ounce-equivalents needed to meet the recommendations for the protein foods group.

HEALTHY VEGETARIAN DIETARY PATTERNS

Table 20.1. Healthy Vegetarian Dietary Pattern for Toddlers Ages 12 through 23 Months Who Are No Longer Receiving Human Milk or Infant Formula, with Daily or Weekly Amounts from Food Groups, Subgroups, and Components

Calorie Level of Pattern[a]	**700**	**800**	**900**	**1,000**
Food Group or Subgroup[b,c]	Daily Amount of Food From Each Group[d] (Vegetable and protein foods subgroup amounts are per week.)			
Vegetables (cup eq/day)	1	1	1	1
	Vegetable Subgroups in Weekly Amounts			
Dark green Vegetables (cup eq/wk)	½	½	½	½
Red and Orange Vegetables (cup eq/wk)	2 ½	2 ½	2 ½	2 ½
Beans, Peas, Lentils (cup eq/wk)	¾	¾	¾	¾
Starchy Vegetables (cup eq/wk)	2	2	2	2

Table 20.1. Continued

Calorie Level of Pattern[a]	**700**	**800**	**900**	**1,000**
Other Vegetables (cup eq/wk)	1 ½	1 ½	1 ½	1 ½
Fruits (cup eq/day)	½	¾	1	1
Grains (ounce eq/day)	1 ¾	2 ¼	2 ¾	3
Whole Grains (ounce eq/day)	1 ¼	1 ¾	2	2
Refined Grains (ounce eq/day)	½	½	¾	1
Dairy (cup eq/day)	1 ½	1 ¾	1 ¾	2
Protein Foods (ounce eq/day)	1	1	1	1
	Protein Foods Subgroups in Weekly Amounts			
Eggs (ounce eq/wk)	3 ½	3 ½	3 ½	3 ½
Nuts, Seeds, Soy Products (ounce eq/wk)	4	4	4	4
Oils (grams/day)	9	8 ½	10	15

[a]***Calorie level ranges:*** *Energy levels are calculated based on median length and body weight reference individuals. Calorie needs vary based on many factors. The DRI Calculator for healthcare professionals available at (nal.usda.gov/fnic/dri-calculator/) can be used to estimate calorie needs based on age, sex, and weight.*

[b]*Definitions for each food group and subgroup and quantity (i.e., cup or ounce) equivalents are provided here: Food group amounts shown in cup equivalents (cup eq) or ounce-equivalents (ounce eq). Oils are shown in grams. Quantity equivalents for each food group are:*

Vegetables, fruits (1 cup eq). *1 cup raw or cooked vegetable or fruit; 1 cup vegetable or fruit juice; 2 cups leafy salad greens; ½ cup dried fruit or vegetable.*

Grains (1 ounce-eq). *½ cup cooked rice, pasta, or cereal; 1 ounce dry pasta or rice; 1 medium (1 ounce) sliced bread, tortilla, or flatbread; 1 ounce of ready-to-eat cereal (about 1 cup of flaked cereal).*

Dairy (1 cup eq). *1 cup milk, yogurt, or fortified soymilk; 1½ ounces natural cheese, such as cheddar cheese or 2 ounces of processed cheese.*

Protein foods (1 ounce-eq). *1 ounce lean meats, poultry, or seafood; 1 egg; ¼ cup cooked beans or tofu; 1 tbsp. nut or seed butter; ½ ounce nuts or seeds.*

[c]*All foods are assumed to be in nutrient-dense forms and prepared with minimal added sugars, refined starches (which are a source of calories but few or no other nutrients), or sodium. Food are also lean or in low-fat forms with the exception of dairy which includes whole-fat fluid milk, reduced-fat plain yogurts, and reduced-fat cheese. There are no calories available for additional added sugars, saturated fat, or to eat more than the recommended amount of food in a food group.*

[d]*In some cases, food subgroup amounts are greatest at the lower calorie levels to help achieve nutrient adequacy when a relatively small number of calories are required.*

Table 20.2. Healthy Vegetarian Dietary Pattern for Ages 2 and Older, with Daily or Weekly Amounts from Food Groups, Subgroups, and Components

Calorie Level of Pattern[a]	1,000	1,200	1,400	1,600	1,800	2,000	2,200	2,400	2,600	2,800	3,000	3,200
Food Group or Subgroup[b]	Daily Amount[c] of Food from Each Group (Vegetable and protein foods subgroup amounts[b] are per week.)											
Vegetables (cup eq/day)	1	1 ½	1 ½	2	2 ½	2 ½	3	3	3 ½	3 ½	4	4
	Vegetable Subgroups in Weekly Amounts											
Dark green Vegetables (cup eq/wk)	½	1	1	1 ½	1 ½	1 ½	2	2	2 ½	2 ½	2 ½	2 ½
Red and Orange Vegetables (cup eq/wk)	2 ½	3	3	4	5 ½	5 ½	6	6	7	7	7½	7½
Beans, Peas, Lentils (cup eq/wk)[d]	½	½	½	1	1 ½	1 ½	2	2	2 ½	2 ½	3	3
Starchy Vegetables (cup eq/wk)	2	3 ½	3 ½	4	5	5	6	6	7	7	8	8
Other Vegetables (cup eq/wk)	1 ½	2 ½	2 ½	3 ½	4	4	5	5	5 ½	5 ½	7	7
Fruits (cup eq/day)	1	1	1 ½	1 ½	1 ½	2	2	2	2	2 ½	2 ½	2 ½
Grains (ounce eq/day)	3	4	5	5 ½	6 ½	6 ½	7 ½	8 ½	9 ½	10 ½	10 ½	10 ½
Whole Grains (ounce eq/day)	1 ½	2	2 ½	3	3 ½	3 ½	4	4 ½	5	5 ½	5 ½	5 ½
Refined Grains (ounce eq/day)	1 ½	2	2 ½	2 ½	3	3	3 ½	4	4 ½	5	5	5
Dairy (cup eq/day)	2	2 ½	2 ½	3	3	3	3	3	3	3	3	3
Protein Foods (ounce eq/day)	1	1 ½	2	2 ½	3	3 ½	3 ½	4	4 ½	5	5 ½	6
	Protein Foods Subgroups in Weekly Amounts											
Eggs (ounce eq/wk)	2	3	3	3	3	3	3	3	3	4	4	4
Beans, Peas, Lentils (cup eq/wk)[d]	1	2	4	4	6	6	6	8	9	10	11	12
Soy Products (ounce eq/wk)	2	3	4	6	6	8	8	9	10	11	12	13

Table 20.2. Continued

Calorie Level of Pattern[a]	1,000	1,200	1,400	1,600	1,800	2,000	2,200	2,400	2,600	2,800	3,000	3,200
Nuts, Seeds, Soy Products (ounce eq/wk)	2	2	3	5	6	7	7	8	9	10	12	13
Oils (grams/day)	15	17	17	22	24	27	29	31	34	36	44	51
Limit on Calories for Other Uses (kcal/day)[e]	170	140	160	150	150	250	290	350	350	350	390	500
Limit on Calories for Other Uses (%/day)	17%	12%	11%	9%	8%	13%	13%	15%	13%	13%	13%	16%

[a]*Patterns at 1,000, 1,200, and 1,400 kcal levels are designed to meet the nutritional needs of children ages 2 through 8 years. Patterns from 1,600 to 3,200 kcal are designed to meet the nutritional needs of children 9 years and older and adults. If a child 4 through 8 years of age needs more energy and, therefore, is following a pattern at 1,600 calories or more, her or his recommended amount from the dairy group should be 2½ cup eq per day. The amount of dairy for children ages 9 through 18 is 3 cup eq per day regardless of calorie level. The 1,000 and 1,200 kcal level patterns are not intended for children 9 and older or adults. The 1,400 kcal level is not intended for children ages 10 and older or adults.*

[b]*Foods in each group and subgroup are:*

Vegetables (dark green vegetables, red and orange vegetables, beans, peas, lentils, starchy vegetables, other vegetables), fruits, grains (whole grains, refined grains) dairy, protein foods (meats, poultry, eggs, seafood, nuts, seeds, soy products)

[c]*Food group amounts shown in cup equivalents (cup eq) or ounce-equivalents (ounce eq). Oils are shown in grams. Quantity equivalents for each food group are:*

Vegetables, fruits (1 cup eq). *1 cup raw or cooked vegetable or fruit; 1 cup vegetable or fruit juice; 2 cups leafy salad greens; ½ cup dried fruit or vegetable.*

Grains (1 ounce-eq). *½ cup cooked rice, pasta, or cereal; 1 ounce dry pasta or rice; 1 medium (1 ounce) sliced bread, tortilla, or flatbread; 1 ounce of ready-to-eat cereal (about 1 cup of flaked cereal).*

Dairy (1 cup eq). *1 cup milk, yogurt, or fortified soymilk; 1½ ounces natural cheese such as cheddar cheese or 2 ounces of processed cheese.*

Protein foods (1 ounce-eq). *1 ounce lean meats, poultry, or seafood; 1 egg; ¼ cup cooked beans or tofu; 1 tbsp. nut or seed butter; ½ ounce nuts or seeds.*

[d]*About half of beans, peas, lentils are shown as vegetables, in cup eq, and half as protein foods, in ounce eq. Beans, peas, lentils in the patterns, in cup eq, is the amount in the vegetable group plus the amount in protein foods group (in ounce eq) divided by four.*

[e]*The U.S. Food and Drug Administration (FDA) and the U.S. Environmental Protection Agency (EPA) provide joint advice regarding seafood consumption to limit methylmercury exposure for women who might become or are pregnant or breastfeeding, and children. Depending on body weight, some women and many children should choose seafood lowest in methylmercury or eat less seafood than the amounts in the Healthy U.S.-Style Eating Pattern.*

Note: *The total dietary pattern should not exceed Dietary Guidelines limits for added sugars, saturated fat, and alcohol; be within the acceptable macronutrient distribution ranges for protein, carbohydrate, and total fats; and stay within calorie limits. Values are rounded.*

VEGETARIAN DIET FOR WOMEN

A vegetarian is someone who does not eat meat. Some vegetarians, called "vegans," do not eat any animal products, such as eggs or milk. If you are a vegetarian or vegan, you may need to take a dietary supplement, especially if you are pregnant or breastfeeding.

What Is a Healthy Eating Plan for Women Who Are Vegetarian?

A healthy eating pattern for women who are vegetarian is the same as for any woman. Because vegetarians eat mostly plant-based foods, they usually get more fiber-rich foods and low-cholesterol foods than nonvegetarians do. But, women who are vegetarians still need to make sure they are eating healthy, which includes foods with calcium and protein.

Do Women Who Are Vegetarian Need to Take a Dietary Supplement?

Not always. You can get all the nutrients you need from a vegetarian eating plan by eating a variety of foods from all of the food groups. But, you may need to take extra steps to get enough protein, iron, calcium, vitamin B_{12}, and zinc.

The extra steps you need to take depend on what type of vegetarian you are. For example, low-fat and fat-free milk and milk products are good sources of calcium, vitamin B_{12}, and complete protein. Eggs are a good source of vitamin B_{12}, choline, and complete protein. So if you do not drink milk or eat eggs, you need to get these nutrients from other foods.

Do Vegetarians Need More Nutrients during Pregnancy?

Yes. Just like all women, your body needs more nutrients, such as folic acid, during pregnancy to help your baby grow and develop. In general, though, choosing a variety of healthy foods from each of the food groups will help you get the nutrients you need during pregnancy. Be sure to get enough protein, found in beans, nuts, nut butter, and eggs if you eat them.

Use the MyPlate Plan tool (www.myplate.gov/myplate-plan) to find out how many calories you need based on your age, sex, height, weight, and physical activity level.

Chapter 21 | Healthy Eating at Home

Chapter Contents

Section 21.1 | **The Importance of Family Mealtime**

This section contains text excerpted from the following sources: Text in this section begins with excerpts from "Healthy Eating for Families," MyPlate, U.S. Department of Agriculture (USDA), December 31, 2020; Text beginning with the heading "The Benefits of Sharing Family Meals" is excerpted from "Benefits of Family Meals," U.S. Department of Homeland Security (DHS), August 25, 2020.

Family schedules may be hectic, but you can still eat well together. Use these tips to make healthy choices with your family.

HEALTHY EATING FOR FAMILIES

Connect at Mealtimes

Sit down together for a meal when you can. Turn off the TV and put away screens and devices, so you can unplug, interact, and focus on each other.

Plan Your Meals

Reduce stress at mealtimes by planning out meals before the week starts. Include quick and easy dishes, or leftovers, on nights that are extra busy.

Let Everyone Help

Kids learn by doing. Younger ones can mix ingredients, wash produce, or set the table; while older kids can help with ingredients. Everyone can help clean up.

Serve a Variety of Foods

Include choices from each food group – fruits, vegetables, grains, protein foods, and dairy and fortified soy alternatives – in meals and snacks throughout the week.

Let Kids Choose

Get kids engaged with meal preparation at home. Serve meals "family style" this will encourage kids to be creative with their plates.

Offer Nonfood Rewards

Foods are not the only rewards that kids like. Younger kids may enjoy gathering points toward a special outing, and older kids could earn extra free time or an allowance.

THE BENEFITS OF SHARING FAMILY MEALS

Work, school, and other responsibilities can make it challenging for families to spend mealtime together. While many of you and your families are home during the COVID-19 pandemic, and it may seem like you are together all the time, prioritizing sharing meals with loved ones in your home can have benefits.

- **Better family relationships.** Mealtime provides an opportunity for the whole family to be together. Use your time together to talk about the day's events, catch up, and simply spend time with each other.
- **Everyone eats healthier meals.** When families share a meal, they tend to eat more vegetables and fruits, fewer fried foods and snacks, and drink less soda. Children who eat family meals are also less likely to become overweight or obese.
- **Improved grades in school.** Studies have proven that there is a link between family dinners and academic performance.
- **Less stress and tension at home.** If you have a demanding job, finding time to eat with your family is a good way to reduce work-related stress and may relieve family tension.

TIPS FOR PLANNING FAMILY MEALS

If you are not regularly eating together as a family, start small and choose a few meals each week – breakfast, lunch, or dinner. Which meal you choose is not important; your goal is to carve out quality time to spend together.

- **Keep it simple.** Family meals do not have to be elaborate. Stick to recipes that you are comfortable with that your family enjoys.

- **Get the family involved.** Let kids help plan for meals, including creating shopping lists, cooking, setting the table, and helping clean up.
- **Make it enjoyable.** Family meals are for nourishment, comfort, and support. Leave the serious discussions for another time.
- **Make it screen-free.** Agree that mealtime is for listening and sharing the day's stories. Leave phones on mute and out of reach.

Section 21.2 | **Healthy Cooking and Snacking**

This section includes text excerpted from "Healthy Cooking and Snacking," National Heart, Lung, and Blood Institute (NHLBI), February 13, 2013. Reviewed May 2021.

Food does not have to be high in fat to be good. Get the whole family to help slice, dice, and chop, and learn how to cut fat and calories in some foods. You would be surprised how easy heart-healthy cooking and snacking can be.

In this section, you will find ideas for healthy snacks, tips for healthy cooking, and food options with less fat and fewer calories.

HEALTHY FAMILY SNACKS

Try these tips for quick and easy snacks:

- Toss sliced apples, berries, bananas, or whole-grain cereal on top of fat-free or low-fat yogurt.
- Put a slice of fat-free or low-fat cheese on top of whole-grain crackers.
- Make a whole-wheat pita pocket with hummus, lettuce, tomato, and cucumber.
- Pop some fat-free or low-fat popcorn.
- Microwave or toast a soft whole-grain tortilla with fat-free or low-fat cheese and sliced peppers and mushrooms to make a mini-burrito or quesadilla.

- Drink fat-free or low-fat chocolate milk (blend it with a banana or strawberries and some ice for a smoothie).

HEALTHY COOKING TIPS

Make a few changes in the kitchen and you will be eating healthy in no time.

Tips for Reducing Fat

- Instead of frying, try baking, broiling, boiling, or microwaving.
- Choose fat-free or low-fat milk products, salad dressings, and mayonnaise.
- Add salsa on a baked potato instead of butter or sour cream.
- Remove skin from poultry (such as chicken or turkey) and do not eat it.
- Cool soups and gravies and skim off fat before reheating them.

Tips for Reducing Sugar

- Serve fruit instead of cookies or ice cream for dessert.
- Eat fruits canned in their own juice rather than syrup.
- Reduce sugar in recipes by 1/4 to 1/3. If a recipe says one cup, use 2/3 cup.
- To enhance the flavor when sugar is reduced, add vanilla, cinnamon, or nutmeg.

HEALTHY BAKING AND COOKING SUBSTITUTES

Cut the fat and sugar in your meals by using these substitutes.

Table 21.1. Food Substitutes

Instead Of	Substitute
1 cup cream	1 cup evaporated fat-free milk
1 cup butter, margarine, or oil	1/2 cup apple butter or applesauce
1 egg	2 egg whites or 1/4 cup egg substitute
Pastry dough	Graham cracker crumb crust
Butter, margarine, or vegetable oil for sautéing	Cooking spray, chicken broth, or a small amount of olive oil
Bacon	Lean turkey bacon
Ground beef	Extra lean ground beef or ground turkey breast
Sour cream	Fat-free sour cream
1 cup chocolate chips	1/4–1/2 cup mini chocolate chips
1 cup sugar	3/4 cup sugar (this works with nearly everything except yeast breads)
1 cup mayonnaise	1 cup fat-free or reduced-fat mayonnaise
1 cup whole milk	1 cup fat-free milk
1 cup cream cheese	1/2 cup ricotta cheese pureed with 1/2 cup fat-free cream cheese
Oil and vinegar dressing with 3 parts oil to 1 part vinegar	1 part olive oil + 1 part vinegar (preferably a flavored vinegar, such as balsamic) + 1 part orange juice
Unsweetened baking chocolate (1 ounce)	3 tablespoons unsweetened cocoa powder + 1 tablespoon vegetable oil or margarine

Note: *Substitute the ingredients in your own favorite recipes to lower the amounts of fat, added sugar, and calories.*

Chapter 22 | The Health Benefits of Eating Breakfast

WHY IS BREAKFAST THE MOST IMPORTANT MEAL OF THE DAY?

Almost everyone is familiar with the idea that breakfast is the most important meal of the day, but the reasons behind that idea may not be so well-known. For most people, the time between yesterday's evening meal and this morning's breakfast is the longest period of time that the body goes without food each day. This means that breakfast has a physical effect on the body that is different than any other meal. Eating breakfast within two hours of waking helps the body's metabolism to operate more efficiently, provides a burst of energy to begin the day's activities, helps to curb appetite throughout the day, and can aid in weight management.

Eating a healthy breakfast that contains a variety of foods, such as whole grains, dairy, cereal, and fruit makes a difference in the way the body processes blood sugar levels. Sometimes called the "second-meal effect," breakfast kick-starts the metabolism and makes it easier for the body to absorb nutrients and regulate blood sugar throughout the rest of the day. Without breakfast, the body experiences prolonged fasting that triggers a spike in hunger-related hormones, which in turn leads to fluctuating blood sugar levels throughout the day. These fluctuations can cause people to feel tired, irritable, and unable to concentrate on tasks. People who eat a healthy breakfast every day tend to maintain better diets overall and weigh less than people who do not eat breakfast. This is because when the metabolism gets moving with breakfast, the body begins to burn more calories converting food to energy.

Breakfast is especially important for school-aged children. Eating breakfast boosts brain function, enhances memory, and improves concentration, attention span, reasoning, creativity, and learning abilities. Eating a healthy breakfast every day has also been linked to improved academic performance. Children who eat breakfast tend to be more active, have fewer health problems, and fewer absences from school. As with adults, children who eat breakfast also tend to consume fewer calories later in the day. Those who skip breakfast are more likely to overeat during lunch due to excessive hunger.

WHAT IS A HEALTHY BREAKFAST?

A healthy breakfast that provides the most physical and mental benefits includes whole grains, dairy, cereal, and fruit, and a balance of carbohydrates, protein, and fiber. Carbohydrates from whole grain bread, muffins, cereals, fruits, and vegetables provide immediate energy that is processed quickly by the body. Longer-term energy from the protein in dairy products, lean meats, eggs, nuts, and beans is accessed by the body after the carbohydrates. The fiber in whole-grain breads, waffles, cereals, bran, fruits, vegetables, nuts, and beans helps people feel full longer and discourages overeating.

A healthy breakfast is not limited to traditional breakfast foods. As long as a nutritional balance is achieved, breakfast can include leftovers from the previous night's dinner, sandwiches, or vegetables and nuts. A healthy breakfast that provides the most physical and mental benefits includes whole grains, dairy, cereal, and fruit, and a balance of carbohydrates, protein, and fiber. Carbohydrates from whole-grain bread, muffins, cereals, fruits, and vegetables provide immediate energy that is processed quickly by the body.

Some ideas for a healthy breakfast include:

- Fruit and yogurt
- Fruit and whole-grain cereal with milk
- Whole-grain muffins, pancakes, or waffles with fruit and milk
- Egg omelet with vegetables

- Mixed nuts and dried fruit
- Hard-cooked eggs with whole-wheat bread
- Oatmeal with fruit, nuts, or spices and milk
- Whole-grain toast with peanut butter and fruit and milk
- Cucumbers and hummus with whole-wheat bread or crackers
- Lean turkey with tomato on whole-wheat bread
- Cheese with whole-wheat bread or crackers
- Cheese pizza

Some traditional breakfast items are best avoided, at least on a daily basis. Donuts, pastries, toaster pastries, and certain breakfast bars contain as much fat, sugar, and calories as a regular candy bar. Sugary cereals can be mixed with regular whole-grain cereals to add flavor and fun without the poor nutritional profile of a whole bowl of sugared cereal.

BREAKFAST PLANNING

Many people skip breakfast because they do not have time to prepare and eat a meal every morning. A healthy breakfast does not have to be complicated or time-consuming, and breakfast can even be planned and prepared the previous night. Rising just ten minutes earlier than usual can provide enough time for everyone to enjoy a bowl of cereal or oatmeal before heading out for the day. Breakfast can be streamlined by stocking the pantry and refrigerator with grab-and-go options, such as whole fruit, yogurt parfaits, and individual containers of whole-grain cereals or snack mixes. Peanut butter and whole wheat sandwiches made the night before are another good option.

References

1. Gavin, Mary L, MD. "Breakfast Basics," KidsHealth, July 2015.
2. "Why Eating the Right Breakfast Is So Important," Consumer Reports, August 26, 2015.

3. "Healthy Breakfasts for Kids," U.S. Food and Drug Administration (FDA), August 13, 2015.
4. Agan, Cathy; Terri Crawford. "Smart Choices: Nutrition News for Seniors," Louisiana State University Agricultural Center, n.d.
5. "Why Is Breakfast Important?" Agriculture and Horticulture Development Board (AHDB), 2016.
6. Bar-Dayan, Alisa. "The Importance of a Healthy Breakfast," April 19, 2010.

Chapter 23 | Healthy Eating Out

Chapter Contents

Section 23.1 | **Tips for Eating Out**

This section contains text excerpted from the following sources: Text in this section begins with excerpts from "Eating Healthy When Eating Out," National Heart, Lung, and Blood Institute (NHLBI), February 13, 2013. Reviewed May 2021; Text under the heading "Avoid Food Poisoning: Tips for Eating at Restaurants" is excerpted from "Food Safety and Eating Out," Centers for Disease Control and Prevention (CDC), April 6, 2021.

Staying in energy balance can be tough when you and your family go out to eat. But, you can still eat healthy and enjoy your meal. Do not be afraid to ask questions about the ingredients and how the food was cooked. You also can ask to leave some items out or replace them with healthier choices.

ORDER HEALTHY

When you are choosing foods, choose items that have less fat or added sugar or ask for a healthier substitution. When you order:

- Choose foods that are steamed, broiled, baked, roasted, poached, or lightly sautéed or stir-fried.
- Ask for fat-free or low-fat milk instead of cream for coffee or tea.
- Pick food without butter, gravy, or sauces – or ask to have the food without it.
- Choose a lower-calorie salad dressing.
- Ask for salad dressing on the side, and use only some of it.
- Pick drinks without added sugar, such as water, fat-free or low-fat milk, unsweetened tea, or diet iced-tea, lemonade, or soda.

EAT HEALTHY

You can make healthy choices throughout your meal, just:

- Trim visible fat from poultry or meat.
- Do not eat the skin on chicken or turkey.
- Share your meal, or take half home for later.
- Skip dessert or order fruit.
- Split dessert with a friend.

AVOID FOOD POISONING: TIPS FOR EATING AT RESTAURANTS

- **Check inspection scores.** Check a restaurant's score at your health department's website (www.cdc.gov/publichealthgateway/sitesgovernance/index.html), ask the health department for a copy of the report, or look for it when you get to the restaurant.
- **Look for certificates that show kitchen managers have completed food safety training.** Proper food safety training can help improve practices that reduce the chance of spreading foodborne germs and illnesses.
- **Look for safe food-handling practices.** Sick food workers can spread their illness to customers. If you can see food being prepared, check to make sure workers are using gloves or utensils to handle foods that will not be cooked further, such as deli meats and salad greens.
- **Order food that is properly cooked.** Certain foods, including meat, poultry, and fish, need to be cooked to a temperature high enough to kill harmful germs that may be present. If a restaurant serves you undercooked meat, poultry, seafood, or eggs, send them back to be cooked until they are safe to eat.
- **Avoid food served lukewarm.** Cold food should be served cold, and hot food should be served hot. If you are selecting food from a buffet or salad bar, make sure the hot food is steaming and the cold food is chilled. Germs that cause food poisoning grow quickly when food is in the danger zone, between 40 °F and 140 °F.
- **Ask your server.** Enquire if they use pasteurized eggs in foods such as Caesar salad dressing, custards, tiramisu, or hollandaise sauce. Raw or undercooked eggs can make you sick unless they are pasteurized to kill germs.
- **Take care of your leftovers quickly.** Refrigerate leftovers within two hours of eating out. If it is above 90 °F outside, refrigerate leftovers within one hour. Eat leftovers within three to four days. Throw them out after that time.

Report a Foodborne Illness

If you think you or someone you know got sick from food, please report it to your local health department. Report it even if you do not know what food made you sick. Reporting an illness can help public-health officials identify a foodborne disease outbreak and keep others from getting sick.

Section 23.2 | Food Safety Tips for Holidays

This section includes text excerpted from "Food Safety Tips for the Holidays," Centers for Disease Control and Prevention (CDC), October 14, 2020.

SIMPLE TIPS TO HELP PREVENT FOOD POISONING

Cook Food Thoroughly

Meat, chicken, turkey, seafood, and eggs can carry germs that cause food poisoning. Use a food thermometer to ensure these foods have been cooked to a safe internal temperature. Roasts, chops, steaks, and fresh ham should rest for three minutes after you remove them from the oven or grill.

Keep Food Out of the "Danger Zone"

Bacteria can grow rapidly in the danger zone between 40 °F and 140 °F. After food is cooked, keep hot food hot and cold food cold. Refrigerate or freeze any perishable food within two hours. The temperature in your refrigerator should be set at or below 40 °F and the freezer at or below 0 °F.

Use Pasteurized Eggs for Dishes Containing Raw Eggs

Salmonella and other harmful germs can live on both the outside and inside of normal-looking eggs. Many holiday favorites contain raw eggs, including eggnog, tiramisu, hollandaise sauce, and Caesar dressing. Always use pasteurized eggs when making these and other foods made with raw eggs.

Do Not Eat Raw Dough or Batter

Dough and batter made with flour or eggs can contain harmful germs, such as *Escherichia coli* (*E. coli*) and *Salmonella*. Do not taste or eat raw dough or batter that is meant to be baked or cooked. This includes dough or batter for cookies, cakes, pies, biscuits, pancakes, tortillas, pizza, or crafts. Do not let children taste raw dough or batter or play with dough at home or in restaurants. Some companies and stores offer edible cookie dough that uses heat-treated flour and pasteurized eggs or no eggs. Read the label carefully to make sure the dough is meant to be eaten without baking or cooking.

Keep Foods Separated

Keep meat, chicken, turkey, seafood, and eggs separate from all other foods at the grocery store and in the refrigerator. Prevent juices from meat, chicken, turkey, and seafood from dripping or leaking onto other foods by keeping them in containers or sealed plastic bags. Store eggs in their original carton in the main compartment of the refrigerator.

Thaw Your Turkey Safely

Thaw turkey in the refrigerator, in a sink of cold water (change the water every 30 minutes), or in the microwave. Avoid thawing foods on the counter. A turkey must thaw at a safe temperature to prevent harmful germs from growing rapidly.

Wash Your Hands

Wash your hands with soap and water during these key times when you are likely to get and spread germs:

- Before, during, and after preparing food
- Before eating food
- After handling pet food or pet treats or touching pets
- After using the toilet
- After changing diapers or cleaning up a child who has used the toilet
- After touching garbage

- Before and after caring for someone who is sick
- Before and after treating a cut or wound
- After blowing your nose, coughing, or sneezing

PREGNANCY AND FOOD

Pregnant women are at increased risk of food poisoning, so take extra care if you are pregnant or preparing food for someone who is.

- **Do not eat or drink raw or unpasteurized milk and products made with it, such as soft cheeses.** They can contain harmful germs, including *Listeria*. Do not eat soft cheeses such as queso fresco, Brie, Camembert, feta, goat cheese, or blue-veined cheese if they are made from raw or unpasteurized milk.
    - Be aware that Hispanic-style cheeses made from pasteurized milk, such as queso fresco, also have caused *Listeria* infections, most likely because they were contaminated during cheese-making.
    - Processed cheeses, cream cheese, mozzarella, and hard cheeses are safer choices.
- Do not drink raw or unpasteurized juice and cider.
- **Be careful with seafood.** Do not eat smoked seafood that was sold refrigerated unless it is in a cooked dish, such as a casserole. Instead, choose shelf-stable smoked seafood in pouches or cans that do not need refrigeration.
- **Take care with holiday beverages.** Drinking any type of alcohol can affect your baby's growth and development and cause fetal alcohol spectrum disorders (FASDs). Do not drink holiday punches and eggnogs that contain alcohol. Avoid eggnog entirely unless you know it does not contain alcohol and is pasteurized or made with pasteurized eggs and milk.

Chapter 24 | Alcohol Use

Chapter Contents

Section 24.1 | **Drink Alcohol Only in Moderation**

This section includes text excerpted from "Drink Alcohol Only in Moderation," Office of Disease Prevention and Health Promotion (ODPHP), U.S. Department of Health and Human Services (HHS), October 15, 2020.

THE BASICS

If you do not drink alcohol, there is no reason to start. If you choose to drink, it is important to have only a moderate (limited) amount. And, some people should not drink at all, such as women who are pregnant or trying to get pregnant and people with certain health conditions.

What Is a Moderate Amount of Alcohol?

A moderate amount of alcohol means:

- Up to one drink in a day for women
- Up to two drinks in a day for men

What Is One Drink Equal To?

Different types of beer, wine, and liquor have different amounts of alcohol. In general, one drink is equal to a:

- Bottle of regular beer (12 ounces)
- A glass of wine (5 ounces)
- Shot of liquor or spirits, such as gin, rum, or vodka (1.5 ounces)

Different drinks have different amounts of calories, too. These calories add up and can make you gain weight. For example, a 12-ounce bottle of beer has about 150 calories.

TAKE ACTION: GET HELP

If You Think You Might Have a Drinking Problem, Ask for Help

Ask your friends and loved ones to support you. Talk to a doctor or nurse if you are having a hard time cutting down on your drinking.

If one type of treatment does not work for you, you can try another. Do not give up!

- Find a doctor or treatment program near you.
- Call 800-662-HELP (800-662-4357) for information about treatment.
- Use the National Institute on Alcohol Abuse and Alcoholism (NIAAA) alcohol treatment to explore treatment options.

WHAT ABOUT COST

The Affordable Care Act (ACA), the healthcare reform law passed in 2010, requires most healthcare plans to cover screening and counseling for alcohol misuse. Depending on your insurance, you may be able to get these services at no cost to you. Check with your insurance provider to find out what is included in your plan.

Are You Worried about a Loved One Drinking?

Use these tips to talk with someone about cutting back or quitting drinking.

It takes courage to talk to a family member or friend about a drinking problem. These tips can help you get started.

BE HONEST ABOUT HOW YOU FEEL

- "I care about you."
- "I am worried about your health. Drinking too much puts you at risk for heart disease, stroke, liver problems, and some cancers."
- "Your drinking is affecting our relationship."

OFFER TIPS ON HOW TO CUT BACK OR QUIT

- "Set a drinking limit. Stick to your limit by writing down every drink you have."
- "Try taking a night or two off from drinking each week."
- "When we go out, we can stay away from bars or other places that make you want to drink."
- "If you are having trouble sticking to your limits, consider joining a support group or talking to a doctor."

SUPPORT MAKING A CHANGE

- "How can I support you?"
- "Talk to me when you want a drink. Whenever you feel the urge to drink, you can call me instead."
- "Let us do things that do not involve drinking – such as seeing a movie or going for a walk."

Section 24.2 | Red Wine's Health Claims

This section includes text excerpted from "Revisiting Resveratrol's Health Claims," National Institutes of Health (NIH), May 20, 2014. Reviewed May 2021.

Over the past decade or so, a lot of us have been led to believe that certain indulgences – such as a glass of Pinot noir or a piece of dark chocolate – can actually be health-promoting. That is because a number of studies had suggested that red wine, chocolate, and other foods containing the antioxidant resveratrol might lower the risk of heart disease, cancer, and other age-related maladies. But, now comes word that a diet rich in resveratrol may not automatically translate into better health.

In a prospective study of nearly 800 people living in Italy, a team from Johns Hopkins University School of Medicine in Baltimore and National Institutes of Health's (NIH) National Institute on Aging (NIA) found no significant differences in heart disease, cancer, or longevity between those who consumed a diet high in resveratrol and those who consumed very little.

Science's fascination with resveratrol dates back to the early 1990s when researchers reported this paradox: the French eat a diet rich in butter, cheese, pork, and other foods high in saturated fat and cholesterol, yet they have relatively low levels of coronary heart disease. Why? It was hypothesized that the cardiovascular protection might have to do with something else the French love: red wine. A powerful antioxidant, called "resveratrol," was eventually isolated from red wine, as well as cocoa, red grapes, and a variety of other berries and roots. After that, a steady stream of studies in cells and various animal models showed that resveratrol reduced inflammation and seemed to protect against the unhealthy effects of a high-fat diet.

While some studies have looked at the health of small numbers of humans who consumed high-dose resveratrol supplements over relatively short periods of time, NIA's Luigi Ferrucci, Johns Hopkins' Richard Semba, and their colleagues wanted to see if the health benefits attributed to resveratrol would hold true in a larger study that tracked the health of people eating normal diets over a much longer time span.

In 1998, while still with the Italian NIA, Ferrucci launched the aging in the Chianti Region (InCHIANTI) study, involving 783 men and women 65 years of age or older from a famed wine-making area of central Italy. Over the past 16 years, these volunteers have donated blood and urine, undergone regular medical exams, and answered dietary and lifestyle questionnaires – all part of an effort to better understand a wide range of factors involved in healthy aging.

For another study, researchers examined levels of resveratrol-derived metabolites in urine collected from InCHIANTI participants in 1998 and then frozen for future analysis. Researchers expected that higher levels of resveratrol might be associated with better health. However, they detected no substantial differences in health status (as measured by medical exams and four biomarkers associated with inflammation and disease risk) between people with high or low resveratrol levels. What is more, researchers found that levels of resveratrol varied widely among the 268 volunteers who died between 1998 and 2009. All told, the researchers say their findings suggest that a diet high in resveratrol did not protect against disease or extend lifespan.

More work is needed to determine why resveratrol's impact on health in the real world does not appear to be as encouraging as results from more controlled settings. One possible explanation is dosage. It is possible that the doses of resveratrol found in regular foods – a single glass of wine contains about 1mg – are too small to pack a big punch. Some previous human studies involving high-dose resveratrol supplements (250 or 500mg) have shown that the antioxidant lowers blood glucose, low-density lipoprotein (LDL) cholesterol, and inflammation; however, other studies (including a randomized, double-blind, placebo-controlled trial) using high-dose resveratrol supplements have found few, if any, beneficial effects. In addition, red wine is known to contain more than four dozen compounds similar to resveratrol, so perhaps one or more of those may be responsible for the heart-protective effects seen in the French Paradox.

Part 5 | Nutrition-Related Health and Safety Concerns

Chapter 25 | **Diet and Metabolic Syndrome**

WHAT IS METABOLIC SYNDROME

Metabolic syndrome is the name for a group of risk factors that raises your risk for heart disease and other health problems, such as diabetes and stroke.

The term "metabolic" refers to the biochemical processes involved in the body's normal functioning. Risk factors are traits, conditions, or habits that increase your chance of developing a disease.

In this chapter, "heart disease" refers to ischemic heart disease (IHD), a condition in which a waxy substance called "plaque" builds up inside the arteries that supply blood to the heart.

Plaque hardens and narrows the arteries, reducing blood flow to your heart muscle. This can lead to chest pain, a heart attack, heart damage, or even death.

WHAT ARE THE CAUSES?

Metabolic syndrome has several causes that act together. You can control some of the causes, such as overweight and obesity, an inactive lifestyle, and insulin resistance.

You cannot control other factors that may play a role in causing metabolic syndrome, such as growing older. Your risk for metabolic syndrome increases with age.

This chapter contains text excerpted from the following sources: Text beginning with the heading "What Is Metabolic Syndrome?" is excerpted from "Metabolic Syndrome," National Heart, Lung, and Blood Institute (NHLBI), December 28, 2020; Text under the heading "The Role of Diet in Metabolic Syndrome" is excerpted from "The Role of Diet in Metabolic Syndrome," National Institutes of Health (NIH), February 25, 2008. Reviewed May 2021.

You also cannot control genetics (ethnicity and family history), which may play a role in causing the condition. For example, genetics can increase your risk for IR, which can lead to metabolic syndrome.

People who have metabolic syndrome often have two other conditions: excessive blood clotting and constant, low-grade inflammation throughout the body. Researchers do not know whether these conditions cause metabolic syndrome or worsen it.

Researchers continue to study conditions that may play a role in metabolic syndromes, such as:

- A fatty liver (excess triglycerides and other fats in the liver)
- Polycystic ovarian syndrome (a tendency to develop cysts on the ovaries)
- Gallstones
- Breathing problems during sleep (such as sleep apnea)

RISK FACTORS OF METABOLIC SYNDROME

People at greatest risk for metabolic syndrome have these underlying causes:

- Abdominal obesity (a large waistline)
- An inactive lifestyle
- Insulin resistance

Some people are at risk for metabolic syndrome because they take medicines that cause weight gain or changes in blood pressure, blood cholesterol, and blood sugar levels. These medicines most often are used to treat inflammation, allergies, HIV, and depression, and other types of mental illness.

Populations Affected

Some racial and ethnic groups in the United States are at higher risk for metabolic syndrome than others. Mexican Americans have the highest rate of metabolic syndrome, followed by whites and Blacks.

Other groups at increased risk for metabolic syndrome include:

- People who have a personal history of diabetes

- People who have a sibling or parent who has diabetes
- Women when compared with men
- Women who have a personal history of polycystic ovarian syndrome (PCOS) (a tendency to develop cysts on the ovaries)

Heart Disease Risk

Metabolic syndrome increases your risk for IHD. Other risk factors, besides metabolic syndrome, also increase your risk for heart disease. For example, a high LDL (bad) cholesterol level and smoking are major risk factors for heart disease.

Even if you do not have metabolic syndrome, you should find out your short-term risk for heart disease. The National Cholesterol Education Program (NCEP) divides short-term heart disease risk into four categories. Your risk category depends on which risk factors you have and how many you have.

Your risk factors are used to calculate your 10-year risk of developing heart disease. The NCEP has an online calculator that you can use to estimate your 10-year risk of having a heart attack.

- **High risk.** You are in this category if you already have heart disease or diabetes, or if your 10-year risk score is more than 20 percent.
- **Moderately high risk.** You are in this category if you have two or more risk factors and your 10-year risk score is 10 percent to 20 percent.
- **Moderate risk.** You are in this category if you have two or more risk factors and your 10-year risk score is less than 10 percent.
- **Lower risk.** You are in this category if you have zero or one risk factor.

Even if your 10-year risk score is not high, metabolic syndrome will increase your risk for coronary heart disease (CHD) over time.

SCREENING AND PREVENTION OF METABOLIC SYNDROME

The best way to prevent metabolic syndrome is to adopt heart-healthy lifestyle changes. Make sure to schedule routine doctor visits to keep track of your cholesterol, blood pressure, and blood sugar levels. Speak with your doctor about a blood test called a "lipoprotein panel," which shows your levels of total cholesterol, LDL cholesterol, HDL cholesterol, and triglycerides.

SIGNS, SYMPTOMS, AND COMPLICATIONS OF METABOLIC SYNDROME

Metabolic syndrome is a group of risk factors that raises your risk for heart disease and other health problems, such as diabetes and stroke. These risk factors can increase your risk for health problems even if they are only moderately raised (borderline-high risk factors).

Most of the metabolic risk factors have no signs or symptoms, although a large waistline is a visible sign.

Some people may have symptoms of high blood sugar if diabetes – especially type 2 diabetes – is present. Symptoms of high blood sugar often include increased thirst; increased urination, especially at night; fatigue (tiredness); and blurred vision.

High blood pressure (HBP) usually has no signs or symptoms. However, some people in the early stages of HBP may have dull headaches, dizzy spells, or more nosebleeds than usual.

HOW IS IT DIAGNOSED?

Your doctor will diagnose metabolic syndrome based on the results of a physical exam and blood tests. You must have at least three of the five metabolic risk factors to be diagnosed with metabolic syndrome.

Metabolic Risk Factors

A LARGE WAISTLINE

Having a large waistline means that you carry excess weight around your waist (abdominal obesity). This is also called having an "apple-shaped" figure. Your doctor will measure your waist to find out whether you have a large waistline.

A waist measurement of 35 inches or more for women or 40 inches or more for men is a metabolic risk factor. A large waistline means you are at increased risk for heart disease and other health problems.

A HIGH TRIGLYCERIDE LEVEL

Triglycerides are a type of fat found in the blood. A triglyceride level of 150 mg/dL or higher (or being on medicine to treat high triglycerides) is a metabolic risk factor. (The mg/dL is milligrams per deciliter – the units used to measure triglycerides, cholesterol, and blood sugar.)

A LOW HDL CHOLESTEROL LEVEL

HDL cholesterol sometimes is called "good cholesterol." This is because it helps remove cholesterol from your arteries.

An HDL cholesterol level of less than 50 mg/dL for women and less than 40 mg/dL for men (or being on medicine to treat low HDL cholesterol) is a metabolic risk factor.

HIGH BLOOD PRESSURE

A blood pressure of 130/85 mmHg or higher (or being on medicine to treat HBP) is a metabolic risk factor. (The mmHg is millimeters of mercury – the units used to measure blood pressure.)

If only one of your two blood pressure numbers is high, you are still at risk for metabolic syndrome.

HIGH FASTING BLOOD SUGAR

A normal fasting blood sugar level is less than 100 mg/dL. A fasting blood sugar level between 100–125 mg/dL is considered prediabetes. A fasting blood sugar level of 126 mg/dL or higher is considered diabetes.

A fasting blood sugar level of 100 mg/dL or higher (or being on medicine to treat high blood sugar) is a metabolic risk factor.

About 85 percent of people who have type 2 diabetes – the most common type of diabetes – also have metabolic syndrome. These people have a much higher risk for heart disease than the 15 percent of people who have type 2 diabetes without metabolic syndrome.

TREATMENT OPTIONS OF METABOLIC SYNDROME

Heart-healthy lifestyle changes are the first line of treatment for metabolic syndrome. If heart-healthy lifestyle changes are not enough, your doctor may prescribe medicines. Medicines are used to treat and control risk factors, such as HBP, high triglycerides, low HDL ("good") cholesterol, and high blood sugar.

Goals of Treatment

The major goal of treating metabolic syndrome is to reduce the risk of IHD. Treatment is directed first at lowering LDL cholesterol and HBP and managing diabetes (if these conditions are present).

The second goal of treatment is to prevent the onset of type 2 diabetes if it has not already developed. Long-term complications of diabetes often include heart and kidney disease, vision loss, and foot or leg amputation. If diabetes is present, the goal of treatment is to reduce your risk for heart disease by controlling all of your risk factors.

Heart-Healthy Lifestyle Changes

Heart-healthy lifestyle changes include heart-healthy eating, aiming for a healthy weight, managing stress, physical activity, and quitting smoking.

Medicines

Sometimes lifestyle changes are not enough to control your risk factors for metabolic syndrome. For example, you may need statin medications to control or lower your cholesterol. By lowering your blood cholesterol level, you can decrease your chance of having a heart attack or stroke. Doctors usually prescribe statins for people who have:

- Diabetes

- Heart disease or had a prior stroke
- High LDL cholesterol levels

Doctors may discuss beginning statin treatment with those who have an elevated risk for developing heart disease or having a stroke.

Your doctor also may prescribe other medications to:

- Decrease your chance of having a heart attack or dying suddenly
- Lower your blood pressure
- Prevent blood clots, which can lead to heart attack or stroke
- Reduce your heart's workload and relieve symptoms of coronary heart disease

Take all medicines regularly, as your doctor prescribes. Do not change the amount of your medicine or skip a dose unless your doctor tells you to. You should still follow a heart-healthy lifestyle, even if you take medicines to treat your risk factors for metabolic syndrome.

LIVING WITH METABOLIC SYNDROME

Metabolic syndrome is a lifelong condition. However, lifestyle changes can help you control your risk factors and reduce your risk for IHD and diabetes.

If you already have heart disease or diabetes, lifestyle changes can help you prevent or delay related problems. Examples of these problems include heart attack, stroke, and diabetes-related complications (e.g., damage to your eyes, nerves, kidneys, feet, and legs).

Heart-healthy lifestyle changes may include:

- Heart-healthy eating
- Aiming for a healthy weight
- Managing stress
- Physical activity
- Quitting smoking

If lifestyle changes are not enough, your doctor may recommend medicines. Take all of your medicines as prescribed by your doctor. Make realistic short- and long-term goals for yourself when you begin to make healthy lifestyle changes. Work closely with your doctor, and seek regular medical care.

THE ROLE OF DIET IN METABOLIC SYNDROME

A study has implicated meat, fried food, and diet soda in the development of metabolic syndrome. More research will now be needed to confirm and explain these intriguing findings.

Metabolic syndrome is a cluster of conditions that increases the risk for heart disease and stroke. Doctors consider someone to have metabolic syndrome when they have 3 or more risk factors, which include elevated blood pressure, low HDL (good cholesterol) levels, and diabetes or prediabetes..

Various aspects of diet have been linked to metabolic syndrome in previous studies, but the diet's role in the syndrome's genesis is not well understood. Dr. Lyn M. Steffen at the University of Minnesota's School of Public Health and her colleagues set out to take a broad look at the relationship between metabolic syndrome and dietary intake. They used data from 9,514 middle-aged adults enrolled in the multicenter Atherosclerosis Risk in Communities (ARIC) study. The study was initiated by NIH's National Heart, Lung and Blood Institute (NHLBI) to investigate the factors that contribute to atherosclerosis (the buildup of cholesterol and fat in the walls of arteries) and the incidence of cardiovascular diseases.

The study found that a Western dietary pattern characterized by high intakes of refined grains, processed meat, fried foods and red meat was associated with a greater risk of developing metabolic syndrome. Upon closer analysis, the researchers found that those who ate the most meat were more likely to develop metabolic syndrome. In particular, hamburgers, hot dogs and processed meats were each associated with higher rates of metabolic syndrome. Fried foods were also associated with an increased risk.

The researchers did not find any association, positive or negative, between metabolic syndrome and whole grains, refined grains, nuts, coffee or fruits and vegetables. On the other hand, they found that those who ate more dairy were less likely to develop metabolic syndrome.

Strikingly, diet soda was strongly associated with an increased risk for metabolic syndrome, although sweetened beverages, such as juices and regular soda were not. Other recent studies have found links between diet soda and metabolic syndrome as well as weight gain. As a possible explanation, findings in rodents suggest that artificial sweeteners may lead to increased intake because they may interfere with the body's ability to properly assess how many calories are in foods.

These findings, however intriguing, are not conclusive. Whole grains have been found in previous studies to lower the risk of metabolic syndrome, but this study did not. Certain foods in themselves may not play a role in causing metabolic syndrome, but rather may serve as markers for other behaviors that do lead to metabolic syndrome. More research into what causes metabolic syndrome will hopefully clear up the confusion.

Chapter 26 | The Truths about Natural, Artificial, and Added Sugars

Chapter Contents

Section 26.1 | How Sugars and Sweeteners Affect Your Health

This section includes text excerpted from "Sweet Stuff," *NIH News in Health*, National Institutes of Health (NIH), October 2014. Reviewed May 2021.

Most of us love sweet foods and drinks. But, after that short burst of sweetness, you may worry about how sweets affect your waistline and your overall health. Is sugar really bad for us? How about artificial or low-calorie sweeteners? What have scientists learned about the sweet things that most of us eat and drink every day?

Our bodies need one type of sugar, called "glucose," to survive. "Glucose is the number one food for the brain, and it is an extremely important source of fuel throughout the body," says Dr. Kristina Rother, an National Institutes of Health (NIH) pediatrician and expert on sweeteners. But, there is no need to add glucose to your diet, because your body can make the glucose it needs by breaking down food molecules, such as carbohydrates, proteins, and fats.

Some sugars are found naturally in foods, such as fruits, vegetables, and milk. "These are healthful additions to your diet," says Dr. Andrew Bremer, a pediatrician and NIH expert on sweeteners. "When you eat an orange, for instance, you are getting a lot of nutrients and dietary fiber along with the natural sugars."

Although sugar itself is not bad, says Rother, "sugar has a bad reputation that is mostly deserved because we consume too much of it. It is now in just about every food we eat."

Experts agree that Americans eat and drink way too much sugar, and it is contributing to the obesity epidemic. Much of the sugar we eat is not found naturally in food but is added during processing or preparation.

About 15 percent of the calories in the American adult diet come from added sugars. That is about 22 teaspoons of added sugar a day. Sugars are usually added to make foods and drinks taste better. But, such foods can be high in calories and offer none of the healthful benefits of fruits and other naturally sweet foods.

Sugar-sweetened beverages, such as soda, energy drinks, and sports drinks are the leading source of added sugars in the American diet. Juices naturally contain a lot of sugar. But, sometimes, even more is added to make them taste sweeter.

"Juices offer some vitamins and other nutrients, but I think those benefits are greatly offset by the harmful effects of too much sugar," says Bremer.

Over time, excess sweeteners can take a toll on your health. "Several studies have found a direct link between excess sugar consumption and obesity and cardiovascular problems worldwide," Bremer says.

Because of these harmful effects, many health organizations recommend that Americans cut back on added sugars. But, added sugars can be hard to identify. On a list of ingredients, they may be listed as sucrose (table sugar), corn sweetener, high-fructose corn syrup, fruit-juice concentrates, nectars, raw sugar, malt syrup, maple syrup, fructose sweeteners, liquid fructose, honey, molasses, anhydrous dextrose, or other words ending in "-ose," the chemical suffix for sugars. If any of these words are among the first few ingredients on a food label, the food is likely high in sugar. The total amount of sugar in a food is listed under "Total Carbohydrate" on the Nutrition Facts label.

Many people try cutting back on calories by switching from sugar-sweetened to diet foods and drinks that contain low- or no-calorie sweeteners. These artificial sweeteners – also known as "sugar substitutes" – are many times sweeter than table sugar, so smaller amounts are needed to create the same level of sweetness.

People have debated the safety of artificial sweeteners for decades. To date, researchers have found no clear evidence that any artificial sweeteners approved for use in the United States cause cancer or other serious health problems in humans.

But, can they help with weight loss? Scientific evidence is mixed. Some studies suggest that diet drinks can help you drop pounds in the short term, but weight tends to creep back up over time. Rother and other NIH-funded researchers are now working to better understand the complex effects that artificial sweeteners can have on the human body.

Studies of rodents and small numbers of people suggest that artificial sweeteners can affect the healthful gut microbes that help us digest food. This in turn can alter the body's ability to use glucose, which might then lead to weight gain. But, until larger studies are done in people, the long-term impact of these sweeteners on gut microbes and weight remains uncertain.

"There is much controversy about the health effects of artificial sweeteners and the differences between sugars and sweeteners," says Dr. Ivan de Araujo of Yale University. "Some animal studies indicate that sweeteners can produce physiological effects. But, depending on what kind of measurement is taken, including in humans, the outcomes may be conflicting."

De Araujo and others have been studying the effects that sugars and low-calorie sweeteners might have on the brain. His animal studies found that sugar and sweeteners tap differently into the brain's reward circuitry, with sugars having a more powerful and pleasurable effect.

"The part of the brain that mediates the 'I cannot stop' kinds of behaviors seems to be especially sensitive to sugars and largely insensitive to artificial sweeteners," de Araujo says. "Our long-term goal is really to understand if sugars or caloric sweeteners drive persistent intake of food. If exposed to too much sugar, does the brain eventually change in ways that lead to excess consumption? That is what we would like to know."

Some research suggests that the intensely sweet taste of artificial, low-calorie sweeteners can lead to a "sweet tooth," or a preference for sweet things. This in turn might lead to overeating. But, more studies are needed to confirm the relative effects of caloric versus noncaloric sweeteners.

"In the long run, if you want to lose weight, you need to establish a healthy lifestyle that contains unprocessed foods, moderate calories, and more exercise," Rother says.

When kids grow up eating a lot of sweet foods, they tend to develop a preference for sweets. But, if you give them a variety of healthy foods, such as fruits and vegetables early in life, they will develop a liking for them too.

"It is important for parents to expose children to a variety of tastes early on, but realize that it often takes several attempts to get a child to eat such foods," says Bremer. "Do not give up too soon."

The key to good health is eating a well-balanced diet with a variety of foods and getting plenty of physical activity. Focus on nutrition-rich whole foods without added sugars.

Section 26.2 | **Cutting Down on Added Sugars**

This section contains text excerpted from the following sources: Text in this section begins with excerpts from "Get the Facts: Added Sugars," Centers for Disease Control and Prevention (CDC), April 6, 2021; Text under the heading "Limiting Calories from Added Sugars" is excerpted from "*Dietary Guidelines for Americans, 2020-2025,*" *Dietary Guidelines for Americans* (*DGA*), U.S. Department of Agriculture (USDA), December 2020.

Americans are eating and drinking too much added sugars which can lead to health problems, such as weight gain and obesity, type 2 diabetes, and heart disease. To live healthier, longer lives, most need to move more and eat better including getting fewer calories from added sugars.

WHAT ARE ADDED SUGARS?

- Added sugars include sucrose, dextrose, table sugar, syrups, honey, and sugars from concentrated fruit or vegetable juices.
- The leading sources of added sugars in the U.S. diet are sugar-sweetened beverages and desserts and sweet snacks. Examples of desserts and sweet snacks are cookies, brownies, cakes, pies, ice cream, frozen dairy desserts, doughnuts, sweet rolls, and pastries.

AMERICANS SHOULD LIMIT THEIR ADDED SUGARS CONSUMPTION

The *Dietary Guidelines for Americans 2020–2025* recommends that:

- Americans 2 years and older keep their intake of added sugars to less than 10 percent of their total daily calories. For example, in a 2,000 calorie diet, no more than 200 calories should come from added sugars (about 12 teaspoons).
- Children younger than 2 years should not be fed foods and beverages with added sugars at all.
- One of the healthy people 2030 objectives is "reduce the consumption of calories from added sugars by persons aged 2 years and over."

LIMITING CALORIES FROM ADDED SUGARS

A healthy dietary pattern limits added sugars to less than 10 percent of calories per day. Added sugars can help with preservation; contribute to functional attributes such as viscosity, texture, body, color, and browning capability, and/or help improve the palatability of some nutrient-dense foods. In fact, the nutrient-dense choices included in the Healthy U.S.-Style Dietary Pattern are based on availability in the U.S. food supply and include 17–50 calories from added sugars or 1.5–2 percent of total calories.

Foods and beverages high in calories from added sugars should be limited to help achieve healthy dietary patterns within calorie limits. When added sugars in foods and beverages exceed 10 percent of calories, a healthy dietary pattern within calorie limits is very difficult to achieve. Most Americans have less than 8 percent of calories available for added sugars, including the added sugars inherent to a healthy dietary pattern. The limit for added sugars is based on the following assumptions:

- Most calorie levels have less than 15 percent of calories remaining after meeting food group recommendations through nutrient-dense choices.
- Approximately half of remaining calories are consumed as saturated fat and half consumed as added sugars.
- Total saturated fat intakes meet the recommendation for less than 10 percent of total calorie intake.
- No alcoholic beverages are consumed
- Overall calorie intake does not exceed the intake needs to maintain or achieve a healthy weight.

Based on the assumptions above, an individual who needs 2,000 calories per day (based on age, sex, and physical activity level) has less than 7 percent of calories available for added sugars. Individuals who need 2,800 calories per day or less have less than 8 percent of calories available for added sugars. Individuals who need more than 3,000 calories may have a total of 9 to 10 percent of calories available for added sugars. In this portion of the population that requires high-calorie intake, an upper limit of 10 percent of calories from added sugars may be consumed while still meeting

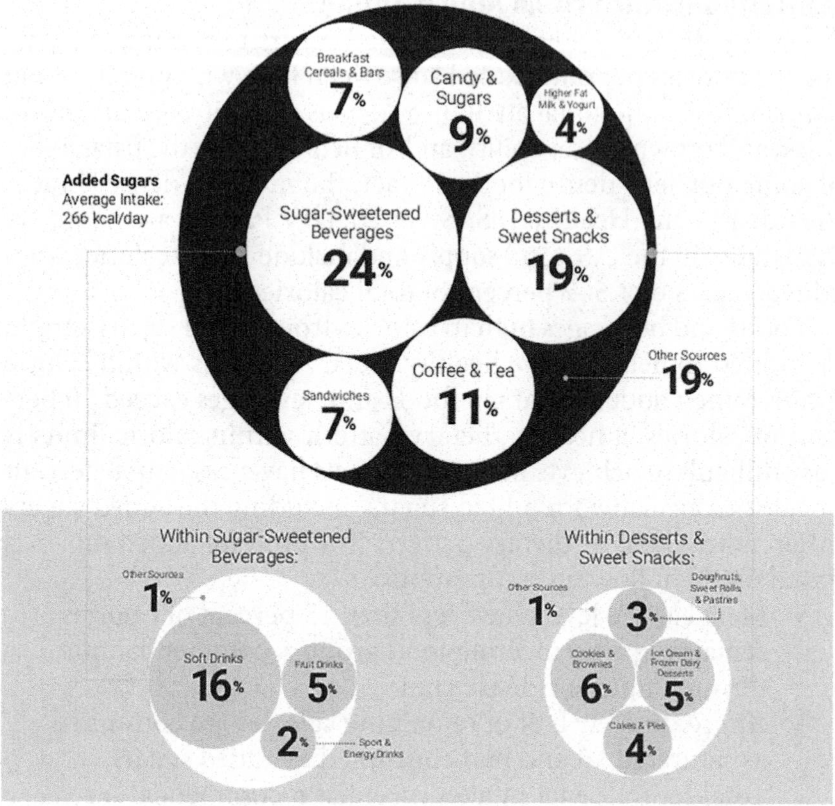

Figure 26.1. Top Sources and Average Intakes of Added Sugars: U.S. Population Ages 1 and Older *(Source: Analysis of What We Eat in America, National Health and Nutrition Examination Survey (NHANES), 2013–2016, ages 1 and older, 2 days dietary intake data, weighted.)*

food group recommendations in nutrient-dense forms. The 10 percent added sugar limit allows for flexibility in food choices over time but also requires careful planning. For example, if one chooses to eat less than the allotted amount of calories for saturated fat, 10 percent of added sugars may fit in a healthy dietary pattern.

Added sugars account on average for almost 270 calories – or more than 13 percent of total calories – per day in the United States population. As shown in Figure 26.1, the major sources of added sugars in typical U.S. diets are sugar-sweetened beverages, desserts, and sweet snacks, sweetened coffee and tea, and candy.

Together, these food categories make up more than half of the intake of all added sugars while contributing very little to food group recommendations.

Individuals have many potential options for reducing the intake of added sugars, including reducing the intake of major sources of added sugars. Strategies include reducing portions, consuming these items less often, and selecting options low in added sugars. For those with a weight loss goal, limiting the intake of foods and beverages high in added sugars is a strategy to help reduce calorie intake.

It should be noted that replacing added sugars with low- and no-calorie sweeteners may reduce calorie intake in the short-term and aid in weight management, yet questions remain about their effectiveness as a long-term weight management strategy.

Section 26.3 | **Artificial Sweeteners: Good or Bad?**

This section includes text excerpted from "Additional Information about High-Intensity Sweeteners Permitted for Use in Food in the United States," U.S. Food and Drug Administration (FDA), February 8, 2018.

High-intensity sweeteners are commonly used as sugar substitutes or sugar alternatives because they are many times sweeter than sugar but contribute only a few to no calories when added to foods. High-intensity sweeteners, such as all other ingredients added to food in the United States, must be safe for consumption.

SACCHARIN

Saccharin is approved for use in food as a nonnutritive sweetener. Saccharin brand names include Sweet and Low®, Sweet Twin®, Sweet'N Low®, and Necta Sweet®. It is 200 to 700 times sweeter than table sugar (sucrose), and it does not contain any calories.

First discovered and used in 1879, saccharin is currently approved for use, under certain conditions, in beverages, fruit juice drinks, and bases or mixes when prepared for consumption in accordance with directions, as a sugar substitute for cooking or table use, and in processed foods. Saccharin is also approved for use for certain technological purposes.

In the early 1970s, saccharin was linked with the development of bladder cancer in laboratory rats, which led Congress to mandate additional studies of saccharin and the presence of a warning label on saccharin-containing products until such warning could be shown to be unnecessary. Since then, more than 30 human studies demonstrated that the results found in rats were not relevant to humans and that saccharin is safe for human consumption. In 2000, the National Toxicology Program (NTP) of the National Institutes of Health (NIH) concluded that saccharin should be removed from the list of potential carcinogens. Products containing saccharin no longer have to carry the warning label.

ASPARTAME

Aspartame is approved for use in food as a nutritive sweetener. Aspartame brand names include Nutrasweet®, Equal®, and Sugar Twin®. It does contain calories, but because it is about 200 times sweeter than table sugar, consumers are likely to use much less of it.

The U.S. Food and Drug Administration (FDA) approved aspartame in 1981 (46 FR 38283) for uses, under certain conditions, as a tabletop sweetener, in chewing gum, cold breakfast cereals, and dry bases for certain foods (i.e., beverages, instant coffee and tea, gelatins, puddings, and fillings, and dairy products and toppings). In 1983 (48 FR 31376), the FDA approved the use of aspartame in carbonated beverages and carbonated beverage syrup bases, and in 1996, the FDA approved it for use as a "general purpose sweetener." It is not heat stable and loses its sweetness when heated, so it typically is not used in baked goods.

Aspartame is one of the most exhaustively studied substances in the human food supply, with more than 100 studies supporting its safety.

The FDA scientists have reviewed scientific data regarding the safety of aspartame in food and concluded that it is safe for the general population under certain conditions. However, people with a rare hereditary disease known as "phenylketonuria" (PKU) have a difficult time metabolizing phenylalanine, a component of aspartame, and should control their intake of phenylalanine from all sources, including aspartame. Labels of aspartame-containing foods and beverages must include a statement that informs individuals with PKU that the product contains phenylalanine.

ACESULFAME POTASSIUM (ACE-K)

Acesulfame potassium is approved for use in food as a nonnutritive sweetener. It is included in the ingredient list on the food label as acesulfame K, acesulfame potassium, or Ace-K. Acesulfame potassium is sold under the brand names Sunett® and Sweet One®. It is about 200 times sweeter than sugar and is often combined with other sweeteners.

The FDA approved acesulfame potassium for use in specific food and beverage categories in 1988 (53 FR 28379), and in 2003 approved it as a general purpose sweetener and flavor enhancer in food, except in meat and poultry, under certain conditions of use. It is heat stable, meaning that it stays sweet even when used at high temperatures during baking, making it suitable as a sugar substitute in baked goods.

Acesulfame potassium is typically used in frozen desserts, candies, beverages, and baked goods. More than 90 studies support its safety.

SUCRALOSE

Sucralose is approved for use in food as a nonnutritive sweetener. Sucralose is sold under the brand name Splenda®. Sucralose is about 600 times sweeter than sugar.

The FDA approved sucralose for use in 15 food categories in 1998 and for use as a general purpose sweetener for foods in 1999, under certain conditions of use. Sucralose is a general purpose sweetener that can be found in a variety of foods including baked goods, beverages, chewing gum, gelatins, and frozen dairy desserts. It is heat stable, meaning that it stays sweet even when used at high temperatures during baking, making it suitable as a sugar substitute in baked goods.

Sucralose has been extensively studied and more than 110 safety studies were reviewed by the FDA in approving the use of sucralose as a general purpose sweetener for food.

NEOTAME

Neotame is approved for use in food as a nonnutritive sweetener. Neotame is sold under the brand name Newtame® and is approximately 7,000 to 13,000 times sweeter than table sugar.

The FDA approved neotame for use as a general purpose sweetener and flavor enhancer in foods (except in meat and poultry), under certain conditions of use, in 2002. It is heat stable, meaning that it stays sweet even when used at high temperatures during baking, making it suitable as a sugar substitute in baked goods.

In determining the safety of neotame, the FDA reviewed data from more than 113 animal and human studies designed to identify possible toxic effects, including effects on the immune system, reproductive system, and nervous system.

ADVANTAME

Advantame is approved for use in food as a nonnutritive sweetener. It is approximately 20,000 times sweeter than table sugar (sucrose).

The FDA approved advantame for use as a general purpose sweetener and flavor enhancer in foods (except in meat and poultry), under certain conditions of use, in 2014. It is heat stable, meaning that it stays sweet even when used at high temperatures during baking, making it suitable as a sugar substitute in baked goods.

In determining the safety of advantame, the FDA reviewed data from 37 animal and human studies designed to identify possible toxic effects, including effects on the immune system, reproductive and developmental systems, and nervous system. The FDA also reviewed pharmacokinetic and carcinogenicity studies, as well as several additional exploratory and screening studies.

STEVIOL GLYCOSIDES

Steviol glycosides are natural constituents of the leaves of *Stevia rebaudiana* Bertoni, a plant native to parts of South America and commonly known as "Stevia." They are nonnutritive sweeteners and are reported to be 200 to 400 times sweeter than table sugar.

The FDA has received many GRAS Notices for the use of high-purity (95 percent minimum purity) steviol glycosides including rebaudioside A (also known as "Reb A"), stevioside, rebaudioside D, or steviol glycoside mixture preparations with rebaudioside A and/or stevioside as predominant components. The FDA has not questioned the notifiers' GRAS determinations for these high-purity stevia derived sweeteners under the intended conditions of use identified in the GRAS notices submitted to the FDA.

The use of stevia leaf and crude stevia extracts is not considered GRAS and their import into the United States is not permitted for use as sweeteners.

LUO HAN GUO FRUIT EXTRACTS

Siraitia grosvenorii Swingle fruit extract (SGFE) contains varying levels of mogrosides, which are the nonnutritive constituents of the fruit primarily responsible for the characteristic sweetness of SGFE. SGFE, depending on the mogroside content, is reported to be 100 to 250 times sweeter than sugar. Siraitia grosvenorii Swingle, commonly known as "Luo Han Guo" or "monk fruit," is a plant native to Southern China.

The FDA has received GRAS Notices for SGFE. The FDA has not questioned the notifiers' GRAS determination for SGFE under the intended conditions of use identified in the GRAS notices submitted to the FDA. The FDA's response letters on SGFE are available at the agency's GRAS Notice Inventory website (www.cfsanappsexternal.fda.gov/scripts/fdcc/index.cfm?set=GRASNotices).

Table 26.1. Sweeteners Permitted for Use in Food

Sweetener	Regulatory Status	Examples of Brand Names Containing Sweetener	Multiplier of Sweetness Intensity Compared to Table Sugar (Sucrose)	Acceptable Daily Intake (ADI) Milligrams per Kilogram Body Weight per Day (Mg/Kg Bw/D)	Number of Tabletop Sweetener Packets Equivalent to ADI*
Acesulfame Potassium (Ace-K)	Approved as a sweetener and flavor enhancer in foods generally (except in meat and poultry)	Sweet One® Sunett®	200 x	15	23
Advantame	Approved as a sweetener and flavor enhancer in foods generally (except in meat and poultry)		20,000 x	32.8	4,920
Aspartame	Approved as a sweetener and flavor enhancer in foods generally	Nutrasweet® Equal® Sugar Twin®	200 x	50	75
Neotame	Approved as a sweetener and flavor enhancer in foods generally (except in meat and poultry)	Newtame®	7,000–13,000 x	0.3	23 (sweetness intensity at 10,000 x sucrose)
Saccharin	Approved as a sweetener only in certain special dietary foods and as an additive used for certain technological purposes	Sweet and Low® Sweet Twin® Sweet'N Low® Necta Sweet®	200–700 x	15	45 (sweetness intensity at 400 x sucrose)

Table 26.1. Continued

Sweetener	Regulatory Status	Examples of Brand Names Containing Sweetener	Multiplier of Sweetness Intensity Compared to Table Sugar (Sucrose)	Acceptable Daily Intake (ADI) Milligrams per Kilogram Body Weight per Day (Mg/Kg Bw/D)	Number of Tabletop Sweetener Packets Equivalent to ADI*
Siraitia grosvenorii Swingle (Luo Han Guo) fruit extracts (SGFE)	SFGE containing 25%, 45% or 55% Mogroside V is the subject of GRAS notices for specific conditions of use	Nectresse® Monk Fruit in the Raw® PureLo®	100–250 x	NS***	ND
Certain high purity steviol glycosides purified from the leaves of *Stevia rebaudiana* (Bertoni) Bertoni	≥95% pure glycosides subject of GRAS notices for specific conditions of use	Truvia® PureVia® Enliten®	200–400 x	4**	9 (sweetness intensity at 300 x sucrose)

Table 26.1. Continued

Sweetener	Regulatory Status	Examples of Brand Names Containing Sweetener	Multiplier of Sweetness Intensity Compared to Table Sugar (Sucrose)	Acceptable Daily Intake (ADI) Milligrams per Kilogram Body Weight per Day (Mg/Kg Bw/D)	Number of Tabletop Sweetener Packets Equivalent to ADI*
Sucralose	Approved as a sweetener in foods generally	Splenda®	600 x	5	23

**Number of Tabletop Sweetener Packets a 60 kg (132 pounds) person would need to consume to reach the ADI. Calculations assume a packet of high-intensity sweetener is as sweet as two teaspoons of sugar.*

***ADI established by the Joint FAO/WHO Expert Committee on Food Additives (JECFA)*

****NS means not specified. A numerical ADI may not be deemed necessary for several reasons, including evidence of the ingredient's safety at levels well above the amounts needed to achieve the desired effect (e.g., as a sweetener) in food.*

WHAT IS THE DIFFERENCE BETWEEN NUTRITIVE AND NONNUTRITIVE HIGH-INTENSITY SWEETENERS?

Nutritive sweeteners add caloric value to the foods that contain them, while nonnutritive sweeteners are very low in calories or contain no calories at all. Specifically, aspartame, the only approved nutritive high-intensity sweetener, contains more than two percent of the calories in an equivalent amount of sugar, as opposed to nonnutritive sweeteners that contain less than two percent of the calories in an equivalent amount of sugar.

WHY DO THE INTENDED CONDITIONS OF USE OF HIGH-INTENSITY SWEETENERS SOMETIMES NOT INCLUDE USE IN MEAT AND POULTRY PRODUCTS?

The intended conditions of use of some high-intensity sweeteners approved for use as food additives do not include use in meat and poultry products because the companies that sought the FDA's approval for these substances did not request these uses. In the case of the high-intensity sweeteners that are subjects of GRAS notices (i.e., certain high-purity steviol glycosides and SGFE), the notifiers did not include use in meat and poultry products as an intended condition of use in the GRAS notices that they submitted for the FDA's evaluation.

If a high-intensity sweetener is proposed for use in a meat or poultry product through a food additive petition, the FDA would be responsible for reviewing the safety of the high-intensity sweetener under the proposed conditions of use, and the Food Safety and Inspection Service (FSIS) of the U.S. Department of Agriculture (USDA) would be responsible for evaluating its suitability. If the FDA is notified under the GRAS Notification Program that a high-intensity sweetener is GRAS for use in a meat or poultry product, the FDA would evaluate whether the notice provides a sufficient basis for a GRAS determination and whether information in the notice or otherwise available to the FDA raises issues that lead the agency to question whether the use of the high-intensity sweetener is GRAS. The FDA would also forward the GRAS notice to FSIS to evaluate whether the intended use of the substance in meat or poultry products complies with the relevant statutes that are administered by FSIS.

Chapter 27 | Food Ingredients: Additives and Colors

For centuries, ingredients have served useful functions in a variety of foods. Our ancestors used salt to preserve meats and fish, added herbs and spices to improve the flavor of foods, preserved fruit with sugar, and pickled cucumbers in a vinegar solution. Today, consumers demand and enjoy a food supply that is flavorful, nutritious, safe, convenient, colorful, and affordable. Food additives and advances in technology help make that possible.

There are thousands of ingredients used to make foods. The U.S. Food and Drug Administration (FDA) maintains a list of over 3,000 ingredients in its database "Everything Added to Food in the United States," many of which we use at home every day (e.g., sugar, baking soda, salt, vanilla, yeast, spices, and colors).

Still, some consumers have concerns about additives because they may see the long, unfamiliar names and think of them as complex chemical compounds. In fact, every food we eat – whether a just-picked strawberry or a homemade cookie – is made up of chemical compounds that determine flavor, color, texture, and nutrient value. All food additives are carefully regulated by federal authorities and various international organizations to ensure that foods are safe to eat and are accurately labeled.

This chapter includes text excerpted from "Overview of Food Ingredients, Additives & Colors," U.S. Food and Drug Administration (FDA), February 6, 2018.

WHY ARE FOOD AND COLOR INGREDIENTS ADDED TO FOOD?

Additives perform a variety of useful functions in foods that consumers often take for granted. Some additives could be eliminated if we were willing to grow our own food, harvest and grind it, spend many hours cooking and canning, or accept increased risks of food spoilage. But, most consumers today rely on the many technological, aesthetic, and convenient benefits that additives provide.

Following are some reasons why ingredients are added to foods:

- **To maintain or improve safety and freshness.** Preservatives slow product spoilage caused by mold, air, bacteria, fungi, or yeast. In addition to maintaining the quality of the food, they help control contamination that can cause foodborne illness, including life-threatening botulism. One group of preservatives – antioxidants – prevents fats and oils and the foods containing them from becoming rancid or developing an off-flavor. They also prevent cut fresh fruits such as apples from turning brown when exposed to air.
- **To improve or maintain nutritional value.** Vitamins and minerals (and fiber) are added to many foods to make up for those lacking in a person's diet or lost in processing or to enhance the nutritional quality of a food. Such fortification and enrichment have helped reduce malnutrition in the U.S. and worldwide. All products containing added nutrients must be appropriately labeled.
- **Improve taste, texture, and appearance.** Spices, natural and artificial flavors, and sweeteners are added to enhance the taste of food. Food colors maintain or improve appearance. Emulsifiers, stabilizers, and thickeners give foods the texture and consistency consumers expect. Leavening agents allow baked goods to rise during baking. Some additives help control the acidity and alkalinity of foods, while other ingredients help maintain the taste and appeal of foods with reduced fat content.

WHAT IS A FOOD ADDITIVE?

In its broadest sense, a food additive is any substance added to food. Legally, the term refers to "any substance the intended use of which results or may reasonably be expected to result – directly or indirectly – in its becoming a component or otherwise affecting the characteristics of any food." This definition includes any substance used in the production, processing, treatment, packaging, transportation, or storage of food. The purpose of the legal definition, however, is to impose a premarket approval requirement. Therefore, this definition excludes ingredients whose use is generally recognized as safe (where government approval is not needed), those ingredients approved for use by the FDA or the U.S. Department of Agriculture (USDA) prior to the food additives provisions of law, and color additives and pesticides where other legal premarket approval requirements apply.

Direct food additives are those that are added to a food for a specific purpose in that food. For example, xanthan gum – used in salad dressings, chocolate milk, bakery fillings, puddings, and other foods to add texture – is a direct additive. Most direct additives are identified on the ingredient label of foods.

Indirect food additives are those that become part of the food in trace amounts due to its packaging, storage, or other handlings. For instance, minute amounts of packaging substances may find their way into foods during storage. Food packaging manufacturers must prove to the FDA that all materials coming in contact with food are safe before they are permitted for use in such a manner.

WHAT IS A COLOR ADDITIVE?

A color additive is any dye, pigment, or substance which when added or applied to a food, drug, or cosmetic, or to the human body, is capable (alone or through reactions with other substances) of imparting color. The FDA is responsible for regulating all color additives to ensure that foods containing color additives are safe to eat, contain only approved ingredients and are accurately labeled.

Color additives are used in foods for many reasons: 1) to offset color loss due to exposure to light, air, temperature extremes, moisture and storage conditions; 2) to correct natural variations in color; 3) to enhance colors that occur naturally; and 4) to provide color to colorless and "fun" foods. Without color additives, colas would not be brown, margarine would not be yellow and mint ice cream would not be green. Color additives are now recognized as an important part of practically all processed foods we eat.

The FDA's permitted colors are classified as subject to certification or exempt from certification, both of which are subject to rigorous safety standards prior to their approval and listing for use in foods.

Certified colors are synthetically produced (or human-made) and used widely because they impart an intense, uniform color, are less expensive, and blend more easily to create a variety of hues. There are nine certified color additives approved for use in the U.S. Certified food colors generally do not add undesirable flavors to foods.

Colors that are exempt from certification include pigments derived from natural sources such as vegetables, minerals or animals. Nature derived color additives are typically more expensive than certified colors and may add unintended flavors to foods. Examples of exempt colors include annatto extract (yellow), dehydrated beets (bluish-red to brown), caramel (yellow to tan), beta-carotene (yellow to orange) and grape skin extract (red, green).

HOW ARE ADDITIVES APPROVED FOR USE IN FOODS?

Today, food and color additives are more strictly studied, regulated, and monitored than at any other time in history. The FDA has the primary legal responsibility for determining their safe use. To market a new food or color additive (or before using an additive already approved for one use in another manner not yet approved), a manufacturer or other sponsor must first petition the FDA for its approval. These petitions must provide evidence that the substance is safe for the ways in which it will be used. As a result of recent legislation, since 1999, indirect additives have been approved via a premarket notification process requiring the same data as was previously required by petition.

When evaluating the safety of a substance and whether it should be approved, the FDA considers: 1) the composition and properties of the substance, 2) the amount that would typically be consumed, 3) immediate and long-term health effects, and 4) various safety factors. The evaluation determines an appropriate level of use that includes a built-in safety margin – a factor that allows for uncertainty about the levels of consumption that are expected to be harmless. In other words, the levels of use that gain approval are much lower than what would be expected to have any adverse effect.

Because of inherent limitations of science, the FDA can never be absolutely certain of the absence of any risk from the use of any substance. Therefore, the FDA must determine – based on the best science available – if there is a reasonable certainty of no harm to consumers when an additive is used as proposed.

If an additive is approved, the FDA issues regulations that may include the types of foods in which it can be used, the maximum amounts to be used, and how they should be identified on food labels. In 1999, procedures changed so that the FDA now consults with the USDA during the review process for ingredients that are proposed for use in meat and poultry products. Federal officials then monitor the extent of Americans' consumption of the new additive and results of any new research on its safety to ensure its use continues to be within safe limits.

If new evidence suggests that a product already in use may be unsafe, or if consumption levels have changed enough to require another look, federal authorities may prohibit its use or conduct further studies to determine if the use can still be considered safe.

Regulations known as "Good Manufacturing Practices" (GMPs) limit the amount of food ingredients used in foods to the amount necessary to achieve the desired effect.

FOOD PRESERVATION

Food ingredients have been used for many years to preserve, flavor, blend, thicken, and color foods, and have played an important role in reducing serious nutritional deficiencies among consumers. These ingredients also help ensure the availability of flavorful, nutritious, safe, convenient, colorful, and affordable foods that meet consumer expectations year-round.

Food and color additives are strictly studied, regulated, and monitored. Federal regulations require evidence that each substance is safe at its intended level of use before it may be added to foods. Furthermore, all additives are subject to ongoing safety review as scientific understanding and methods of testing continue to improve. Consumers should feel safe about the foods they eat.

QUESTIONS AND ANSWERS ABOUT FOOD AND COLOR ADDITIVES

How Are Ingredients Listed on a Product Label?

Food manufacturers are required to list all ingredients in the food on the label. On a product label, the ingredients are listed in order of predominance, with the ingredients used in the greatest amount first, followed in descending order by those in smaller amounts. The label must list the names of any FDA-certified color additives (e.g., FD&C Blue No. 1 or the abbreviated name, Blue 1). But, some ingredients can be listed collectively as "flavors," "spices," "artificial flavoring," or in the case of color additives exempt from certification, "artificial colors," without naming each one. Declaration of an allergenic ingredient in a collective or single color, flavor, or spice could be accomplished by simply naming the allergenic ingredient in the ingredient list.

What Are Dyes and Lakes in Color Additives?

Certified color additives are categorized as either dyes or lakes. Dyes dissolve in water and are manufactured as powders, granules, liquids, or other special-purpose forms. They can be used in beverages, dry mixes, baked goods, confections, dairy products, pet foods, and a variety of other products.

Lakes are the water-insoluble form of dye. Lakes are more stable than dyes and are ideal for coloring products containing fats and oils or items lacking sufficient moisture to dissolve dyes. Typical uses include coated tablets, cake and donut mixes, hard candies, and chewing gums.

Do Additives Cause Childhood Hyperactivity?

Although this hypothesis was popularized in the 1970s, results from studies on this issue either have been inconclusive, inconsistent, or difficult to interpret due to inadequacies in study design. A Consensus Development Panel (CDP) of the National Institutes of Health (NIH) concluded in 1982 that for some children with attention deficit hyperactivity disorder (ADHD) and confirmed food allergy, dietary modification has produced some improvement in behavior. Although the panel said that elimination diets should not be used universally to treat childhood hyperactivity, since there is no scientific evidence to predict which children may benefit, the panel recognized that initiation of a trial of dietary treatment or continuation of a diet in patients whose families and physicians perceive benefits may be warranted.

However, a 1997 review published in the *Journal of the American Academy of Child & Adolescent Psychiatry* noted there is minimal evidence of efficacy and extreme difficulty inducing children and adolescents to comply with restricted diets. Thus, dietary treatment should not be recommended, except possibly with a small number of preschool children who may be sensitive to tartrazine, known commonly as "FD&C Yellow No.5." In 2007, synthetic certified color additives again came under scrutiny following publication of a study commissioned by the U.K. Food Standards Agency (FSA) to investigate whether certain color additives cause hyperactivity in children. Both the FDA and the European Food Safety Authority (EFSA) independently reviewed the results from this study and each has concluded that the study does not substantiate a link between the color additives that were tested and behavioral effects.

What Is the Difference between Natural and Artificial Ingredients? Is a Naturally Produced Ingredient Safer than an Artificially Manufactured Ingredient?

Natural ingredients are derived from natural sources (e.g., soybeans and corn provide lecithin to maintain product consistency; beets provide beet powder used as food coloring). Other ingredients are not found in nature and therefore must be synthetically produced as artificial ingredients. Also, some ingredients found in nature can be manufactured artificially and produced more economically, with greater purity and more consistent quality, than their natural counterparts. For example, vitamin C or ascorbic acid may be derived from an orange or produced in a laboratory. Food ingredients are subject to the same strict safety standards regardless of whether they are naturally or artificially derived.

Are Certain People Sensitive to FD&C Yellow No. 5 in Foods?

FD&C Yellow No. 5, is used to color beverages, dessert powders, candy, ice cream, custards and other foods. The FDA's Committee on Hypersensitivity to Food Constituents concluded in 1986 that FD&C Yellow No. 5 might cause hives in fewer than one out of 10,000 people. It also concluded that there was no evidence the color additive in food provokes asthma attacks. The law now requires Yellow No. 5 to be identified on the ingredient line. This allows the few who may be sensitive to the color to avoid it.

Do Low-Calorie Sweeteners Cause Adverse Reactions?

No. Food safety experts generally agree there is no convincing evidence of a cause and effect relationship between these sweeteners and negative health effects in humans. The FDA has monitored consumer complaints of possible adverse reactions for more than 15 years.

For example, in carefully controlled clinical studies, aspartame has not been shown to cause adverse or allergic reactions. However, persons with a rare hereditary disease known as "phenylketonuria" (PKU) must control their intake of phenylalanine from all sources, including aspartame. Although aspartame contains only a small amount of phenylalanine, labels of aspartame-containing foods and beverages must include a statement advising phenylketonurics of the presence of phenylalanine.

Individuals who have concerns about possible adverse effects from food additives or other substances should contact their physicians.

How Do They Add Vitamins and Minerals to Fortified Cereals?

Adding nutrients to cereal can cause taste and color changes in the product. This is especially true with added minerals. Since no one wants cereal that tastes like a vitamin supplement, a variety of techniques are employed in the fortification process. In general, those nutrients that are heat stable (such as vitamins A and E and various minerals) are incorporated into the cereal itself (they are baked right in). Nutrients that are not stable to heat (such as B-vitamins) are applied directly to the cereal after all heating steps are completed. Each cereal is unique – some can handle more nutrients than others can. This is one reason why fortification levels are different across all cereals.

What Is the Role of Modern Technology in Producing Food Additives?

Many new techniques are being researched that will allow the production of additives in ways not previously possible. One approach is the use of biotechnology, which can use simple organisms to produce food additives. These additives are the same as food components found in nature. In 1990, the FDA approved the first bioengineered enzyme, rennin, which traditionally had been extracted from calves' stomachs for use in making cheese.

TYPES OF FOOD INGREDIENTS

The following summary lists the types of common food ingredients, why they are used, and some examples of the names that can be found on product labels. Some additives are used for more than one purpose.

Table 27.1. Types of Common Food Ingredients

Types of Ingredients	What They Do	Examples of Uses	Names Found on Product Labels
Preservatives	Prevent food spoilage from bacteria, molds, fungi, or yeast (antimicrobials); slow or prevent changes in color, flavor, or texture and delay rancidity (antioxidants); maintain freshness	Fruit sauces and jellies, beverages, baked goods, cured meats, oils and margarines, cereals, dressings, snack foods, fruits, and vegetables	Ascorbic acid, citric acid, sodium benzoate, calcium propionate, sodium erythorbate, sodium nitrite, calcium sorbate, potassium sorbate, BHA, BHT, EDTA, tocopherols (Vitamin E)
Sweeteners	Add sweetness with or without the extra calories	Beverages, baked goods, confections, table-top sugar, substitutes, many processed foods	Sucrose (sugar), glucose, fructose, sorbitol, mannitol, corn syrup, high fructose corn syrup, saccharin, aspartame, sucralose, acesulfame potassium (acesulfame-K), neotame
Color Additives	Offset color loss due to exposure to light, air, temperature extremes, moisture, and storage conditions; correct natural variations in color; enhance colors that occur naturally; provide color to colorless and "fun" foods	Many processed foods, (candies, snack foods margarine, cheese, soft drinks, jams/jellies, gelatins, pudding, and pie fillings)	FD&C Blue Nos. 1 and 2, FD&C Green No. 3, FD&C Red Nos. 3 and 40, FD&C Yellow Nos. 5 and 6, Orange B, Citrus Red No. 2, annatto extract, beta-carotene, grape skin extract, cochineal extract or carmine, paprika oleoresin, caramel color, fruit and vegetable juices, saffron (**Note:** Exempt color additives are not required to be declared by name on labels but may be declared simply as colorings or color added)

Table 27.1. Continued

Types of Ingredients	What They Do	Examples of Uses	Names Found on Product Labels
Flavors and Spices	Add specific flavors (natural and synthetic)	Pudding and pie fillings, gelatin dessert mixes, cake mixes, salad dressings, candies, soft drinks, ice cream, BBQ sauce	Natural flavoring, artificial flavor, and spices
Flavor Enhancers	Enhance flavors already present in foods (without providing their own separate flavor)	Many processed foods	Monosodium glutamate (MSG), hydrolyzed soy protein, autolyzed yeast extract, disodium guanylate, or inosinate
Fat Replacers (and components of formulations used to replace fats)	Provide expected texture and a creamy "mouth-feel" in reduced-fat foods	Baked goods, dressings, frozen desserts, confections, cake, and dessert mixes, dairy products	Olestra, cellulose gel, carrageenan, polydextrose, modified food starch, microparticulated egg white protein, guar gum, xanthan gum, whey protein concentrate
Nutrients	Replace vitamins and minerals lost in processing (enrichment), add nutrients that may be lacking in the diet (fortification)	Flour, breads, cereals, rice, macaroni, margarine, salt, milk, fruit beverages, energy bars, instant breakfast drinks	Thiamine hydrochloride, riboflavin (Vitamin B_2), niacin, niacinamide, folate or folic acid, beta carotene, potassium iodide, iron or ferrous sulfate, alpha tocopherols, ascorbic acid, Vitamin D, amino acids (L-tryptophan, L-lysine, L-leucine, L-methionine)

Table 27.1. Continued

Types of Ingredients	What They Do	Examples of Uses	Names Found on Product Labels
Emulsifiers	Allow smooth mixing of ingredients, prevent separation Keep emulsified products stable, reduce stickiness, control crystallization, keep ingredients dispersed, and to help products dissolve more easily	Salad dressings, peanut butter, chocolate, margarine, frozen desserts	Soy lecithin, mono- and diglycerides, egg yolks, polysorbates, sorbitan monostearate
Stabilizers and Thickeners, Binders, Texturizers	Produce uniform texture, improve "mouth-feel"	Frozen desserts, dairy products, cakes, pudding and gelatin mixes, dressings, jams and jellies, sauces	Gelatin, pectin, guar gum, carrageenan, xanthan gum, whey
pH Control Agents and Acidulants	Control acidity and alkalinity, prevent spoilage	Beverages, frozen desserts, chocolate, low acid canned foods, baking powder	Lactic acid, citric acid, ammonium hydroxide, sodium carbonate
Leavening Agents	Promote rising of baked goods	Breads and other baked goods	Baking soda, monocalcium phosphate, calcium carbonate
Anti-caking Agents	Keep powdered foods free-flowing, prevent moisture absorption	Salt, baking powder, confectioner's sugar	Calcium silicate, iron ammonium citrate, silicon dioxide
Humectants	Retain moisture	Shredded coconut, marshmallows, soft candies, confections	Glycerin, sorbitol

Table 27.1. Continued

Types of Ingredients	What They Do	Examples of Uses	Names Found on Product Labels
Yeast Nutrients	Promote growth of yeast	Breads and other baked goods	Calcium sulfate, ammonium phosphate
Dough Strengtheners and Conditioners	Produce more stable dough	Breads and other baked goods	Ammonium sulfate, azodicarbonamide, L-cysteine
Firming Agents	Maintain crispness and firmness	Processed fruits and vegetables	Calcium chloride, calcium lactate
Enzyme Preparations	Modify proteins, polysaccharides and fats	Cheese, dairy products, meat	Enzymes, lactase, papain, rennet, chymosin
Gases	Serve as propellant, aerate, or create carbonation	Oil cooking spray, whipped cream, carbonated beverages	Carbon dioxide, nitrous oxide

Chapter 28 | Safety of Irradiated Food

Irradiation does not make foods radioactive, compromise nutritional quality, or noticeably change the taste, texture, or appearance of food. In fact, any changes made by irradiation are so minimal that it is not easy to tell if a food has been irradiated.

Food irradiation (the application of ionizing radiation to food) is a technology that improves the safety and extends the shelf life of foods by reducing or eliminating microorganisms and insects. Like pasteurizing milk and canning fruits and vegetables, irradiation can make food safer for the consumer. The U.S. Food and Drug Administration (FDA) is responsible for regulating the sources of radiation that are used to irradiate food. The FDA approves a source of radiation for use on foods only after it has determined that irradiating the food is safe.

WHY IRRADIATE FOOD?

Irradiation can serve many purposes:

- Prevention of foodborne illness – to effectively eliminate organisms that cause foodborne illness, such as *Salmonella* and *Escherichia coli (E. coli)*.
- Preservation – to destroy or inactivate organisms that cause spoilage and decomposition and extend the shelf life of foods.
- Control of insects – to destroy insects in or on tropical fruits imported into the United States. Irradiation also

This chapter includes text excerpted from "Food Irradiation: What You Need to Know," U.S. Food and Drug Administration (FDA), January 4, 2018.

decreases the need for other pest-control practices that may harm the fruit.

- Delay of sprouting and ripening – to inhibit sprouting (e.g., potatoes) and delay ripening of fruit to increase longevity.
- Sterilization – irradiation can be used to sterilize foods, which can then be stored for years without refrigeration. Sterilized foods are useful in hospitals for patients with severely impaired immune systems, such as patients with acquired immunodeficiency syndrome (AIDS) or undergoing chemotherapy. Foods that are sterilized by irradiation are exposed to substantially higher levels of treatment than those approved for general use.

How Is Food Irradiated?

There are three sources of radiation approved for use on foods:

- Gamma rays are emitted from radioactive forms of the element cobalt (Cobalt 60) or of the element cesium (Cesium 137). Gamma radiation is used routinely to sterilize medical, dental, and household products and is also used for the radiation treatment of cancer.
- X-rays are produced by reflecting a high-energy stream of electrons off a target substance (usually one of the heavy metals) into food. X-rays are also widely used in medicine and industry to produce images of internal structures.
- Electron beam (or e-beam) is similar to x-rays and is a stream of high-energy electrons propelled from an electron accelerator into food.

IS IRRADIATED FOOD SAFE TO EAT?

The FDA has evaluated the safety of irradiated food for more than 30 years and has found the process to be safe. The World Health Organization (WHO), the Centers for Disease Control and Prevention (CDC), and the U.S. Department of Agriculture (USDA) have also endorsed the safety of irradiated food.

The FDA has approved a variety of foods for irradiation in the United States including:

- Beef and pork
- Crustaceans (e.g., lobster, shrimp, and crab)
- Fresh fruits and vegetables
- Lettuce and spinach
- Poultry
- Seeds for sprouting (e.g., for alfalfa sprouts)
- Shell eggs
- Shellfish or molluscan (e.g., oysters, clams, mussels, and scallops)
- Spices and seasonings

HOW WILL YOU KNOW IF YOUR FOOD HAS BEEN IRRADIATED?

The FDA requires that irradiated foods bear the international symbol for irradiation. Look for the radura symbol along with the statement "treated with radiation" or "treated by irradiation" on the food label. Bulk foods, such as fruits and vegetables, are required to be individually labeled or to have a label next to the sale container. The FDA does not require that individual ingredients in multi-ingredient foods (e.g., spices) be labeled. It is important to remember that irradiation is not a replacement for proper food handling practices by producers, processors, and consumers. Irradiated foods need to be stored, handled, and cooked in the same way as nonirradiated foods because they could still become contaminated with disease-causing organisms after irradiation if the rules of basic food safety are not followed.

Chapter 29 | Excess Sodium

Chapter Contents

Section 29.1 | **The Role of Sodium in Your Food**

This section contains text excerpted from the following sources: Text under the heading "What Do the 2020–2025 Guidelines Say about Sodium?" is excerpted from "*Dietary Guidelines for Americans, 2020-2025*," *Dietary Guidelines for Americans* (*DGA*), U.S. Department of Agriculture (USDA), December 2020; Text beginning with the heading "Sodium Can Add Up Quickly" is excerpted from "Get the Facts: Sodium and the Dietary Guidelines," Centers for Disease Control and Prevention (CDC), October 2017. Reviewed May 2021; Text beginning with the heading "Where Does Dietary Sodium Come From?" is excerpted from "The Role of Sodium in Your Food," Centers for Disease Control and Prevention (CDC), September 8, 2020.

WHAT DO THE 2020–2025 GUIDELINES SAY ABOUT SODIUM?

The number of adults exceeding the chronic disease risk reduction (CDRR) level for sodium during this life stage is concerning given that 45 percent of adults ages 18 and older are living with hypertension. During adulthood, the prevalence of hypertension increases from about 22 percent of adults ages 18 through 39 to about 55 percent of adults ages 40 through 59. Changing this trend is important because hypertension is a preventable risk factor for cardiovascular disease and stroke. Unlike other factors that cannot be changed, such as genetics and family history, reduced dietary intake of sodium is a modifiable risk factor that can help improve blood pressure control and reduce the risk of hypertension.

SODIUM CAN ADD UP QUICKLY

The first thing to know is that the salt you use at the dinner table is not the biggest sodium contributor in the American diet. In fact, the majority of the sodium Americans consume – more than 70 percent – are found in processed food and restaurant meals.

And, do not let your taste buds fool you. Foods, such as grains, baked goods, and meats may not taste salty, but they add up to major sources of daily sodium because they are eaten so often.

The majority of Americans' daily sodium intake comes from grains and meat, and other top contributors include processed poultry, soups, and sandwiches.

Depending on your food choices, it does not take much to consume more sodium than recommended.

- One slice of bread can contain anywhere from 80 to 230 mg of sodium, and a slice of frozen pizza can contain between 370 and 730 mg.
- Some breakfast cereals contain 150 to 300 mg of sodium before milk is added.
- Canned soups and soups served in restaurants can contribute high amounts of sodium.
- Processed tomato products and salad dressings often include salt and other ingredients that contain sodium.
- Many snack foods – chips, crackers, and pretzels – contain several hundred milligrams of sodium per serving.

TIPS FOR SHOPPING SMARTER

The more you know about the food you eat, the better the decisions you can make for yourself and your family.

- Eat more fresh fruits and vegetables and low-fat dairy. Research shows that foods low in sodium and high in potassium can help reduce blood pressure and the risk for other serious conditions. Examples include bananas, dried apricots, and spinach. Low- or no-fat yogurt, beans other than green beans, and potatoes are also low in sodium and high in potassium.
- When eating frozen and canned vegetables, choose no salt added or low sodium versions, or choose frozen varieties without sauce.
- When buying processed foods, read nutrition labels and choose products with less sodium.
    - Note how many milligrams of sodium is in each serving – and how many servings are in the package.
    - Foods that contain 35 mg or less per serving are very low in sodium. Foods that contain 140 mg or less per serving are defined as low sodium.
- Check processed meat and poultry, which are often "enhanced" with salt water or saline.
- Opt for lower sodium or no salt added bread, crackers, and cereals.

TIPS FOR COOKING AT HOME

- Use lemon juice and salt-free herbs and spices, such as garlic and pepper, to flavor your food instead of sauces and prepackaged seasonings.
- Limit added salt while cooking, and taste food first before salting at the table.

WHERE DOES DIETARY SODIUM COME FROM?

Although many people are quick to blame the salt shaker, only a small amount of dietary sodium is added during home cooking and at the table. Most of the sodium that Americans consume - about 70 percent - comes from restaurant, prepackaged, and processed foods, including many products that do not even taste salty. For consumers to make informed decisions about what they eat, it is helpful to understand the role sodium plays in different foods.

WHY IS SODIUM ADDED TO PROCESSED FOOD?

Sodium plays many roles in our foods, mainly:

To Enhance Flavor

- Adds a salty taste
- Boosts flavor balance and can enhance the sweetness of sugary items
- Masks "off notes," such as bitterness and strange tastes, that can result from food processing
- Makes some types of processed foods more palatable

To Preserve Freshness

- Increases shelf life
- Helps prevent growth of bacteria and other disease-causing agents

To Improve Texture and Appearance

- Makes the product seem thicker or fuller

- Enhances color and hue
- Helps retain moisture in processed meat products as a trade-off for saturated fat
- Stabilizes texture, allowing bread to rise and cheese to stick together
- Prevents unwanted chemical changes to other ingredients in many baked items

WHY IS EATING TOO MUCH SODIUM A PROBLEM?

- Our bodies require only a small amount of sodium each day to function normally. Eating too much sodium can lead to increased blood pressure, which can raise the risk of heart attack, stroke, and other cardiovascular conditions.
- Most adults in the United States exceed their recommended daily limit of sodium.
- Reducing your sodium intake can help lower your blood pressure and improve the health of your heart.

IS ALL OF THIS SODIUM NECESSARY?

- In many cases, no. For many products, sodium's technical functions can be accomplished with lower levels than are currently being used.
- Many familiar products already contain lower amounts of sodium in other countries. This international variability indicates that these companies could readily introduce lower sodium versions of popular products in the United States.
- Sodium levels in similar U.S. products vary greatly across – and even within – brands, indicating consumers' willingness to buy less salty products.
- Although many food manufacturers express concern about the altered taste of lower sodium products, salt is an acquired taste. Some research indicates that consumers – and their taste buds – can adapt to the taste of lower sodium foods.

- Certain studies found that when a reduced-sodium version of a popular food is served, the typical consumer adds less than 20 percent of the removed sodium back. This behavior suggests that individuals are relatively comfortable with gradual reductions of sodium in products.

Section 29.2 | **How the Body Regulates Salt Levels**

This section includes text excerpted from "How the Body Regulates Salt Levels," National Institutes of Health (NIH), May 2, 2017. Reviewed May 2021.

Sodium chloride, commonly called "dietary salt," is essential to our body. But, a high salt intake can raise blood pressure, which can damage the body in many ways over time. High blood pressure (HBP) has been linked to heart disease, stroke, kidney failure, and other health problems. However, not everyone is equally sensitive to high levels of salt.

Researchers have long believed that the way the level of salt inside our bodies is controlled is fairly straightforward: when levels are too high, our brains are stimulated to make us thirsty. We drink more and excrete more urine, through which the body expels excess salt.

To gain insight into this process, a team led by Dr. Jens Titze at the University of Erlangen-Nuremberg in Germany took the opportunity to study men participating in a simulated space flight program. Between 2009 and 2011, they tightly controlled the daily salt intake of 10 men simulating a flight to Mars: four in a 105-day preflight phase and six others for 205 days. The men were given 12 grams of salt per day, 9 g/day, or 6 g/day for 30–60 days. The researchers collected all the men's urine for testing.

The scientists were surprised to find that, whatever the level of salt consumed, sodium was stored and released from the men's bodies in roughly weekly and monthly patterns. The team uncovered similar rhythms for the hormones aldosterone, which regulates sodium excretion from the kidney, and glucocorticoids, which help regulate metabolism.

Titze, now at Vanderbilt University Medical Center, continued to examine the long-term control of sodium and water balance in the men. To better understand the mechanisms at work, his team also performed experiments in mice.

Changing salt intake affected levels of both aldosterone and glucocorticoids, the hormones found to rhythmically control the body's salt and water balance. These, in turn, had a number of interesting effects on the body. Increasing salt intake increased sodium excretion, but also unexpectedly caused the kidney to conserve water. Excess sodium was thus released in concentrated urine. This method of protecting the body's water was so efficient that the men actually drank less when their salt intake was highest.

These results show that the body regulates its salt and water balance not only by releasing excess sodium in urine but by actively retaining or releasing water in urine. The advantage of this mechanism is that the long-term maintenance of body fluids is not as dependent on external water sources as once believed.

The researchers found that the kidney conserves or releases water by balancing levels of sodium, potassium, and the waste product urea. This may be what ties glucocorticoid levels to salt intake. A high salt diet increased glucocorticoid levels, causing muscle and liver to burn more energy to produce urea, which was then used in the kidney for water conservation. That also led the mice to eat more. These salt-driven changes in metabolism may thus partly explain why high salt diets have been linked to diabetes, heart disease, and other health problems that can result from the condition known as "metabolic syndrome."

"We have always focused on the role of salt in arterial hypertension. Our findings suggest that there is much more to know – a high salt intake may predispose to metabolic syndrome," Titze says. More work will be needed to better understand these mechanisms.

Section 29.3 | **How to Reduce Sodium**

This section includes text excerpted from "How to Reduce Sodium," Centers for Disease Control and Prevention (CDC), September 8, 2020.

The majority of sodium in our diets comes from packaged and restaurant food (not the salt shaker) and is a direct result of food processing. Even foods that may not taste salty can be major sources of sodium. Foods with only moderate amounts of sodium, such as bread, can be major sources in our diets because we eat so much of them.

TIPS FOR REDUCING SODIUM

Things you or the person who purchases and prepares your food can do to reduce sodium:

At the Grocery Store

- Buy fresh, frozen, or canned vegetables with no salt or sauce added.
- Choose packaged foods labeled "low sodium," "reduced sodium," or "no salt added" when available.
- Read food labels and compare the amount of sodium in different products, then choose the options with the lowest amounts of sodium.
- When buying prepared meals, look for those with less than 600 milligrams (mg) of sodium per meal, which is the upper limit set by the U.S. Food and Drug Administration (FDA) for a meal or main dish to be labeled "healthy."
- Check the amount of sodium per serving, and do not forget to check the number of servings per container.
- When possible, purchase fresh poultry, fish, pork, and lean meat, rather than cured, salted, smoked, and other processed meats. For fresh items, check to see whether saline or salt solution has been added – if so, choose another brand.

- Ask your grocer if they have a low sodium shopping list available.
- Ask to speak to the registered dietitian at your local grocery store to learn more about buying low sodium products. If your grocer does not have a registered dietitian, ask your doctor for a referral. A registered dietitian can provide valuable guidance on reducing your family's sodium intake and managing blood pressure.

At Home

- When cooking, use alternatives to replace or reduce the amount of salt you use, such as garlic, citrus juice, salt-free seasonings, or spices.
- Prepare rice, pasta, beans, and meats from their most basic forms (dry and fresh) when possible.
- Eat more fruits and vegetables.
- Limit sauces, mixes, and "instant" products, including flavored rice and ready-made pasta.

Dining Out

- Ask for nutrition information before you order, and select a lower sodium meal.
- Ask that no salt be added to your meal.
- Split a meal with a friend or family member.
- Keep takeout and fast food to an occasional treat.

The *2015–2020 Dietary Guidelines for Americans* recommend that Americans consume less than 2,300 mg of sodium each day as part of a healthy eating pattern. For individuals with hypertension or prehypertension, further reduction to 1,500 mg of sodium per day can result in greater blood pressure reduction. Ask your doctor whether you have any of these conditions.

CHOOSE A HEART-HEALTHY DIET

The DASH (Dietary Approaches to Stop Hypertension) eating plan is a simple, heart-healthy diet that can help prevent or lower high blood pressure. The DASH diet is low in sodium, cholesterol, and saturated and total fats, and it is high in fruits and vegetables, fiber, potassium, and low-fat dairy products.

If you follow the DASH eating plan and also make other healthy lifestyle changes, such as getting more physical activity, you will see the biggest benefits.

Chapter 30 | Health Effects of Commercial Beverages

Chapter Contents

Section 30.1 | **Making Healthy Beverage Choices**

This section includes text excerpted from "Rethink Your Drink," Centers for Disease Control and Prevention (CDC), February 10, 2021.

Most of us eat and drink too many added sugars, which can lead to significant health problems. Sugary drinks are the leading source of added sugars in the American diet.

WHAT ARE SUGARY DRINKS?

Sugary drinks, also known as "sugar-sweetened beverages" are any liquids that are sweetened with added sugars. Beverages, such as regular soda (not sugar-free), fruit drinks, sports drinks, energy drinks, sweetened waters, and coffee and tea beverages with added sugars are sugary drinks.

WHY SHOULD YOU BE CONCERNED ABOUT SUGARY DRINKS?

People who often drink sugary drinks are more likely to face health problems, such as weight gain, obesity, type 2 diabetes, heart disease, kidney diseases, nonalcoholic liver disease, cavities, and gout, a type of arthritis.

Limiting sugary drinks can help you maintain a healthy weight and have a healthy diet. Many people do not realize just how much sugar and how many calories are in their drinks:

Table 30.1. Calories in Drinks

Drink (12 Ounce Serving)	Teaspoons of Sugar	Calories
Tap or Bottled Water	0 teaspoons	0
Unsweetened Tea	0 teaspoons	0
Sports Drinks	2 teaspoons	75
Lemonade	6 ¼ teaspoons	105
Sweet Tea	8 ½ teaspoons	120

Table 30.1. Continued

Drink (12 Ounce Serving)	Teaspoons of Sugar	Calories
Cola	10 ¼ teaspoons	150
Fruit Punch	11 ½ teaspoons	195
Root Beer	11 ½ teaspoons	170
Orange Soda	13 teaspoons	210

TRICKS TO RETHINK YOUR DRINK

Choose water (tap, bottled, or sparkling) over sugary drinks.

- Need more flavor? Add berries or slices of lime, lemon, or cucumber to water.
- Missing fizzy drinks? Add a splash of 100 percent juice to plain sparkling water for a refreshing, low-calorie drink.
- Need help breaking the habit? Do not stock up on sugary drinks. Instead, keep a jug or bottles of cold water in the fridge.
- Water just will not do? Reach for drinks that contain important nutrients, such as low-fat or fat-free milk, fortified milk alternatives, or 100 percent fruit or vegetable juice first.
- At the coffee shop? Skip the flavored syrups or whipped cream. Ask for a drink with low-fat or fat-free milk, a milk alternative, such as soy or almond, or get back to basics with black coffee.
- At the store? Read the Nutrition Facts label to choose drinks that are low in calories, added sugars, and saturated fat.
- On the go? Carry a reusable water bottle with you and refill it throughout the day.
- Still thirsty? Start drinking more water.

Section 30.2 | Energy Drinks, Caffeine, and Health

This section contains text excerpted from the following sources: Text in this section begins with excerpts from "Energy Drinks," National Center for Complementary and Integrative Health (NCCIH), July 2018; Text under the heading "Dangers of Mixing Alcohol and Energy Drinks" is excerpted from "Alcohol and Caffeine," Centers for Disease Control and Prevention (CDC), February 4, 2020.

Energy drinks are widely promoted as products that increase energy and enhance mental alertness and physical performance. Next to multivitamins, energy drinks are the most popular dietary supplement consumed by American teens and young adults. Men between 18 and 34 years of age consume the most energy drinks, and almost one-third of teens between 12 and 17 years of age drink them regularly.

There are two kinds of energy drink products. One is sold in containers similar in size to those of ordinary soft drinks, such as a 16-oz. bottle. The other kind, called "energy shots," is sold in small containers holding 2 to 2½ oz. of concentrated liquid. Caffeine is a major ingredient in both types of energy drink products – at levels of 70 to 240 mg in a 16-oz. drink and 113 to 200 mg in an energy shot. (For comparison, a 12-oz. can of cola contains about 35 mg of caffeine, and an 8-oz. cup of coffee contains about 100 mg.) Energy drinks also may contain other ingredients, such as guarana (another source of caffeine sometimes called "Brazilian cocoa"), sugars, taurine, ginseng, B vitamins, glucuronolactone, yohimbe, carnitine, and bitter orange.

ENERGY DRINKS AND GROWING CONCERNS

Bottom Line

- A growing body of scientific evidence shows that energy drinks can have serious health effects, particularly in children, teenagers, and young adults.
- In several studies, energy drinks have been found to improve physical endurance, but there is less evidence of any effect on muscle strength or power. Energy drinks may enhance alertness and improve reaction time, but they may also reduce the steadiness of the hands.

- The amounts of caffeine in energy drinks vary widely, and the actual caffeine content may not be identified easily. Some energy drinks are marketed as beverages and others as dietary supplements. There is no requirement to declare the amount of caffeine on the label of either type of product.

Safety

- Large amounts of caffeine may cause serious heart and blood vessel problems, such as heart rhythm disturbances and increases in heart rate and blood pressure. Caffeine also may harm children's developing cardiovascular and nervous systems.
- Caffeine use may also be associated with anxiety, sleep problems, digestive problems, and dehydration.
- Guarana, commonly included in energy drinks, contains caffeine. Therefore, the addition of guarana increases the drink's total caffeine content.
- People who combine caffeinated drinks with alcohol may not be able to tell how intoxicated they are; they may feel less intoxicated than they would if they had not consumed caffeine, but their motor coordination and reaction time may be just as impaired.
- Excessive energy drink consumption may disrupt teens' sleep patterns and may be associated with increased risk-taking behavior.
- A single 16-oz. container of an energy drink may contain 54 to 62 grams of added sugar; this exceeds the maximum amount of added sugars recommended for an entire day.

DANGERS OF MIXING ALCOHOL AND ENERGY DRINKS

- Energy drinks typically contain caffeine, plant-based stimulants, simple sugars, and other additives.
- Mixing alcohol with energy drinks is a popular practice, especially among young people in the United States. In 2017, 10.6 percent of students in grades 8, 10, and 12 and

31.8 percent of young adults 19 to 28 years of age reported consuming alcohol mixed with energy drinks at least once in the past year.

- In a study among Michigan high-school students, those who binge drank were more than twice as likely to mix alcohol with energy drinks as nonbinge drinkers (49.0 percent vs. 18.2 percent). Liquor was the usual type of alcohol consumed by students who reported mixing alcohol and energy drinks (52.7 percent).
- Drinkers 15 to 23 years of age who mix alcohol with energy drinks are four times more likely to binge drink at a high intensity (i.e., consume six or more drinks per binge episode) than drinkers who do not mix alcohol with energy drinks.
- Drinkers who mix alcohol with energy drinks are more likely than drinkers who do not mix alcohol with energy drinks to report unwanted or unprotected sex, driving drunk or riding with a driver who was intoxicated, or sustaining alcohol-related injuries.

Chapter 31 | How Safe Are Dietary Supplements for Exercise and Athletic Performance?

WHAT ARE DIETARY SUPPLEMENTS FOR EXERCISE AND ATHLETIC PERFORMANCE AND WHAT DO THEY DO?

If you get regular exercise – and especially if you are an athlete and compete in sporting events – you know that a nutritionally adequate diet and plenty of fluids are important for maximizing your physical performance. But, you may wonder if dietary supplements could help you train harder, improve performance, or gain a competitive edge.

This chapter describes what is known about the effectiveness and safety of many ingredients in dietary supplements that are promoted to improve exercise and athletic performance. These products are sometimes called "ergogenic aids," but it simply refers to them as "performance supplements." Sellers of these supplements might claim that their products improve strength or endurance, help you achieve a performance goal more quickly, or increase your tolerance for more intense training. They might also claim that their supplements can help prepare your body for exercise, reduce the chance of injury during training, or assist with recovery after exercise.

This chapter includes text excerpted from "Dietary Supplements for Exercise and Athletic Performance: Fact Sheet for Consumers," Office of Dietary Supplements (ODS), National Institutes of Health (NIH), October 4, 2017. Reviewed May 2021.

Performance supplements cannot substitute for a healthy diet, but some of them may have value, depending on the type and intensity of your activity. Other supplements do not seem to work, and a few might be harmful.

If you are thinking about taking a performance supplement, talk to your healthcare provider. If you have a trainer or coach with knowledge of sports medicine, ask them about performance supplements. Talking to an expert is important if you are a teenager or have any medical conditions. It is also important to find out whether the medications you take might interact with the performance supplements you are considering.

WHAT ARE INGREDIENTS IN SUPPLEMENTS FOR EXERCISE AND ATHLETIC PERFORMANCE?

Performance supplements can contain many ingredients – such as vitamins and minerals, protein, amino acids, and herbs – in different amounts and in many combinations. These products are sold in various forms, such as capsules, tablets, liquids, and powders.

This chapter describes ingredients in performance supplements below in alphabetical order. You will learn whether each ingredient is effective and safe and get expert advice about using it. But, keep in mind that many performance supplements in the marketplace contain more than one ingredient, and ingredients can work differently when they are combined. Because most ingredient combinations have not been studied, we do not know how effective or safe they are in improving performance.

You may be surprised to learn that makers of performance supplements usually do not carry out studies in people to find out whether their products really work and are safe. When studies on performance supplement ingredients and ingredient combinations are done (mainly by researchers at colleges and universities), they often involve small numbers of people taking the supplement for just a few days, weeks, or months. Much of the research is done in young healthy men, but not women, middle-aged and older adults, or teenagers. And often, studies have not looked at the use of supplement ingredients or combinations in people involved in the same athletic activity as you. For example, the results from a study in weightlifters might not apply to you if you are a distance runner.

INGREDIENTS IN SUPPLEMENTS FOR EXERCISE AND ATHLETIC PERFORMANCE

Antioxidants (Vitamin C, Vitamin E, and Coenzyme Q_{10})

You breathe in more oxygen when you exercise. As a result, free radicals form and damage muscle cells. Because antioxidants can reduce free-radical damage to muscle, some people think that taking them in a supplement might reduce muscle inflammation, soreness, and fatigue.

DO THEY WORK?

No. The free radicals that form when you exercise seem to help muscle fibers grow and produce more energy. Antioxidant supplements might actually reduce some of the benefits of exercise, including muscle growth and power output. Also, they have little effect on aerobic fitness and performance in endurance activities such as distance running.

ARE THEY SAFE?

Everyone needs adequate amounts of vitamin C and vitamin E for good health. Getting too much of these nutrients can be harmful, but the amounts of vitamin C (about 1,000 milligrams) and vitamin E (about 500 IU) typically used in studies of performance supplements are below safe upper limits. The side effects from coenzyme Q_{10} can include tiredness, insomnia, headaches, and some gastrointestinal (GI) discomfort, but these effects tend to be mild.

BOTTOM LINE

There is little scientific evidence to support taking supplements containing vitamins C and E or coenzyme Q_{10} to improve performance if you are getting adequate amounts of these nutrients from a nutritious diet.

Arginine

Arginine is an amino acid in foods that contain protein, such as meat, poultry, fish, eggs, dairy products, and legumes. A nutritious diet supplies about 4 to 5 grams a day. Supplement sellers claim that taking larger amounts of arginine in supplements improves performance, partly because the body converts it into nitric oxide, which expands blood vessels and increases blood flow. Increased blood flow helps deliver oxygen and nutrients to exercising muscles and speeds up the removal of waste products that cause muscle fatigue.

DOES IT WORK?

Although the research is limited, arginine supplements seem to have little to no effect on strengthening and muscle-building exercises (such as bodybuilding) or aerobic activities (such as running and cycling). Studies have used 2 to 20 grams a day of arginine for up to three months.

IS IT SAFE?

Arginine supplements seem safe when users take up to 9 grams a day for several days or weeks. Taking more can cause GI discomfort and can slightly lower blood pressure.

BOTTOM LINE

There is little scientific evidence to support taking arginine supplements to increase strength, improve performance, or help tired and sore muscles recover after exercise.

Beetroot or Beet Juice

Beets and beet juice are among the best food sources of nitrate. Beet juice might improve athletic performance because the body converts some of this nitrate to nitric oxide, which expands blood vessels. This blood vessel expansion increases blood flow and the delivery of oxygen and nutrients to exercising muscles. The expanded blood vessels also speed up the removal of waste products that cause muscle fatigue.

DOES IT WORK?

Many, but not all, studies have found that beet juice can improve performance and endurance in aerobic activities, such as running, swimming, cycling, and rowing. But, whether it helps with strengthening and bodybuilding exercises is not known. Beet juice is more likely to improve the performance of recreational exercisers than highly-trained athletes. The usual approach in studies is for participants to drink two cups of beet juice about 2.5 to 3 hours before exercise.

IS IT SAFE?

Drinking moderate amounts of beet juice is safe, but it can turn your urine pink or red.

BOTTOM LINE

Beet juice might improve aerobic exercise performance if you are recreationally active. But, whether dietary supplements containing beetroot powder have the same effects as beet juice is not known.

Beta-Alanine

Beta-alanine is an amino acid in foods such as meat, poultry, and fish. People get up to about 1 gram a day of beta-alanine, depending on their diet. Your body uses beta-alanine to make carnosine in skeletal muscles. When you exercise intensely for several minutes, your muscles produce lactic acid, which reduces muscular force and causes tiredness. Carnosine reduces the buildup of lactic acid. Beta-alanine supplements increase muscle carnosine levels by different amounts, depending on the person.

DOES IT WORK?

Some, but not all, studies have shown that beta-alanine produces small performance improvements in swimming and team sports, such as hockey and football, that require high-intensity, intermittent effort over short periods. Whether beta-alanine helps with endurance activities, such as cycling is not clear. It is also not clear whether beta-alanine mainly benefits trained athletes or recreational exercisers. In most studies, participants took 1.6 to 6.4 grams a day of beta-alanine for 4 to 8 weeks.

IS IT SAFE?

Taking 800 milligrams or more beta-alanine can cause moderate-to-severe paresthesia, a tingling, prickling, or burning sensation in your face, neck, back of the hands, and upper trunk. This effect can last 60 to 90 minutes but is not considered serious or harmful. Taking divided doses or a sustained-release form of beta-alanine can reduce or eliminate this paresthesia. It is not known whether it is safe to take beta-alanine supplements daily for more than several months.

BOTTOM LINE

Sports-medicine experts disagree on the value of taking beta-alanine supplements to enhance performance in high-intensity, intermittent activities. The International Society of Sports Nutrition (ISSN) recommends that if you are healthy and want to try beta-alanine supplements, take a daily loading dose of 4 to 6 grams per day (in divided doses with meals) for at least 2 weeks to see if it helps.

Beta-Hydroxy-Betamethylbutyrate

Your body converts a small amount of leucine, one of the amino acids in foods and protein powders, to beta-hydroxy-betamethylbutyrate (HMB). Your liver then converts the HMB into another compound that experts think helps muscle cells restore their structure and function after exercise. HMB also helps build protein in muscle and reduces muscle-protein breakdown.

DOES IT WORK?

It is hard to know whether you might benefit from using HMB supplements because the research on these supplements has included adults of very different ages and fitness levels who took widely varying doses for different amounts of time. Overall, HMB seems to speed up recovery from exercise that is intense enough and long enough to cause muscle damage. Therefore, if you are a trained athlete, you will need to exert yourself more than recreationally active people to cause the muscle damage that HMB might help treat.

IS IT SAFE?

Studies have not reported any side effects in adults taking 3 grams per day of HMB for up to eight weeks.

BOTTOM LINE

It is not clear whether taking HMB supplements will improve athletic performance. The ISSN recommends that if you are a healthy adult who wants to try HMB supplements, to take 3 grams per day in three equal servings of 1 gram for at least two weeks to see if it helps. HMB comes in two forms: one with calcium and one without. A dose of 3 grams of the type with calcium supplies about 400 milligrams of calcium.

Betaine

Your body makes betaine, and it is also found in foods such as beets, spinach, and whole-grain bread. You get about 100 to 300 milligrams a day of betaine when you eat a nutritious diet. How betaine supplements might affect or improve your performance is not known.

DOES IT WORK?

Only a few, mostly small, studies have evaluated betaine as a performance supplement. Most of these studies examined the use of betaine supplements to improve strength and power performance in bodybuilders. The studies found either no performance improvements or only modest ones. Participants in these studies took 2 to 5 grams a day of betaine for up to 15 days.

IS IT SAFE?

The few studies in which athletes took betaine supplements did not find any side effects. But, there has not been enough research to know for sure whether it is really safe.

BOTTOM LINE

There is little scientific evidence to support taking betaine supplements to improve performance if you eat a nutritious diet.

Branched-Chain Amino Acids

The amino acids leucine, isoleucine, and valine are known as "branched-chain amino acids" (BCAAs). Animal foods, such as meat, fish, and milk, contain BCAAs. Your muscles can use these three amino acids to provide energy during exercise. Leucine might also help build muscle.

DO THEY WORK?

There is little evidence that BCAA supplements improve performance in endurance activities such as distance running. BCAA supplements might help increase your muscle size and strength together with a weight-training program. But, it is not clear whether taking BCAA supplements will help you build more muscle than just eating enough high-quality protein foods.

ARE THEY SAFE?

A nutritious diet with enough protein can easily provide 10 to 20 grams a day of the BCAAs. Taking up to another 20 grams a day of BCAAs in supplements seems to be safe.

BOTTOM LINE

There is not much scientific evidence to support taking BCAA supplements to improve performance, build muscle, or help tired and sore muscles to recover after exercise. Eating foods containing protein automatically increases your intake of BCAAs.

Caffeine

Caffeine is a stimulant in beverages (such as coffee, tea, and energy drinks) and in herbs (such as guarana and kola nut). Caffeine is also added to some dietary supplements. Moderate amounts of caffeine might increase your energy levels and reduce fatigue for several hours.

DOES IT WORK?

Caffeine might improve endurance, strength, and power in team sports. It is most likely to help with endurance activities (such as distance running) and sports that require intense, intermittent effort (such as soccer and tennis). Caffeine does not help with short, intense exercise, such as sprinting or weightlifting. People have different responses to caffeine. It does not boost performance in everyone, or may only slightly boost performance. The usual dose of caffeine to aid performance is 2 to 6 milligrams per kilogram of body weight or about 210 to 420 mg caffeine for a 154-pound person. (By comparison, a cup of coffee has about 85 to 100 milligrams of caffeine.) Taking more probably does not improve performance further and can increase the risk of side effects.

IS IT SAFE?

Caffeine intakes of up to 400 to 500 milligrams a day seem safe in adults. Teenagers should limit their caffeine intake to no more than 100 milligrams a day. Taking 500 milligrams or more a day can reduce rather than improve physical performance, disturb sleep, and cause irritability and anxiety. Taking 10,000 milligrams or more in a single dose (one tablespoon of pure caffeine powder) can be fatal.

BOTTOM LINE

Sports-medicine experts agree that caffeine can help you exercise at the same intensity level for longer and reduce feelings of fatigue. They suggest taking 2 to 6 milligrams per kilogram of body weight 15 to 60 minutes before you exercise. The National

Collegiate Athletic Association (NCAA) and International Olympic Committee limit the amount of caffeine that athletes can take before a competition.

Citrulline

Citrulline is an amino acid that your body produces; it is also present in some foods. Your kidneys convert most citrulline into another amino acid, arginine. Your body then transforms the arginine into nitric oxide, which expands blood vessels. This expansion increases blood flow and the delivery of oxygen and nutrients to exercising muscles and speeds up the removal of waste products that cause muscle fatigue.

DOES IT WORK?

The research on citrulline as a performance supplement is limited. A few studies find that citrulline might help improve, hinder, or have no effect on performance. In these studies, participants took up to 9 grams of citrulline for one day or 6 grams per day for up to 16 days.

IS IT SAFE?

There is not enough research on citrulline to know for sure whether it is safe. Some users have reported that it can cause stomach discomfort.

BOTTOM LINE

There is not much scientific evidence to support taking citrulline supplements to improve exercise or athletic performance.

Creatine

Creatine is a compound that is stored in your muscles and supplies them with energy. Your body produces some creatine (about 1 gram a day), and you get some creatine from eating animal-based foods, such as beef and salmon (about 500 milligrams in a 4-ounce serving). But, it is only when you take much larger amounts of creatine from dietary supplements that it might improve certain types of performance.

DOES IT WORK?

Creatine supplements can increase strength, power, and the ability to contract muscles for maximum effort. But, the extent of performance improvements from creatine supplements differs among individuals. The use of creatine supplements for several weeks or months can help with training. Overall, creatine enhances performance during repeated short bursts of intense, intermittent activity (lasting up to about 2.5 minutes at a time), such as sprinting and weight lifting. Creatine seems to have little value for endurance activities, such as distance running, cycling, or swimming.

IS IT SAFE?

Creatine is safe for healthy adults to take for several weeks or months. It also seems safe for long-term use over several years. Creatine usually causes some weight gain because it increases water retention. Rare individual reactions to creatine include some muscle stiffness and cramps as well as GI distress.

BOTTOM LINE

Sports-medicine experts agree that creatine supplements can improve performance in activities that involve intense effort followed by short recovery periods. It can also be valuable in training for certain athletic competitions. In studies, people often took a loading dose of about 20 grams per day of creatine (in four equal portions) for 5 to 7 days and then 3 to 5 grams a day. Creatine monohydrate is the most widely used and studied form of creatine in supplements.

Deer Antler Velvet

Deer antler velvet supplements are made from the antlers of deer or elk before the antlers turn into bone. Deer antlers might contain growth factors that could promote muscle growth.

DOES IT WORK?

There has been little research on use of deer antler velvet to improve performance in either strength or endurance activities. The few published studies have found no benefit from taking the supplement.

IS IT SAFE?

Deer antler velvet has not been studied enough to know whether taking it is safe.

BOTTOM LINE

There is no scientific evidence to support taking deer antler velvet supplements to improve exercise or athletic performance.

Dehydroepiandrosterone

Dehydroepiandrosterone (DHEA) is a steroid hormone produced by the adrenal glands. Your body converts some DHEA into testosterone, the male hormone that enhances muscle size and strength.

DOES IT WORK?

There has been little study of the use of DHEA supplements to improve performance. The few published studies (all in men) have found no benefit from taking the supplement. Muscle size or strength and aerobic capacity did not improve, and testosterone levels did not rise.

IS IT SAFE?

Dehydroepiandrosterone has not been studied enough to know whether it is safe to take. Two small studies in men found no side effects. But, in women, taking DHEA supplements for months can increase testosterone levels, which can cause acne and facial hair growth.

BOTTOM LINE

There is no scientific evidence to support taking DHEA to improve exercise or athletic performance. The NCAA and the World

Anti-Doping Agency (WADA) prohibit the use of DHEA in athletic competitions.

Ginseng

Ginseng is the root of a plant used for thousands of years in traditional Chinese medicine. Some experts believe that Panax (also known as "Chinese," "Korean," "Japanese," or "American") ginseng might improve stamina and vitality. Siberian or Russian ginseng has been used to fight fatigue and strengthen the immune system.

DOES IT WORK?

Several small studies have examined whether Panax or Siberian ginseng supplements can improve performance. This research provides little evidence that various doses and preparations of these supplements improve performance in athletes or recreational exercisers.

IS IT SAFE?

Both Panax and Siberian ginseng seem to be safe. However, ginseng supplements can cause headaches or GI effects and disturb sleep.

BOTTOM LINE

There is little scientific evidence to support taking ginseng supplements to improve exercise or athletic performance.

Glutamine

Glutamine is an amino acid that your body uses to produce energy. Adults consume about 3 to 6 grams a day from protein-containing foods such as meat, poultry, fish, eggs, dairy products, and legumes. Your body also makes some glutamine, mainly from branched-chain amino acids (BCAAs).

DOES IT WORK?

Only a few studies have examined the use of glutamine supplements for improving performance in strengthening and muscle-building exercises (such as bodybuilding) and for recovering from these exercises (e.g., by reducing muscle soreness). Glutamine has either no effect or provides only a small benefit.

IS IT SAFE?

Studies have not reported any side effects from the use of up to 45 grams a day of glutamine for several weeks in adults.

BOTTOM LINE

There is little scientific evidence to support taking glutamine supplements to improve exercise or athletic performance.

Iron

Iron is a mineral that delivers oxygen to muscles and tissues throughout your body. Cells also need iron to turn food into energy. Iron deficiency, especially with anemia, limits your ability to exercise and be active because it makes you tired and reduces your performance. The recommended amount of iron to get each day is 11 milligrams for teenage boys, 15 milligrams for teenage girls, 8 milligrams for men to 50 years of age, 18 milligrams for women to 50 years of age, and 8 milligrams for older adults of both sexes. Recommended amounts are even higher for athletes, vegetarians, and vegans. Teenage girls and premenopausal women have the greatest risk of not getting enough iron from their diets.

DOES IT WORK?

For people with iron deficiency anemia, taking an iron supplement will probably improve performance in both strength and endurance activities. But, if you get enough iron from your diet, taking extra iron will not help. It is not clear whether milder iron deficiency without anemia reduces exercise and athletic performance.

IS IT SAFE?

Taking less than 45 milligrams of iron in a supplement is safe for teenagers and adults. Higher doses can cause upset stomach, constipation, nausea, abdominal pain, vomiting, and fainting. However, doctors sometimes prescribe large amounts of iron for a short time to treat iron-deficiency anemia.

BOTTOM LINE

Taking enough iron in supplements to treat iron-deficiency anemia improves exercise capacity. But, a health-care provider should diagnose this condition before you start taking iron supplements. If you want to improve your athletic performance, you should eat a healthy diet containing foods rich in iron, such as lean meats, seafood, poultry, beans, nuts, and raisins. If needed, an iron-containing dietary supplement can help you get the recommended amount of iron.

Protein

Protein helps to build, maintain, and repair your muscles. It improves your body's response to athletic training and helps shorten the time you need to recover after exercise. Protein is made from amino acids. Your body makes some amino acids but needs to get others (known as "essential amino acids" or "EAAs") from food. Animal foods, such as meat, poultry, fish, eggs, and dairy products contain all of the EAAs. Plant foods, such as grains and legumes contain different EAAs, so eating a diet containing different types of plant-based foods is one way to get all EAAs. Most protein powders and drinks contain whey, a protein in milk that provides all the EAAs.

DOES IT WORK?

Adequate protein in your diet provides the EAAs necessary for making muscle proteins and reduces the breakdown of proteins in your muscles. Athletes need about 0.5 to 0.9 grams of protein per pound of bodyweight a day (or about 75 to 135 grams for a person weighing 150 pounds). You might need even more for a short time when you are training intensely or if you reduce your food intake to improve your physique or achieve a competitive weight.

IS IT SAFE?

High intakes of protein seem to be quite safe, but there is no benefit to consuming more than recommended amounts.

BOTTOM LINE

If you are an athlete, you can probably eat enough foods that contain protein to meet your needs for protein. If needed, protein supplements and protein-fortified food and beverage products can help you get enough protein. Sports-medicine experts recommend that athletes consume 0.14 grams of protein per pound of body weight (about 20 grams for a person weighing 150 pounds) of high-quality protein (from animal foods and/or a mix of different plant foods) every three to five hours, including before sleep and within two hours after exercising.

Quercetin

Quercetin is a compound found in fruits, vegetables, and some beverages (such as tea). Some experts suggest that quercetin supplements increase energy production in muscle and improve blood flow throughout your body. A nutritious diet provides up to about 13 milligrams a day of quercetin.

DOES IT WORK?

There is limited research on the use of quercetin supplements to improve performance. The studies found that any benefits when they occur, tend to be small. In these studies, participants took about 1,000 milligrams a day of quercetin for up to eight weeks.

IS IT SAFE?

The studies of quercetin supplements did not find any side effects in the athletes who took them. But, quercetin has not been studied enough to know whether it is really safe.

BOTTOM LINE

There is little scientific evidence to support taking quercetin supplements to improve exercise or athletic performance.

Ribose

Ribose is a natural sugar your body makes that helps with energy production in muscle. Some scientists believe that ribose supplements help muscles produce more energy.

DOES IT WORK?

There has been little study of the use of ribose supplements to improve performance. The few published studies in both trained athletes and occasional exercisers have shown little if any benefit from doses ranging from 625 milligrams to 10,000 milligrams a day for up to eight weeks.

IS IT SAFE?

The studies of athletes taking ribose supplements have found no side effects. But, ribose has not been studied enough to know whether it is really safe when taken in large amounts for several months or more.

BOTTOM LINE

There is very little scientific evidence to support taking ribose supplements to improve exercise or athletic performance.

Sodium Bicarbonate

Sodium bicarbonate is commonly known as "baking soda." Exercising intensely over several minutes causes muscles to produce acids, such as lactic acid, that reduce muscle force and cause tiredness. Sodium bicarbonate can reduce the buildup of these acids.

DOES IT WORK?

Studies show that athletes who take sodium bicarbonate might improve their performance a little in intense, short-term activities (such as sprinting and swimming) and in intermittently intense sports (such as tennis and boxing). But, different athletes respond differently to sodium bicarbonate. Sodium bicarbonate might actually hinder performance in some people. The usual dose taken is 300 milligrams per kilogram of body weight or about four to five teaspoons of baking soda. Some people find this amount of sodium bicarbonate, dissolved in liquid, too salty to drink.

IS IT SAFE?

Sodium bicarbonate can cause GI distress, including nausea and vomiting, and weight gain due to water retention. It is also high in sodium (1,260 milligrams per teaspoon).

BOTTOM LINE

Sodium bicarbonate might provide some performance benefit in strenuous exercise that lasts several minutes and in sports that require intermittent, intense activity, especially for trained athletes. However, in some people, sodium bicarbonate provides no performance benefit, and it can even reduce performance.

Tart or Sour Cherry

Tart or sour cherries of the Montmorency variety contain compounds that might help you recover from strenuous exercise. Specifically, these cherries might help to reduce pain, muscle damage from strength-related activities, and lung trauma from endurance activities that require deep, heavy breathing.

DOES IT WORK?

There is limited research on tart cherry as a performance supplement. The studies that have been done suggest that it might help bodybuilders recover their strength faster and feel less muscle soreness after exercising. The supplements could also help runners race faster and be less likely to develop a cold or respiratory problem after a marathon. The typical dose is about two cups of juice or 500 milligrams of tart-cherry-skin powder for a week before the exercise and for two days afterward.

IS IT SAFE?

Studies of tart-cherry products in athletes have not found any side effects. But, the safety of tart-cherry supplements has not been well studied.

BOTTOM LINE

There is limited scientific evidence to support taking tart-cherry products to improve exercise and athletic performance.

Tribulus terrestris

Tribulus terrestris is a plant containing compounds that some sellers claim can improve performance by increasing levels of several hormones, including the male hormone testosterone.

DOES IT WORK?

There is limited research on the use of *Tribulus terrestris* supplements to increase strength or muscle mass. The few studies investigating it did not find that it had any benefit.

IS IT SAFE?

Tribulus terrestris has not been studied enough to know whether it is safe. Studies in animals show that high doses can cause heart, liver, and kidney damage.

BOTTOM LINE

There is no scientific evidence to support taking *Tribulus terrestris* supplements to improve exercise or athletic performance. Some sports-medicine experts advise against taking any dietary supplements claimed to boost testosterone.

HOW DOES THE U.S. GOVERNMENT REGULATE DIETARY SUPPLEMENTS FOR EXERCISE AND ATHLETIC PERFORMANCE?

The U.S. Food and Drug Administration (FDA) regulates dietary supplements for exercise and athletic performance differently from prescription or over-the-counter (OTC) drugs. As with other dietary supplements, the FDA does not test or approve performance supplements before they are sold. Manufacturers are responsible for making sure that their supplements are safe and that the claims on the product labels are truthful and not misleading.

When the FDA finds an unsafe dietary supplement, it can remove the supplement from the market or ask the supplement maker to recall the product. The FDA and the Federal Trade Commission (FTC) can also take action against companies that make false performance-improvement claims about their supplements; add pharmaceutical drugs or other adulterants to their supplements, or claim that their supplements can diagnose, treat, cure, or prevent disease.

CAN DIETARY SUPPLEMENTS FOR EXERCISE AND ATHLETIC PERFORMANCE BE HARMFUL?

Like all dietary supplements, performance supplements can have side effects and might interact with prescription and over-the-counter medications. Many of these products contain multiple ingredients that have not been adequately tested in combination with each other.

- **Interactions with medications.** Some dietary supplements for improving exercise and athletic performance can interact or interfere with other medications or supplements. For example, ginseng can reduce the blood-thinning effects of warfarin (Coumadin). Cimetidine (Tagamet HB, used to treat duodenal ulcers) can slow the removal of caffeine from the body and thus increase the risk of side effects from caffeine consumption. If you take dietary supplements and medications on a regular basis, tell your healthcare provider.
- **Fraudulent and adulterated products.** The FDA warns that some products marketed as dietary supplements to improve exercise and athletic performance might contain inappropriate, unlabeled, or unlawful stimulants, steroids, hormone-like ingredients, controlled substances, prescription medications, or

unapproved drugs. Using these tainted products can cause health problems and disqualify athletes from competitions.

The FDA prohibits certain ingredients that some performance dietary supplements used to contain. These prohibited ingredients include androstenedione, dimethylamylamine (DMAA), and ephedra. Not only are these ingredients unsafe, but there is no scientific evidence showing that they can improve performance.

Sellers of some performance supplements ask certain companies to evaluate their products and certify that they are free from many banned ingredients and drugs. The major companies providing this certification service are NSF (nsf.org) through its Certified for Sport® program, Informed-Choice (informed-choice.org), and the Banned Substances Control Group (bscg.org). Products that pass these tests may carry the certifier's official logo and are listed on the certifier's website.

CHOOSING A SENSIBLE APPROACH TO IMPROVING EXERCISE AND ATHLETIC PERFORMANCE

If you are a competitive or recreational athlete, you will perform at your best and recover most quickly when you eat a nutritionally adequate diet, drink enough fluids, are physically fit, and are properly trained. Only a few dietary supplements have enough scientific evidence showing that they can improve certain types of exercise and athletic performance. Athletes might use these supplements, if interested, if they already eat a good diet, train properly, and obtain guidance from a healthcare provider or sports medicine expert.

In most cases, only adults should use performance supplements. The American Academy of Pediatrics (AAP) for example, states that performance supplements do not improve the abilities of teenage athletes beyond those that come from proper nutrition and training.

Chapter 32 | Food Safety

Chapter Contents

Section 32.1 | **How Food Gets Contaminated: The Food Production Chain**

This section includes text excerpted from "How Food Gets Contaminated – The Food Production Chain," Centers for Disease Control and Prevention (CDC), September 5, 2017. Reviewed May 2021.

It takes several steps to get food from the farm or fishery to the dining table. We call these steps the food production chain (see Figure 32.1). Contamination can occur at any point along the chain – during production, processing, distribution, or preparation.

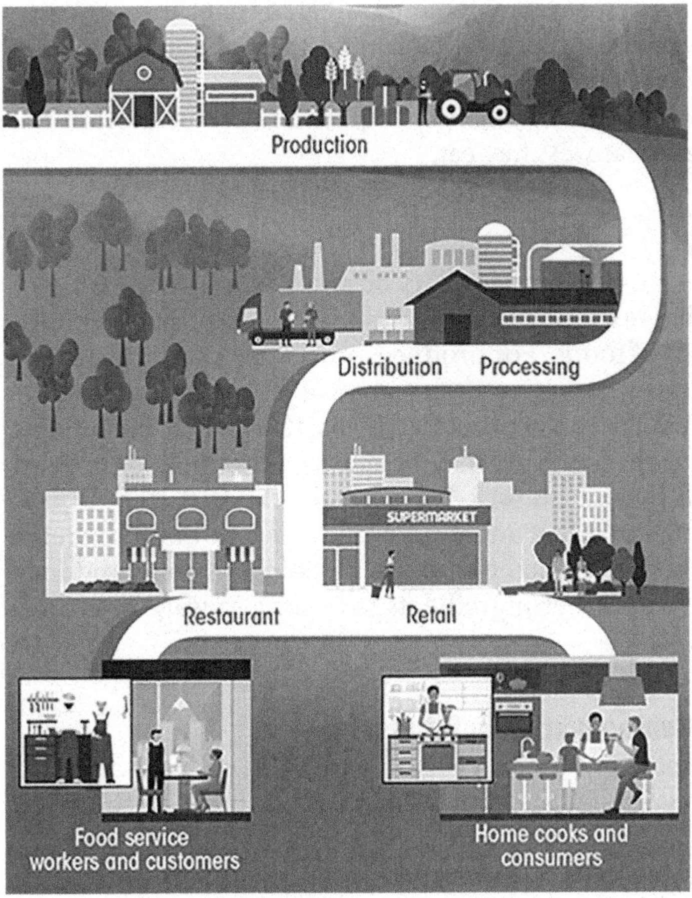

Figure 32.1. The Food Production Chain

PRODUCTION

Production means growing the plants we harvest or raising the animals we use for food. Most food comes from domesticated animals and plants, and their production occurs on farms or ranches. Some foods are caught or harvested from the wild, such as some fish, mushrooms, and game.

Examples of Contamination in Production

- If a hen's reproductive organs are infected, the yolk of an egg can be contaminated in the hen before it is even laid.
- If the fields are sprayed with contaminated water for irrigation, fruits and vegetables can be contaminated before harvest.
- Fish in some tropical reefs may acquire a toxin from the smaller sea creatures they eat.

PROCESSING

Processing means changing plants or animals into what we recognize and buy as food. Processing involves different steps for different kinds of foods. For produce, processing can be as simple as washing and sorting, or it can involve trimming, slicing, or shredding. Milk is usually processed by pasteurizing it; sometimes it is made into cheese. Nuts may be roasted, chopped, or ground (such as with peanut butter). For animals, the first step of processing is slaughter. Meat and poultry may then be cut into pieces or ground. They may also be smoked, cooked, or frozen and may be combined with other ingredients to make a sausage or entrée, such as a potpie.

Examples of Contamination in Processing

- If contaminated water or ice is used to wash, pack, or chill fruits or vegetables, the contamination can spread to those items.
- During the slaughter process, germs on an animal's hide that came from the intestines can get into the final meat product.

- If germs contaminate surfaces used for food processing, such as a processing line or storage bins, germs can spread to foods that touch those surfaces.

DISTRIBUTION

Distribution means getting food from the farm or processing plant to the consumer or a food service facility such as a restaurant, cafeteria, or hospital kitchen. This step might involve transporting foods just once, such as trucking produce from a farm to the local farmers' market. Or it might involve many stages. For instance, frozen hamburger patties might be trucked from a meat processing plant to a large supplier, stored for a few days in the supplier's warehouse, trucked again to a local distribution facility for a restaurant chain, and finally delivered to an individual restaurant.

Examples of Contamination in Distribution

- If refrigerated food is left on a loading dock for a long time in warm weather, it could reach temperatures that allow bacteria to grow.
- Fresh produce can be contaminated if it is loaded into a truck that was not cleaned after transporting animals or animal products.

PREPARATION

Preparation means getting the food ready to eat. This step may occur in the kitchen of a restaurant, home, or institution. It may involve following a complex recipe with many ingredients, simply heating and serving food on a plate, or just opening a package and eating the food.

Examples of Contamination in Preparation

- If a food worker stays on the job while sick and does not wash her or his hands carefully after using the toilet, the food worker can spread germs by touching food.
- If a cook uses a cutting board or knife to cut raw chicken and then uses the same knife or cutting board without

washing it to slice tomatoes for a salad, the tomatoes can be contaminated by germs from the chicken.
- Contamination can occur in a refrigerator if meat juices get on items that will be eaten raw.

MISHANDLING AT MULTIPLE POINTS

Sometimes, by the time a food causes illness, it has been mishandled in several ways along the food production chain. Once contamination occurs, further mishandling, such as undercooking the food or leaving it out on the counter at an unsafe temperature, can make a foodborne illness more likely. Many germs grow quickly in food held at room temperature; a tiny number can grow to a large number in just a few hours. Reheating or boiling food after it has been left at room temperature for a long time does not always make it safe because some germs produce toxins that are not destroyed by heat.

Section 32.2 | **Safe Food Preparation and Handling**

This section includes text excerpted from "Safe Food Handling," U.S. Food and Drug Administration (FDA), November 30, 2017. Reviewed May 2021.

The food supply in the United States is among the safest in the world. However, when certain disease-causing bacteria or pathogens contaminate food, they can cause foodborne illness, often called "food poisoning." The federal government estimates that there are about 48 million cases of foodborne illness annually – the equivalent of sickening 1 in 6 Americans each year. And, each year, these illnesses result in an estimated 128,000 hospitalizations and 3,000 deaths.

KNOW THE SYMPTOMS

Consuming dangerous foodborne bacteria will usually cause illness within 1 to 3 days of eating the contaminated food. However, sickness can also occur within 20 minutes or up to six weeks later.

Symptoms of foodborne illness can include: vomiting, diarrhea, and abdominal pain – and flu-like symptoms, such as fever, headache, and body ache.

HANDLE FOODS SAFELY

Although most healthy people will recover from a foodborne illness within a short period of time, some can develop chronic, severe, or even life-threatening health problems. In addition, some people are at a higher risk for developing foodborne illness, including pregnant women, young children, older adults, and people with weakened immune systems (such as transplant patients and individuals with human immunodeficiency virus (HIV) or acquired immunodeficiency syndrome (AIDS), cancer, or diabetes. To keep your family safer from food poisoning, follow these four simple steps: clean, separate, cook, and chill.

Clean

WASH HANDS AND SURFACES OFTEN

- Wash your hands with warm water and soap for at least 20 seconds before and after handling food and after using the bathroom, changing diapers, and handling pets.
- Wash your cutting boards, dishes, utensils, and counter tops with hot soapy water after preparing each food item.
- Consider using paper towels to clean up kitchen surfaces. If you use cloth towels, launder them often in the hot cycle.
- Rinse fresh fruits and vegetables under running tap water, including those with skins and rinds that are not eaten. Scrub firm produce with a clean produce brush.
- With canned goods, remember to clean lids before opening.

Separate

SEPARATE RAW MEATS FROM OTHER FOODS

- Separate raw meat, poultry, seafood, and eggs from other foods in your grocery shopping cart, grocery bags, and refrigerator.

- Use one cutting board for fresh produce and a separate one for raw meat, poultry, and seafood.
- Never place cooked food on a plate that previously held raw meat, poultry, seafood, or eggs unless the plate has been washed in hot, soapy water.
- Do not reuse marinades used on raw foods unless you bring them to a boil first.

Cook

COOK TO THE RIGHT TEMPERATURE

- Color and texture are unreliable indicators of safety. Using a food thermometer is the only way to ensure the safety of meat, poultry, seafood, and egg products for all cooking methods. These foods must be cooked to a safe minimum internal temperature to destroy any harmful bacteria.
- Cook eggs until the yolk and white are firm. Only use recipes in which eggs are cooked or heated thoroughly.
- When cooking in a microwave oven, cover food, stir, and rotate for even cooking. If there is no turntable, rotate the dish by hand once or twice during cooking. Always allow standing time, which completes the cooking, before checking the internal temperature with a food thermometer.
- Bring sauces, soups, and gravy to a boil when reheating.

Chill

REFRIGERATE FOODS PROMPTLY

- Use an appliance thermometer to be sure the temperature is consistently 40 °F or below and the freezer temperature is 0 °F or below.
- Refrigerate or freeze meat, poultry, eggs, seafood, and other perishables within two hours of cooking or purchasing. Refrigerate within one hour if the temperature outside is above 90 °F.
- Never thaw food at room temperature, such as on the counter top. There are three safe ways to defrost food:

in the refrigerator, in cold water, and in the microwave. Food thawed in cold water or in the microwave should be cooked immediately.

- Always marinate food in the refrigerator.
- Divide large amounts of leftovers into shallow containers for quicker cooling in the refrigerator.

Section 32.3 | Food Safety Mistakes

This section contains text excerpted from the following sources: Text under the heading "Dangerous Food Safety Mistakes" is excerpted from "10 Dangerous Food Safety Mistakes," Centers for Disease Control and Prevention (CDC), March 20, 2020; Text under the heading "Food Safety Steps" is excerpted from "Keep Food Safe," Foodsafety.gov, U.S. Department of Health and Human Services (HHS), May 19, 2020.

DANGEROUS FOOD SAFETY MISTAKES

We all want to keep our families safe and healthy. But, sometimes a simple mistake in the way we handle and prepare food can lead to a serious sickness. With some germs such as *Salmonella*, just a small amount in undercooked food is enough to cause food poisoning. And, just a tiny taste of food with botulism toxin can cause paralysis and even death.

You can protect your family by avoiding these common food safety mistakes.

Eating Risky Foods If You Are More Likely to Get Food Poisoning

WHY IT IS A MISTAKE

Anyone can get food poisoning. But, some people are more likely to get sick and to have a more serious illness. This includes:

- Adults 65 years of age and older
- Children younger than 5 years of age
- People who have health problems or who take medicines that lower the body's ability to fight germs and sickness (weakened immune systems)
- Pregnant women

SOLUTION

People who are more likely to get food poisoning should not eat the following:

- Undercooked or raw animal products (such as meat, chicken, turkey, eggs, or seafood)
- Raw or lightly cooked sprouts
- Unpasteurized (raw) milk and juices
- Soft cheese (such as queso fresco), unless it is labeled as made with pasteurized milk

Not Washing Your Hands

WHY IT IS A MISTAKE

Germs on your hands can get on food and make it unsafe.

SOLUTION

Wash hands the right way – for 20 seconds with soap and running water. Wash hands before, during, and after preparing food; before eating; and after using the toilet or changing a child's diaper.

Washing Meat, Chicken, or Turkey

WHY IT IS A MISTAKE

Washing raw meat, chicken, turkey, or eggs can spread germs to your sink, countertops, and other surfaces in your kitchen. Those germs can get on other foods, such as salads or fruit, and make you sick.

SOLUTION

Do not wash meat, chicken, turkey, or eggs. Cooking them thoroughly will kill harmful germs.

Peeling Fruits and Vegetables without Washing Them First

WHY IT IS A MISTAKE

Fruits and vegetables may have germs on their peeling or skin. It is easy to transfer those germs to the inside of fruits and vegetables when you cut or peel them.

SOLUTION

Wash all fruits and vegetables under running water even if you are going to peel them. Use a clean vegetable brush to scrub firm fruits and vegetables such as melons, avocados, and cucumbers.

Putting Cooked Meat Back on a Plate That Held Raw Meat

WHY IT IS A MISTAKE

Germs from the raw meat can spread to the cooked meat.

SOLUTION

Always use separate plates for raw meat and cooked meat. The same rule applies to chicken, turkey, and seafood.

Not Cooking Meat, Chicken, Turkey, Seafood, or Eggs Thoroughly

WHY IT IS A MISTAKE

Cooked food is safe only after it has been cooked to a high enough temperature to kill germs.

SOLUTION

Use a food thermometer to make sure you cook food to a safe internal temperature.

- 145 °F for whole cuts of beef, pork, veal, and lamb (then allow the meat to rest for three minutes before carving or eating)
- 160 °F for ground meats, such as beef and pork
- 165 °F for all poultry, including ground chicken and turkey
- 165 °F for leftovers and casseroles
- 145 °F for fresh ham (raw)
- 145 °F for seafood, or cook until flesh is opaque

Visit (www.foodsafety.gov/food-safety-charts/safe-minimum-cooking-temperature) to get a detailed list of foods and safe temperatures. Also, if you will not be serving hot food right away, keep it hot (at 140 °F or above) until serving.

Eating Raw Batter or Dough, including Cookie Dough, and Other Foods with Uncooked Eggs or Uncooked Flour

WHY IT IS A MISTAKE

Flour and uncooked eggs may contain *Escherichia coli* (*E. coli*), *Salmonella*, or other harmful bacteria.

SOLUTION

Cook or bake flour and eggs thoroughly. Do not eat foods that contain raw or undercooked eggs, such as runny eggs, or homemade mayonnaise, hollandaise sauce, and eggnog. Do not eat raw (uncooked) dough or batter that contains either flour or eggs. Keep raw dough away from children, including play dough. Wash hands, work surfaces, and utensils thoroughly after contact with flour and raw dough.

Tasting or Smelling Food to See If It Is Still Good

WHY IT IS A MISTAKE

You cannot taste, smell, or see the germs that cause food poisoning. Tasting only a tiny amount can make you very sick.

SOLUTION

Check the storage times chart (www.foodsafety.gov/food-safety-charts/cold-food-storage-charts) to see how long you can store food safely. When the time is up, throw it out.

Thawing or Marinating Food on the Counter

WHY IT IS A MISTAKE

Harmful germs can multiply very quickly at room temperature.

SOLUTION

Thaw food safely. You can thaw it:

- In the refrigerator
- In cold water
- In the microwave

- Always marinate food in the refrigerator no matter what kind of marinade you are using.

Leaving Food out Too Long before Putting It in the Fridge

WHY IT IS A MISTAKE

Harmful germs can grow in perishable foods (including meat, chicken, turkey, seafood, eggs, cut fruit, cooked rice, and left-overs) if you leave them out of the refrigerator for two hours or longer.

SOLUTION

Put perishable foods in the refrigerator within two hours or within one hour if the food is exposed to a temperature over 90 °F (such as in a hot car). Divide roasts and large portions of food, such as pots of stew or chili, into smaller containers so they will chill quickly. It is ok to put warm or hot food into the refrigerator, as long as it is packaged in small enough amounts that will cool quickly.

FOOD SAFETY STEPS

Healthy eating means more than managing calories or choosing a balanced diet of nutrient-rich foods. The best healthy eating plans also involve safe food handling, cooking, and storage practices that help prevent food poisoning and foodborne illness.

In 2020, an estimated 1 in 6 Americans got sick from food poisoning. Find out what you can do to keep you and your family safe.

- **Check your steps.** Following four simple steps – Clean, Separate, Cook, and Chill – can help protect your family from food poisoning at home.
- **Keep food safe by type of food.** Get the latest tips and techniques to keep specific foods safe and prevent food poisoning.
- **Keep food safe by type of events and seasons.** Whether you are planning a small summer cookout or a big holiday celebration, a camping trip or a potluck

dinner, you need to follow special precautions to ensure that you and your guests are safe from food poisoning.

- **Food safety in a disaster or emergency.** Find out how to keep food safe during and after an emergency, such as a hurricane, flood, fire, or loss of power.
- **FoodKeeper app.** Use this app to help you use food while at peak quality and reduce waste.

Section 32.4 | Foodborne Illnesses

This section includes text excerpted from "Food Poisoning," National Digestive Diseases Information Clearinghouse (NDDIC), National Institute of Diabetes and Digestive and Kidney Diseases (NIDDK), June 2019.

WHAT IS FOOD POISONING?

Food poisoning, also called "foodborne illness," is an infection or irritation of your digestive tract that spreads through food or drinks. Viruses, bacteria, and parasites cause most food poisoning. Harmful chemicals may also cause food poisoning.

Food poisoning is most often acute, meaning it happens suddenly and lasts a short time. Most cases of food poisoning last less than a week, and most people get better on their own without treatment. In some cases, food poisoning can last longer or lead to serious complications.

HOW COMMON IS FOOD POISONING?

Each year, about 48 million people in the United States have food poisoning. Food poisoning causes about 3,000 deaths in the United States each year.

WHO IS MORE LIKELY TO GET FOOD POISONING?

Although anyone can get food poisoning, some people are more likely to get food poisoning than others, including:

- Infants and children

- Pregnant women and their fetuses
- Older adults
- People with weak immune systems

People in these groups are also more likely to have severe symptoms or complications of food poisoning. Food safety is especially important for people in these groups.

WHAT ARE THE COMPLICATIONS OF FOOD POISONING?

In some cases, food poisoning can lead to dehydration, hemolytic uremic syndrome (HUS), or other complications. However, serious complications are uncommon. In most cases, food poisoning lasts only a short time, and most people recover without developing complications.

Dehydration

Dehydration is the most common complication of food poisoning. When food poisoning causes you to vomit or have diarrhea, your body loses fluids and electrolytes. If you do not replace those fluids and electrolytes, you may become dehydrated. When you are dehydrated, your body does not have enough fluid and electrolytes to work properly.

Dehydration is especially dangerous in children, older adults, and people with weakened immune systems. If you are dehydrated, see a doctor right away to prevent serious health problems. Without treatment, dehydration can lead to problems such as organ damage, shock, coma, or even death.

Hemolytic Uremic Syndrome

Hemolytic uremic syndrome is a kidney condition that happens when red blood cells (RBCs) are destroyed and block the kidneys' filtering system. If your kidneys stop working, you have acute kidney injury (AKI) – the sudden and temporary loss of kidney function.

The most common cause of HUS is infection with a strain of *Escherichia coli* (*E. coli*) bacterium called "*E. coli O157:H7*," although other bacteria and viruses may also cause this condition. HUS is most common in children younger than 5 years of age.

Other Complications

In some cases, food poisoning may lead to serious health problems such as:

- Health problems during pregnancy and pregnancy complications. Some types of food poisoning during pregnancy can cause complications, such as dehydration, for the pregnant woman or can affect the fetus. For example, food poisoning by the bacterium *Listeria* can cause miscarriage or stillbirth.
- Guillain-Barre syndrome, which may occur after food poisoning caused by bacteria or viruses, most commonly *Campylobacter jejuni*.
- Irritable bowel syndrome (IBS), which may occur after food poisoning caused by various bacteria, viruses, or parasites.
- Problems breathing due to botulism – a rare type of food poisoning caused by *Clostridium botulinum* and sometimes by *Clostridium butyricum* or *Clostridium baratii* – and some forms of fish and shellfish poisoning, which affect the nervous system and may paralyze the muscles that control your breathing.
- Reactive arthritis, which may occur after food poisoning by certain bacteria, viruses, and parasites, including *Campylobacter jejuni* and *Salmonella*.

WHAT ARE THE SYMPTOMS OF FOOD POISONING?

Common symptoms of food poisoning include:

- Diarrhea or bloody diarrhea
- Vomiting
- Pain in your abdomen
- Fever
- Headache

Symptoms range from mild to severe and may last from a few hours to several days.

Less commonly, some types of food poisoning – such as botulism and fish and shellfish poisoning – can affect your nervous system. Symptoms may include:

- Blurred vision
- Headache
- Paralysis
- Tingling or numbness of your skin
- Weakness

People with nervous system symptoms should see a doctor or go to an emergency room right away.

WHAT CAUSES FOOD POISONING

Infections with microbes – viruses, bacteria, and parasites – cause most food poisoning. Harmful chemicals also cause some cases of food poisoning.

Microbes can spread to food at any time while the food is grown, harvested, or slaughtered, processed, stored, shipped, or prepared.

Some harmful microbes may already be present in foods when you buy them. Foods that may contain microbes include:

- Fresh produce
- Raw or undercooked meat, poultry, and eggs
- Dairy products and fruit juices that have not been pasteurized – heated to kill harmful microbes
- Fish and shellfish
- Foods that people handle during preparation, sometimes called "deli foods," such as sliced meat, salads and cut fruit, sandwiches, and baked goods
- Processed and ready-to-eat meats such as hot dogs or deli meat
- Foods that are not properly canned or sealed

If you do not keep raw foods – such as beef, poultry, seafood, and eggs – separate from other foods, microbes from the raw foods can spread to other foods. Microbes can also spread from raw foods to your hands, kitchen utensils, cutting boards, and kitchen surfaces during food preparation. If you do not wash your hands, utensils, cutting boards, and surfaces completely after they have come into contact with raw foods, they can spread microbes to other foods.

Microbes can cause food poisoning if you do not take steps to kill or slow the growth of microbes in food. Microbes can grow if people do not cook food thoroughly, keep cooked food hot, or promptly refrigerate or freeze food that can spoil.

Microbes present in the stool or vomit of people who are infected can also spread to food and cause food poisoning. People may spread these microbes to foods and drinks, especially if they do not wash their hands thoroughly after using the bathroom, after changing a diaper, and before preparing foods and drinks.

WHAT KINDS OF MICROBES CAUSE FOOD POISONING?

Viruses

Viruses invade normal cells in your body. Many viruses cause infections that can be spread from person-to-person.

If water comes into contact with stools of infected people, the water may become contaminated with a virus. The contaminated water can spread the virus to foods. For example, if contaminated water is used to water or wash produce, the virus can spread to the produce. Similarly, shellfish that were living in contaminated water could contain a virus.

If people who are infected with a virus prepare or handle foods, they may spread the virus to the foods.

Common viruses that cause food poisoning include norovirus and hepatitis A.

Bacteria

Bacteria are tiny organisms that can cause infection or disease. Bacteria can enter your body through contaminated food or water.

Bacteria grow quickly when the temperature of food is between 40-140 °F. Keeping food colder than 40 °F in a refrigerator or freezer can slow or stop the growth of bacteria. Cooking food thoroughly often kills bacteria.

Many types of bacteria can cause food poisoning, including:

- Certain types of *Salmonella*
- Certain types of *Clostridium*, including the common *C. perfringens* and the less common *C. botulinum*, which causes an illness called "botulism"
- Certain types of *Campylobacter*, including *C. jejuni*
- *Staphylococcus aureus*, also called "*staph*"
- *Escherichia coli*, also called "*E. coli*"
- Certain types of *Vibrio*
- *Listeria monocytogenes*, also called "*Listeria*"

Parasites

Parasites are tiny organisms that live inside other organisms. Parasites can enter your body through food or water and settle in your digestive tract. In developed countries such as the United States, parasitic infections are rare.

Parasites that cause food poisoning include:

- *Toxoplasma gondii*, which causes an illness called "*toxoplasmosis*"
- *Giardia*
- *Cryptosporidium*, which causes an illness called "*cryptosporidiosis*" or "*crypto*"

Travelers' Diarrhea

People who travel from the United States to developing countries may develop travelers' diarrhea. Eating food or drinking water contaminated with bacteria, parasites, or viruses causes travelers' diarrhea. Although travelers' diarrhea is most often acute, some parasites cause diarrhea that lasts longer.

HOW DO HARMFUL CHEMICALS CAUSE FOOD POISONING?

Harmful chemicals may be present in certain foods, including:

- Fish and shellfish that contain toxins produced by algae or bacteria
- Certain types of wild mushrooms

- Unwashed produce that contains large amounts of chemical pesticides

HOW DO DOCTORS DIAGNOSE FOOD POISONING?

Doctors often diagnose food poisoning based on your symptoms. If your symptoms are mild and last only a short time, you typically will not need tests.

In some cases, a medical history, a physical exam, stool tests, and blood tests can help diagnose food poisoning. Your doctor may perform additional tests to check for complications or to rule out other health problems. Your doctor may need to contact the health department to report your illness.

HOW CAN YOU TREAT FOOD POISONING?

In most cases, people with food poisoning get better on their own without medical treatment. You can treat food poisoning by replacing lost fluids and electrolytes to prevent dehydration. In some cases, over-the-counter (OTC) medicines may help relieve your symptoms.

When you have food poisoning, you may vomit after you eat or lose your appetite for a short time. When your appetite returns, you can most often go back to eating your normal diet, even if you still have diarrhea.

If your child has symptoms of food poisoning, such as vomiting or diarrhea, do not hesitate to call a doctor for advice.

HOW DO DOCTORS TREAT FOOD POISONING?

To treat food poisoning caused by bacteria or parasites, your doctor may prescribe antibiotics or medicines that target parasites, in addition to rehydration solutions.

In some cases, doctors may recommend probiotics. Probiotics are live microbes, most often bacteria, that may be similar to microbes you normally have in your digestive tract. Studies suggest that some probiotics may help shorten a bout of diarrhea. Researchers are still studying the use of probiotics to treat food poisoning. For safety reasons, talk with your doctor before using probiotics or any other complementary or alternative medicines (CAMs) or practices. This is especially important when children, older adults, or those with weak immune systems have diarrhea.

Doctors may need to treat people with life-threatening symptoms and complications – such as severe dehydration, HUS, or paralysis – in a hospital.

HOW CAN YOU PREVENT FOOD POISONING?

You can prevent some food poisoning by properly storing, cooking, cleaning, and handling foods. For example:

- Keep raw meat, poultry, seafood, and eggs separate from other foods.
- Prepare salads and refrigerate them before handling raw meat, poultry, seafood, or eggs.
- Promptly refrigerate or freeze foods that can spoil.
- Wash your hands with soap and water before and after handling food.
- Wash fruits and vegetables before eating, cutting, or cooking.
- Cook foods long enough and at high enough temperatures to kill harmful microbes.
- Wash utensils and surfaces after each use.
- Do not eat foods that can spoil that have been sitting out for more than two hours, or in temperatures over 90 °F, for more than one hour.

WHAT SHOULD YOU EAT IF YOU HAVE FOOD POISONING?

When you have food poisoning, you should drink plenty of liquids to replace lost fluids and electrolytes. You may vomit after you eat or lose your appetite for a short time. When your appetite returns, you can most often go back to eating your normal diet, even if you still have diarrhea.

When children have food poisoning, parents and caretakers should give children what they usually eat as soon as their appetite returns. Parents and caretakers should give infants breast milk or formula as usual.

WHAT SHOULD YOU AVOID EATING IF YOU HAVE FOOD POISONING?

For some people, certain food ingredients may make food poisoning symptoms, such as diarrhea, worse, including:

- Drinks with caffeine, such as coffee and tea, and some soft drinks
- Foods that are high in fat, such as fried foods, pizza, and fast foods
- Foods and drinks that contain large amounts of simple sugars, such as sweetened beverages and some fruit juices
- Milk and milk products, which contain the sugar lactose. Some people recovering from food poisoning have problems digesting lactose for up to a month or more afterward.

Research shows that following a restricted diet does not help treat diarrhea. Most experts do not recommend fasting or following a restricted diet when you have diarrhea.

Section 32.5 | Food Safety Recalls and Outbreaks

This section includes text excerpted from "Recalls and Outbreaks," Foodsafety.gov, U.S. Department of Health and Human Services (HHS), January 13, 2020.

RECALLS

What Is a Food Recall?

A food recall is when a food producer takes a product off the market because there is reason to believe that it may cause consumers to become ill. In some situations, government agencies may request a food recall. Food recalls may happen for many reasons, including but not limited to:

- Discovery of organisms, including bacteria such as *Salmonella* or parasites such as *Cyclospora*.

- Discovery of foreign objects such as broken glass or metal.
- Discovery of a major allergen that does not appear on the product label.

What to Do with a Recalled Product

A food product that has been recalled due to a possible germ contamination or illness, can leave germs around your kitchen and contaminate surfaces, including the drawers and shelves in your refrigerator.

If you have already prepared a recalled food item in your kitchen or still have it in your refrigerator, it is important to throw out the food and clean your kitchen.

- Wash all cookware and utensils (including cutting boards) with hot soapy water.
- Clear off counters and refrigerator drawers and shelves and wash them with hot soapy water.
- Then wipe any surfaces, shelves, or drawers and rinse dishes and cookware with a sanitizing solution and let them air dry. You can use a diluted bleach solution (one tbsp. unscented, liquid chlorine bleach in one gallon of water).
- Products recalled due to an undeclared allergen may be a risk for anyone in your household with an allergy to that substance. If the product has never been served, throw it away or return it for a refund. If the product has been served, wash with soap and water any surfaces – plates, pots and pans, utensils, and counters – with which the product may have had contact.

OUTBREAKS

What Is an Outbreak?

A foodborne outbreak occurs when two or more people get the same illness from the same contaminated food or drink. When an outbreak is detected, public health and regulatory officials work quickly to collect as much information as possible to find out what is causing it so they can take action to prevent more people from getting sick. This action includes warning the public when there is clear and convincing information linking illness to a contaminated food. Federal, state, and local officials may investigate an outbreak, depending on how widespread it is.

Section 32.6 | Food Safety and COVID-19

This section includes text excerpted from "Food and Coronavirus Disease 2019 (COVID-19)," Centers for Disease Control and Prevention (CDC), December 31, 2020.

Coronaviruses, like the one that causes COVID-19, are thought to spread mostly person-to-person through respiratory droplets when someone coughs, sneezes, or talks. It is possible that a person can get COVID-19 by touching a surface or object, including food or food packaging, that has the virus on it and then touching their own mouth, nose, or possibly their eyes. However, this is not thought to be the main way the virus spreads.

After shopping, handling food packages, or before preparing or eating food, it is important to always wash your hands with soap and water for at least 20 seconds. If soap and water are not available, use a hand sanitizer that contains at least 60 percent alcohol. Cover all surfaces of your hands and rub them together until they feel dry. Remember, it is always important to follow good food safety practices to reduce the risk of illness from common foodborne pathogens.

- The risk of getting COVID-19 from food you cook yourself or from handling and consuming food from restaurants and takeout or drive-thru meals is thought to be very low. Currently, there is no evidence that food is associated with spreading the virus that causes COVID-19.
- The risk of infection by the virus from food products, food packaging, or bags is thought to be very low. Currently, no cases of COVID-19 have been identified

where infection was thought to have occurred by touching food, food packaging, or shopping bags.
- Although some people who work in food production and processing facilities have gotten COVID-19, there is no evidence of the virus spreading to consumers through the food or packaging that workers in these facilities may have handled.

FOOD SAFETY IN THE KITCHEN

Use proper food safety practices when handling food and before, during, and after preparing or eating food.

- For now, there is no evidence that the virus that causes COVID-19 spreads to people through food. However, it is important to safely handle and continue to cook foods to their recommended cooking temperatures to prevent foodborne illness.
- The virus that causes COVID-19 has not been found in drinking water. The Environmental Protection Agency (EPA) regulates water treatment plants to ensure that treated water is safe to drink.

HANDLING PACKAGED FOOD

- When unpacking groceries, refrigerate or freeze meat, poultry, eggs, seafood, and other perishables within two hours of purchasing.
- Do not use disinfectants designed for hard surfaces, such as bleach or ammonia, on food packaged in cardboard or plastic wrap.
- If reusable cloth bags become soiled, follow instructions for washing them, and dry them in the warmest appropriate setting.

HANDLING AND CLEANING FRESH PRODUCE

- Do not wash produce with soap, bleach, sanitizer, alcohol, disinfectant, or any other chemical.

- Gently rinse fresh fruits and vegetables under cold, running tap water.
- Scrub uncut firm produce (e.g., potatoes, cucumbers, melons) with a clean brush, even if you do not plan to eat the peel.
- Salt, pepper, vinegar, lemon juice, and lime juice have not been shown to be effective at removing germs on produce.

HANDLING MEAL KITS AND DELIVERY

- Because of the COVID-19 outbreak and increases in demand, some deliveries have been delayed.
- If you have a meal kit or frozen prepared meal delivery, check the temperature of any food that is normally kept in the refrigerator or freezer (such as milk, meat, and eggs) immediately after it is delivered, using a food thermometer and make sure the food is 40 °F or below.
- Refrigerate or freeze your delivery as soon as possible.
- To help prevent the spread of COVID-19, pay online or on the phone when you order (if that is an option) and accept deliveries without in-person contact whenever possible.

HANDLING BULK MEAT, POULTRY, AND SEAFOOD PURCHASING

In response to changes in the food supply chain, some meat and poultry manufacturers, restaurants, and restaurant suppliers have begun selling large amounts of meat, poultry, and seafood directly to consumers. While there is currently no evidence that food can spread the virus that causes COVID-19, there are other important considerations for bulk purchasing.

- Harmful bacteria grow fastest between 41 °F and 140 °F. If you are picking up meat, poultry, or seafood order, bring a cooler and ice packs to keep food at 41 °F or colder during transit.
- Never allow meat, poultry, or seafood that requires refrigeration to sit at room temperature for more than two hours. Never allow meat, poultry, or seafood that requires refrigeration to sit at room temperature for

more than one hour if the air temperature is above 90 °F.

- Once you arrive home, meat, poultry, and seafood items should either be prepared immediately or put in the refrigerator or freezer for safe storage.
- In case of leaks in the packaging, bring a secondary container or place cases of meat, poultry, or seafood in an area of your vehicle that can be easily clean and sanitized. If leaks occur, thoroughly wash the surface with hot, soapy water or a bleach solution after it comes in contact with raw meat, poultry, or seafood, or its juices.

COVID-19 AND NUTRITION FOR HEALTH

- To help cope with the stress that may be related to the pandemic, take care of your body including good nutrition, as part of self-care.
- Dietary supplements are not meant to treat or prevent COVID-19. Certain vitamins and minerals (e.g., Vitamins C and D, zinc) may have effects on how our immune system works to fight off infections, as well as inflammation and swelling.
    - The best way to obtain these nutrients is through foods: Vitamin C in fruits and vegetables, Vitamin D in low-fat milk, fortified milk alternatives, and seafood, and zinc in lean meat, seafood, legumes, nuts, and seeds.
    - In some cases, dietary supplements may have unwanted effects, especially if taken in too large amounts, before surgery, or with other dietary supplements or medicines, or if you have certain health conditions.
    - If you are considering taking vitamins or dietary supplements, talk with your pharmacist, registered dietitian, or other healthcare provider before taking them, especially when combining or substituting them with other foods or medicine.
    - With changes in food availability in some communities, you may be consuming more canned or packaged food.

Tips on purchasing canned and packaged goods using the Nutrition Facts label are available. In addition, helpful food planning is available at MyPlate.

- Getting the right amount of nutritious food like plenty of fruits and vegetables, lean protein, and whole grains is important for health. If you or your household need help in obtaining nutritious food, find additional resources at the USDA Nutrition Assistance Program, or call the USDA National Hunger Hotline at 866-3-HUNGRY or 877-8-HAMBRE to speak with a representative who will find food resources such as meal sites, food banks, and other social services available near your location.
- Managers of food pantries and food distribution sites can consider these steps to help ensure safe access to food for their clients while helping prevent the spread of COVID-19.

Chapter 33 | The Health Consequences of Nutrition Misinformation

WHY IS FOOD AND NUTRITION MISINFORMATION ON THE RISE?

Health fraud takes many forms, and one of the most common examples is nutrition fraud. Nutrition fraud refers to inaccurate, misleading, or exaggerated information about the content, ingredients, or expected results of food and nutritional products, including food items, supplements, diet plans, and devices. In the United States, nutrition fraud is a serious problem. Nutrition fraud is occurring with increasing frequency due to a large number of new food products and herbal, botanical, sports, and dietary supplements entering the market. The rise of food fads has also contributed to the increase of nutrition misinformation. Food fads are themselves based on misinformation and exaggerated claims that certain foods have special health benefits, or that certain foods are harmful and should be eliminated from the diet.

Nutrition misinformation spreads in many ways. Overzealous marketers promote new products through books, television talk shows, articles and advertisements in magazines and newspapers, and direct mail to consumers. Word of mouth also helps to spread misinformation among families, friends, and communities. Nutrition misinformation is difficult to control through government regulation, therefore consumers must thoughtfully evaluate the information they receive about the nutritional properties of food and dietary supplements.

SOURCES OF FOOD AND NUTRITION MISINFORMATION

Consumers get information about food products and dietary supplements from a variety of sources. The media plays a role by providing information via television, newspapers, and magazines. Information reaches consumers directly from the food industry in the form of advertisements, celebrity endorsements, food labels and packaging, and other communications. Information is also passed via more informal means, through word of mouth among friends, coworkers, neighbors, and other community members. The Internet is also a primary source of information for many consumers. Many channels of information about food and nutrition are not well regulated and must be evaluated carefully by consumers. For example, information appearing on websites is generally not governed by any regulatory agency. On the Internet, misleading or false information often appears side-by-side with valid, science-based information. Discussions in Internet chat rooms and forums are a popular source of nutrition information, and these sources may be sponsored or influenced by people or organizations with a vested interest in promoting a certain product. The Internet can facilitate the spread of inaccurate information with alarming speed.

TYPES OF FOOD AND NUTRITION MISINFORMATION

Nutrition misinformation takes many forms. Food fads are a major source of misinformation about individual foods or food ingredients. A certain food, for example, kale, may suddenly become wildly popular and heralded as a "superfood" offering many health benefits. Or a food ingredient such as gluten can suddenly be labeled as bad, unhealthy, and even harmful for people to consume. Fad diets are another source of nutrition misinformation. Fad diets promote rapid weight loss through either eliminating "bad" foods or consuming only "good" foods. Examples of fad diets include low-carbohydrate eating plans and specific-food diets, such as the grapefruit diet. Health fraud can generally be recognized by the use of extravagant claims touting the product or diet as a "miracle cure" or "secret to effortless weight loss." Health fraud usually involves the promotion of a product for financial gain that is unproven or does not work. In a similar way, misdirected health claims are statements intended to encourage consumers to make incorrect judgments about the nutritional content or health benefits of a food or product. One example of a misdirected health claim is a food that is advertised as low fat and therefore healthy when it in fact is high in calories.

CONSEQUENCES OF NUTRITION MISINFORMATION

Consumers spend billions of dollars each year on food and nutrition products, dietary supplements, and weight-loss products. An overwhelming amount of information is circulated about the nutritional value and effects of various foods, supplements, diet products, and so on. In this environment, it can be difficult for consumers to make educated decisions about the potential value and merit of their purchasing decisions. When misinformation leads people to purchase products that do not work, are unproven, or promise unrealistic results, there can be serious health and economic consequences for consumers.

SHORT- AND LONG-TERM COSTS OF FOOD AND NUTRITION MISINFORMATION

Nutrition misinformation can result in both short- and long-term costs for individuals and for society as a whole. These costs can include physical harm if foods contain undocumented ingredients, toxic ingredients, or unknown/undocumented interactions with other substances such as prescription medications. Personal health products can result in physical harm if the use of these products replaces proper medical treatment. This is also the case when remedies fail to work, even if no harm is done. All of these circumstances can also result in economic costs to consumers. The current overall annual cost of health fraud is estimated in billions of dollars. Other costs which cannot be measured in dollars include a loss of faith in traditional sources of health and nutrition information and scientific findings. It is difficult to promote public health and gain public trust in an environment of persistent misinformation.

COMMUNICATING EVIDENCE-BASED NUTRITION INFORMATION

Successful communication of accurate nutrition and health information depends on two factors: how the information is communicated and how well the information is understood. Health and nutrition information must be communicated with a careful balance between providing enough context and background for consumers to make educated decisions and overwhelming consumers with too much scientific detail. Information that is provided in clear, easy-to-understand language can reduce consumer confusion while reinforcing the credibility of the source, whether that is a scientific report, a health professional, or other experts. Agencies and regulatory bodies of the U.S. federal government play a role in communicating nutrition information to consumers through the U.S. Food and Drug Administration's (FDA) food labeling programs. The FDA has implemented standard labeling intended to make it easier for consumers to understand and compare the nutrition information of different products. Government agencies also work with various organizations to communicate health and nutrition information to consumers via websites, publications, and the media. The media has the capability to effectively reach the largest number of consumers through television, radio, newspapers, and magazines.

THE ROLE OF CONSUMERS IN INTERPRETING INFORMATION

Ultimately, consumers bear the burden of evaluating health and nutrition information and making reasoned choices. Consumers must thoughtfully assess claims made in advertisements to determine whether a product will meet their specific needs, keeping in mind the trustworthiness and credibility of the information source. A wise consumer will attempt to validate the information by checking with their doctor or other health professionals, or by contacting the FDA, Better Business Bureau (BBB), or other consumer interest groups. In cases of direct marketing, consumers are wise to avoid making spontaneous purchases. A reputable seller will provide time for consumers to think about their purchase and verify the information. A legitimate product will stand up to consumer evaluation.

HOW TO ASSESS THE CREDIBILITY OF INFORMATION

If in doubt that any product will perform as advertised, consumers should attempt to gather and verify product information. Some points to evaluate include:

- What or who is the source of the information? Is that source trustworthy and credible? Does the person or organization have any credentials, professional license, or certification?
- Is the information current?
- How much information is provided? Does it answer all your questions?
- Are there credible references and reviews of the product? Are there testimonials or case histories?
- Is the information balanced? Are any exceptions or disclaimers noted?
- Does the information promise immediate or guaranteed results for little or no effort? These claims should raise suspicions. Does the information include words, such as "breakthrough," "miracle," or "secret?" Does the product claim to be a "recent discovery" that cannot be found or obtained anywhere else? These claims should raise suspicions.
- Are results described in specific or broad terms? The broader the claims, the less likely they are to be true.
- Does the information attempt to use guilt or fear to sell the product? Are you asked to pay in advance? These tactics indicate a possible scam.
- If it sounds too good to be true, it probably is.

TEN RED FLAGS OF JUNK SCIENCE

1. Recommendations that promise a quick fix
2. Dire warnings of danger from a single product or regimen.
3. Claims that sound too good to be true.
4. Simplistic conclusions drawn from a complex study.
5. Recommendations based on a single study.

6. Dramatic statements that are refuted by reputable scientific organizations.
7. Lists of "good" and "bad" foods.
8. Recommendations made to help sell a product.
9. Recommendations based on studies published without peer review.
10. Recommendations from studies that ignore individual or group differences.

References

1. "Position of the American Dietetic Association: Food and Nutrition Misinformation," American Dietetic Association, April 2006.
2. Bellows, L.; Moore, R. "Nutrition Misinformation: How to Identify Fraud and Misleading Claims," Colorado State University Extension, September 2013.
3. Hermann, Janice R. "Nutritional Misinformation," Oklahoma State University Cooperative Extension Service, n.d.

Chapter 34 | Food Insecurity of U.S. Households

RANGES OF FOOD SECURITY AND FOOD INSECURITY

In 2006, the U.S. Department of Agriculture (USDA) introduced a new language to describe ranges of severity of food insecurity. The USDA made these changes in response to recommendations of an expert panel convened at the USDA's request by the Committee on National Statistics (CNSTAT) of the National Academies. Although new labels were introduced, the methods used to assess households' food security remained unchanged, so statistics for 2005 to now are directly comparable with those for earlier years. The following labels define ranges of food security:

Food Security

- High food security (old label = food security): no reported indications of food-access problems or limitations.
- Marginal food security (old label = food security): one or two reported indications – typically of anxiety over food sufficiency or shortage of food in the house. Little or no indication of changes in diets or food intake.

This chapter contains text excerpted from the following sources: Text beginning with the heading "Ranges of Food Security and Food Insecurity" is excerpted from "Definitions of Food Security," Economic Research Service (ERS), U.S. Department of Agriculture (USDA), September 9, 2020; Text under the heading "Household Food Security in the United States in 2019" is excerpted from "Household Food Security in the United States in 2019," Economic Research Service (ERS), U.S. Department of Agriculture (USDA), September 2020.

Food Insecurity

- Low food security (old label = food insecurity without hunger): reports of reduced quality, variety, or desirability of diet. Little or no indication of reduced food intake.
- Very low food security (old label = food insecurity with hunger): reports of multiple indications of disrupted eating patterns and reduced food intake.

COMMITTEE ON NATIONAL STATISTICS REVIEW AND RECOMMENDATIONS

The USDA requested the review by CNSTAT to ensure that the measurement methods the USDA uses to assess households' access, or lack of access to adequate food and the language used to describe those conditions are conceptually and operationally sound and that they convey relevant information to policy officials and the public. The CNSTAT panel that conducted this study included economists, sociologists, nutritionists, statisticians, and other researchers. One of the central issues the panel addressed was whether the concepts and definitions underlying the measurement methods – especially the concept and definition of hunger and the relationship between hunger and food insecurity were appropriate for the policy context in which food security statistics are used.

The CNSTAT panel:

- Recommended that USDA continue to measure and monitor food insecurity regularly in a household survey
- Affirmed that the general methodology used to measure food insecurity is appropriate
- Suggested several ways refine the methodology (contingent on additional research). The ERS published technical research reports on potential refinements and continues to conduct research on these issues.

The CNSTAT panel also recommended that USDA make a clear and explicit distinction between food insecurity and hunger:

- Food insecurity – the condition assessed in the food security survey and represented in USDA food security

reports – is a household-level economic and social condition of limited or uncertain access to adequate food.
- Hunger is an individual-level physiological condition that may result from food insecurity.

The word "hunger," the panel stated in its final report, " should refer to a potential consequence of food insecurity that, because of prolonged, involuntary lack of food, results in discomfort, illness, weakness, or pain that goes beyond the usual uneasy sensation." To measure hunger in this sense would require collecting more detailed and extensive information on physiological experiences of individual household members than could be accomplished effectively in the Current Population Survey (CPS). The panel recommended, therefore, that new methods be developed to measure hunger and that a national assessment of hunger is conducted using an appropriate survey of individuals rather than a survey of households.

The CNSTAT panel also recommended that USDA consider alternative labels to convey the severity of food insecurity without using the word "hunger," since hunger is not adequately assessed in the food security survey. USDA concurred and introduced the labels "low food security" and "very low food security" in 2006.

HOUSEHOLD FOOD SECURITY IN THE UNITED STATES IN 2019

What Is the Issue?

Most United States households have consistent, dependable access to enough food for active, healthy living – they are food secure. However, some households experience food insecurity at times during the year, meaning their access to adequate food is limited by a lack of money and other resources. USDA's food and nutrition assistance programs aim to increase food security by providing low-income households access to food for a healthful diet, as well as nutrition education. USDA monitors the extent and severity of food insecurity in U.S. households through an annual, nationally representative survey sponsored and analyzed by USDA's Economic Research Service (ERS). This report presents statistics from the survey that cover household food security, food expenditures, and use of federal nutrition assistance programs in 2019. Readers should note that these are 2019 statistics collected in December 2019 and do not reflect the potential impacts of the COVID-19 pandemic that began in 2020.

What Did the Study Find?

MAIN FINDINGS

- The 2019 prevalence of food insecurity, at 10.5 percent, continued to decline from a high of 14.9 percent in 2011 and was significantly below the prerecession level (2007) of 11.1 percent.
- In 2019, 89.5 percent of U.S. households were food secure. The remaining 10.5 percent (13.7 million households) were food insecure. Food-insecure households (those with low and very low food security) had difficulty at some time during the year providing enough food for all their members due to a lack of resources. The decline from 2018 (11.1 percent) was statistically significant.
- In 2019, 4.1 percent of U.S. households (5.3 million households) had very low food security, not significantly different from 4.3 percent in 2018. In this more severe range of food insecurity, the food intake of some household members was reduced and normal eating patterns were disrupted at times during the year due to limited resources.

FINDINGS FOR HOUSEHOLDS WITH CHILDREN

- Children were food insecure at times during 2019 in 6.5 percent of U.S. households with children (2.4 million households), not significantly different from 7.1 percent in 2018. These households with food insecurity among children were unable at times to provide adequate, nutritious food for their children.
- While children are usually shielded from the disrupted eating patterns and reduced food intake that characterize

very low food security, in 2019, both children and adults suffered instances of very low food security in 0.6 percent of households with children (213,000 households), unchanged from 0.6 percent in 2018. These households with very low food security among children reported that children were hungry, skipped a meal, or did not eat for a whole day because there was not enough money for food.

FINDINGS FOR POPULATION SUBGROUPS AND STATES

- Rates of food insecurity were higher than the national average for the following groups: Households with incomes near or below the federal poverty line, including those with incomes below 185 percent of the poverty line; all households with children and particularly households with children headed by single women or single men; women and men living alone; Black and Hispanic-headed households; and households in principal cities and nonmetropolitan areas.
- The prevalence of food insecurity varied considerably from state to state, ranging from 6.6 percent in New Hampshire to 15.7 percent in Mississippi in 2017–19.

FINDINGS FOR FOOD SPENDING AND FEDERAL NUTRITION ASSISTANCE PARTICIPATION

- The typical (median) food-secure household spent 24 percent more for food than the typical food-insecure household of the same size and composition. These estimates include food purchases made with Supplemental Nutrition Assistance Program (SNAP) benefits.
- About 58 percent of food-insecure households in the survey reported that, in the previous month, they had participated in one or more of the three largest federal nutrition assistance programs: SNAP; Special Supplemental Nutrition Program for Women, Infants, and Children (WIC); and National School Lunch Program (NSLP).

Part 6 | Importance of Nutrition in Weight Management

Chapter 35 | The Health Risks of Overweight and Obesity

Chapter Contents

Section 35.1 | Health Problems Associated with Overweight and Obesity

This section includes text excerpted from "Overweight and Obesity," National Heart, Lung, and Blood Institute (NHLBI), January 4, 2021.

Overweight and obesity are increasingly common conditions in the United States. They are caused by the increase in the size and the amount of fat cells in the body. Doctors measure body mass index (BMI) and waist circumference to screen and diagnose overweight and obesity. Obesity is a serious medical condition that can cause complications such as metabolic syndrome, high blood pressure (HBP), atherosclerosis, heart disease, diabetes, high blood cholesterol, cancers and sleep disorders. Treatment depends on the cause and severity of your condition and whether you have complications. Treatments include lifestyle changes, such as heart-healthy eating and increased physical activity, and the U.S. Food and Drug Administration (FDA)-approved weight-loss medicines. For some people, surgery may be a treatment option.

CAUSES OF OVERWEIGHT AND OBESITY

Energy imbalances, some genetic or endocrine medical conditions, and certain medicines are known to cause overweight or obesity.

Energy Imbalances Cause the Body to Store Fat

Energy imbalances can cause overweight and obesity. An energy imbalance means that your energy IN does not equal your energy OUT. This energy is measured in calories. Energy IN is the amount of calories you get from food and drinks. Energy OUT is the amount of calories that your body uses for things such as breathing, digesting, being physically active, and regulating body temperature.

Overweight and obesity develop over time when you take in more calories than you use, or when energy IN is more than your energy OUT. This type of energy imbalance causes your body to store fat.

Your body uses certain nutrients such as carbohydrates or sugars, proteins, and fats from the foods you eat to:

- Make energy for immediate use to power routine daily body functions and physical activity
- Store energy for future use by your body. Sugars are stored as glycogen in the liver and muscles. Fats are stored mainly as triglyceride in fat tissue.

The amount of energy that your body gets from the food you eat depends on the type of foods you eat, how the food is prepared, and how long it has been since you last ate.

The body has three types of fat tissue – white, brown, and beige – that it uses to fuel itself, regulate its temperature in response to cold, and store energy for future use. Learn about the role of each fat type in maintaining energy balance in the body.

- White fat tissue can be found around the kidneys and under the skin in the buttocks, thighs, and abdomen. This fat type stores energy, makes hormone that control the way the body regulates urges to eat or stop eating, and makes inflammatory substances that can lead to complications.
- Brown fat tissue is located in the upper back area of human infants. This fat type releases stored energy as heat energy when a baby is cold. It also can make inflammatory substances. Brown fat can be seen in children and adults.
- Beige fat tissue is seen in the neck, shoulders, back, chest and abdomen of adults and resembles brown fat tissue. This fat type, which uses carbohydrates and fats to produce heat, increases when children and adults are exposed to cold.

Medical Conditions

Some genetic syndromes and endocrine disorders can cause overweight or obesity.

GENETIC SYNDROMES

Several genetic syndromes are associated with overweight and obesity, including the following:

- Prader-Willi syndrome
- Bardet-Biedl syndrome
- Alström syndrome
- Cohen syndrome

The study of these genetic syndromes has helped researchers understand obesity.

ENDOCRINE DISORDERS

Because the endocrine system produces hormones that help maintain energy balances in the body, the following endocrine disorders or tumor affecting the endocrine system can cause overweight and obesity.

- **Hypothyroidism.** People with this condition have low levels of thyroid hormones. These low levels are associated with decreased metabolism and weight gain, even when food intake is reduced. People with hypothyroidism also produce less body heat, have a lower body temperature, and do not efficiently use stored fat for energy.
- **Cushing syndrome.** People with this condition have high levels of glucocorticoids, such as cortisol, in the blood. High cortisol levels make the body feel like it is under chronic stress. As a result, people have an increase in appetite and the body will store more fat. Cushing syndrome may develop after taking certain medicines or because the body naturally makes too much cortisol.
- **Tumors.** Some tumors, such as craneopharingioma, can cause severe obesity because the tumors develop near parts of the brain that control hunger.

Medicines

Medicines such as antipsychotics, antidepressants, antiepileptics, and antihyperglycemics can cause weight gain and lead to overweight and obesity.

Talk to your doctor if you notice weight gain while you are using one of these medicines. Ask if there are other forms of the same medicine or other medicines that can treat your medical condition, but have less of an effect on your weight. Do not stop taking the medicine without talking to your doctor.

Several parts of your body, such as your stomach, intestines, pancreas, and fat tissue, use hormones to control how your brain decides if you are hungry or full. Some of these hormones are insulin, leptin, glucagon-like peptide (GLP-1), peptide YY, and ghrelin.

RISK FACTORS OF OVERWEIGHT AND OBESITY

There are many risk factors for overweight and obesity. Some risk factors can be changed, such as unhealthy lifestyle habits and environments. Other risk factors, such as age, family history and genetics, race and ethnicity, and sex, cannot be changed. Healthy lifestyle changes can decrease your risk for developing overweight and obesity.

Unhealthy Lifestyle Habits

Lack of physical activity, unhealthy eating patterns, not enough sleep, and high amounts of stress can increase your risk for overweight and obesity.

LACK OF PHYSICAL ACTIVITY

Lack of physical activity due to high amounts of TV, computer, videogame or other screen usage has been associated with a high BMI. Healthy lifestyle changes, such as being physically active and reducing screen time, can help you aim for a healthy weight.

UNHEALTHY EATING BEHAVIORS

Some unhealthy eating behaviors can increase your risk for overweight and obesity.

- **Eating more calories than you use.** The amount of calories you need will vary based on your sex, age, and physical activity level. Find out your daily calorie needs or goals with the Body Weight Planner.
- Eating too much saturated and *trans* fats
- Eating foods high in added sugars

NOT ENOUGH SLEEP

Many studies have seen a high BMI in people who do not get enough sleep. Some studies have seen a relationship between sleep and the way our bodies use nutrients for energy and how lack of sleep can affect hormones that control hunger urges.

HIGH AMOUNTS OF STRESS

Acute stress and chronic stress affect the brain and trigger the production of hormones, such as cortisol, that control our energy balances and hunger urges. Acute stress can trigger hormone changes that make you not want to eat. If the stress becomes chronic, hormone changes can make you eat more and store more fat.

Age

Childhood obesity remains a serious problem in the United States, and some populations are more at risk for childhood obesity than others. The risk of unhealthy weight gain increases as you age. Adults who have a healthy BMI often start to gain weight in young adulthood and continue to gain weight until 60 to 65 years old, when they tend to start losing weight.

Unhealthy Environments

Many environmental factors can increase your risk for overweight and obesity:

- Social factors such as having a low socioeconomic status or an unhealthy social or unsafe environment in the neighborhood
- Built environment factors such as easy access to unhealthy fast foods, limited access to recreational facilities or parks, and few safe or easy ways to walk in your neighborhood
- Exposure to chemicals known as "obesogens" that can change hormones and increase fatty tissue in our bodies

Family History and Genetics

Genetic studies have found that overweight and obesity can run in families, so it is possible that our genes or deoxyribonucleic acid (DNA) can cause these conditions. Research studies have found that certain DNA elements are associated with obesity.

Did you know obesity can change your DNA and the DNA you pass on to your children?

Eating too much or eating too little during your pregnancy can change your baby's DNA and can affect how your child stores and uses fat later in life. Also, studies have shown that obese fathers have DNA changes in their sperm that can be passed on to their children.

Race or Ethnicity

Overweight and obesity is highly prevalent in some racial and ethnic minority groups. Rates of obesity in American adults are highest in Blacks, followed by Hispanics, then whites. This is true for men or women. While Asian men and women have the lowest rates of unhealthy BMIs, they may have high amounts of unhealthy fat in the abdomen. Some people may be at risk for overweight and obesity because they may carry a DNA variant that is associated with increased BMI but not with common obesity-related complications.

Sex

In the United States, obesity is more common in Black or Hispanic women than in Black or Hispanic men. A person's sex may also affect the way the body stores fat. For example, women tend to store less unhealthy fat in the abdomen than men do.

Overweight and obesity is also common in women with polycystic ovary syndrome (PCOS). This is an endocrine condition that causes large ovaries and prevents proper ovulation, which can reduce fertility.

SIGNS, SYMPTOMS, AND COMPLICATIONS OF OVERWEIGHT AND OBESITY

There are no specific symptoms of overweight and obesity. The signs of overweight and obesity include a high BMI and an unhealthy body fat distribution that can be estimated by measuring your waist circumference. Obesity can cause complications in many parts of your body.

High Body Mass Index

A high BMI is the most common sign of overweight and obesity.

Table 35.1. BMI Table for Children and Adult

Weight Category	Body Mass Index	
	Children	**Adults**
Underweight	Below 5th percentile*	Below 18.5
Healthy weight	5th percentile to less than 85th percentile	18.5 to 24.9
Overweight	85th percentile to less than 95th percentile	25 to 29.9
Obese	95th percentile or above	30 or above

Body mass index is used to determine if you or your child are underweight, healthy, or overweight, or obese. Children are underweight if their BMI is below the 5th percentile, healthy weight if their BMI is between the 5th to less than the 85th percentile, overweight if their BMI is the 85th percentile to less than the 95th percentile, and obese if their BMI is the 95th percentile or above. Adults are underweight if their BMI is below 18.5, healthy weight if their BMI is 18.5 to 24.9, overweight if their BMI is 25 to 29.9, and obese if their BMI is 30 or above.
**A child's BMI percentile is calculated by comparing your child's BMI to growth charts for children who are the same age and sex as your child.*

Unhealthy Body Fat Distribution

Another sign of overweight and obesity is having an unhealthy body fat distribution. Fatty tissue is found in different parts of your body and has many functions. Having an increased waist circumference suggests that you have increased amounts of fat in your abdomen. An increased waist circumference is a sign of obesity and can increase your risk for obesity-related complications.

Did you know that fatty tissue has different functions depending on its location in your body?

Visceral fat is the fatty tissue inside of your abdomen and organs. While we do not know what causes the body to create and store visceral fat, it is known that this type of fat interferes with the body's endocrine and immune systems and promotes chronic inflammation, and contributes to obesity-related complications.

Complications

Obesity may cause the following complications:

- Metabolic syndrome
- Type 2 diabetes
- High blood cholesterol and high triglyceride levels in the blood
- Diseases of the heart and blood vessels such as HBP, atherosclerosis, heart attacks, and stroke
- Respiratory problems such as obstructive sleep apnea (OSA), asthma, and obesity hypoventilation syndrome (OHS)
- Back pain
- Nonalcoholic fatty liver disease (NAFLD)
- Osteoarthritis, a chronic inflammation that damages the cartilage and bone in or around the affected joint. It can cause mild or severe pain and usually affects weight-bearing joints in people who are obese. It is a major cause of knee replacement surgery in patients who are obese for a long time.
- Urinary incontinence, the unintentional leakage of urine. Chronic obesity can weaken pelvic muscles, making it

harder to maintain bladder control. While it can happen to both sexes, it usually affects women as they age.
- Gallbladder disease
- Emotional health issues such as low self-esteem or depression. This may commonly occur in children.
- Cancers of the esophagus, pancreas, colon, rectum, kidney, endometrium, ovaries, gallbladder, breast, or liver

Did you know inflammation is thought to play a role in the onset of certain obesity-related complications?

Researchers now know more about visceral fat, which is deep in the abdomen of patients who are overweight and obese. Visceral fat releases factors that promote inflammation. Chronic obesity-related inflammation is thought to lead to insulin resistance and diabetes, changes in the liver or NAFLD, and cancers. More research is needed to understand what triggers inflammation in some patients who are obese and to find new treatments.

Section 35.2 | **Portion Size and Obesity**

This section contains text excerpted from the following sources: Text in this section begins with excerpts from "*We Can!*® Community News Feature," National Heart, Lung, and Blood Institute (NHLBI), February 13, 2013. Reviewed May 2021; Text under the heading "Avoiding Portion Size Pitfalls to Manage Weight" is excerpted from "How to Avoid Portion Size Pitfalls to Help Manage Your Weight," Centers for Disease Control and Prevention (CDC), January 11, 2021.

Food portions in America's restaurants have doubled or tripled over the last 20 years, a key factor that is contributing to a potentially devastating increase in obesity among children and adults. Ways to Enhance Children's Activities and Nutrition (*We Can!*), a program from the National Institutes of Health (NIH), offers parents tips to help their families maintain a healthy weight.

"Super-sized portions at restaurants have distorted what Americans consider a normal portion size, and that affects how much we eat at home as well," said Dr. Elizabeth G. Nabel, director of NIH's National Heart, Lung, and Blood Institute (NHLBI). "One way to keep calories in check is to keep food portions no larger than the size of your fist." Larger portions mean more calories, which can easily add up to extra weight.

Consider, for example, if you had today's portions of the following meals:

- **Breakfast.** A bagel (6 inches in diameter) and a 16 ounce coffee with sugar and milk.
- **Lunch.** Two pieces of pepperoni pizza and a 20 ounce soda.
- **Dinner.** A chicken Caesar salad and a 20 ounce soda.

In one day, you would consume 1,595 more calories than if you had the same foods at typical portions served 20 years ago. Over the course of one year, if consumed daily, the larger portions could amount to more than 500,000 extra calories.

Controlling portion sizes and eating smarter can help you and your family avoid extra calories. Here are some tips from the NIH:

- Bring a healthy, low-calorie lunch to work and pack a healthy "brown bag" for your children. When eating out, order an appetizer instead of an entrée, share an entrée or eat half of a meal and bring the rest home.
- Cut high-calorie foods, such as cheese and chocolate into small pieces and eat fewer pieces.
- Substitute a salad for french fries.
- For snacks, serve fruits and vegetables instead of sweets.

We Can! is designed to assist parents in helping children between the ages of 8 and 13 maintain a healthy weight through improving food choices, increasing physical activity and reducing television and recreational computer time.

AVOIDING PORTION SIZE PITFALLS TO MANAGE WEIGHT

When eating at many restaurants, it is hard to miss that portion sizes have gotten larger in the last few years. The trend has also spilled over into the grocery store and vending machines, where a bagel has become a BAGEL and an "individual" bag of chips can easily feed more than one. Research shows that people unintentionally consume more calories when faced with larger portions. This can mean significant excess calorie intake, especially when eating high-calorie foods. Here are some tips to help you avoid some common portion-size pitfalls.

Portion control when eating out. Many restaurants serve more food than one person needs at one meal. Take control of the amount of food that ends up on your plate by splitting an entrée with a friend. Or, ask the waitperson for a "to-go" box and wrap up half your meal as soon as it is brought to the table.

Portion control when eating in. To minimize the temptation of second and third helpings when eating at home, serve the food on individual plates, instead of putting the serving dishes on the table. Keeping the excess food out of reach may discourage overeating.

Portion control in front of the TV. When eating or snacking in front of the TV, put the amount that you plan to eat into a bowl or container instead of eating straight from the package. It is easy to overeat when your attention is focused on something else.

Go ahead, spoil your dinner. We learned as children not to snack before a meal for fear of "spoiling our dinner." Well, it is time to forget that old rule. If you feel hungry between meals, eat a healthy snack, such as a piece of fruit or small salad, to avoid overeating during your next meal.

Be aware of large packages. For some reason, the larger the package, the more people consume from it without realizing it. To minimize this effect:

- Divide up the contents of one large package into several smaller containers to help avoid overconsumption.
- Do not eat straight from the package. Instead, serve the food in a small bowl or container.

Out of sight, out of mind. People tend to consume more when they have easy access to food. Make your home a "portion-friendly zone."

- Replace the candy dish with a fruit bowl.
- Store especially tempting foods, such as cookies, chips, or ice cream, out of immediate eyesight, like on a high

shelf or at the back of the freezer. Move the healthier food to the front at eye level.
- When buying in bulk, store the excess in a place that is not convenient to get to, such as a high cabinet or at the back of the pantry.

Section 35.3 | **Obesity and Cancer Risk**

This section includes text excerpted from "Obesity and Cancer," National Cancer Institute (NCI), January 17, 2017. Reviewed May 2021.

WHAT IS KNOWN ABOUT THE RELATIONSHIP BETWEEN OBESITY AND CANCER?

Nearly all of the evidence linking obesity to cancer risk comes from large cohort studies, a type of observational study. However, data from observational studies can be difficult to interpret and cannot definitively establish that obesity causes cancer. That is because obese or overweight people may differ from people who are lean in ways other than their body fat, and it is possible that these other differences – rather than their body fat – are what explains their different cancer risk.

Despite the limitations of the study designs, there is consistent evidence that higher amounts of body fat are associated with increased risks of a number of cancers, including:

- **Endometrial cancer.** Obese and overweight women are two to about four times as likely as women who are normal weight to develop endometrial cancer (cancer of the lining of the uterus), and extremely obese women are about seven times as likely to develop the more common of the two main types of this cancer. The risk of endometrial cancer increases with increasing weight gain in adulthood, particularly among women who have never used menopausal hormone therapy (MHT).

- **Esophageal adenocarcinoma.** People who are overweight or obese are about twice as likely as people who are normal weight to develop a type of esophageal cancer called "esophageal adenocarcinoma," and people who are extremely obese are more than four times as likely.
- **Gastric cardia cancer.** People who are obese are nearly twice as likely as people who are normal weight to develop cancer in the upper part of the stomach, that is, the part that is closest to the esophagus.
- **Liver cancer.** People who are overweight or obese are up to twice as likely as people who are normal weight to develop liver cancer. The association between overweight/obesity and liver cancer is stronger in men than women.
- **Kidney cancer.** People who are overweight or obese are nearly twice as likely as people who are normal weight to develop renal cell cancer, the most common form of kidney cancer. The association of renal cell cancer with obesity is independent of its association with high blood pressure (HBP), a known risk factor for kidney cancer.
- **Multiple myeloma.** Compared with normal weight individuals, overweight and obese individuals have a slight (10 to 20 percent) increase in the risk of developing multiple myeloma.
- **Meningioma.** The risk of this slow-growing brain tumor that arises in the membranes surrounding the brain and the spinal cord is increased by about 50 percent in people who are obese and about 20 percent in people who are overweight.
- **Pancreatic cancer.** People who are overweight or obese are about 1.5 times as likely to develop pancreatic cancer as people who are normal weight.
- **Colorectal cancer.** People who are obese are slightly (about 30 percent) more likely to develop colorectal cancer than people who are normal weight.

A higher BMI is associated with increased risks of colon and rectal cancers in both men and in women, but the increases are higher in men than in women.

- **Gallbladder cancer.** Compared with people who are normal weight, people who are overweight have a slight (about 20 percent) increase in risk of gallbladder cancer, and people who are obese have a 60 percent increase in risk of gallbladder cancer. The risk increase is greater in women than men.
- **Breast cancer.** Many studies have shown that, in postmenopausal women, a higher BMI is associated with a modest increase in risk of breast cancer. For example, a 5-unit increase in BMI is associated with a 12 percent increase in risk. Among postmenopausal women, those who are obese have a 20 to 40 percent increase in risk of developing breast cancer compared with women who are normal weight. The higher risks are seen mainly in women who have never used MHT and for tumors that express hormone receptors. Obesity is also a risk factor for breast cancer in men.

In premenopausal women, by contrast, overweight and obesity have been found to be associated with a 20 percent decreased risk of breast tumors that express hormone receptors.

- **Ovarian cancer.** Higher BMI is associated with a slight increase in the risk of ovarian cancer, particularly in women who have never used menopausal hormone therapy. For example, a 5-unit increase in BMI is associated with a 10 percent increase in risk among women who have never used MHT.
- **Thyroid cancer.** Higher BMI (specifically, a 5-unit increase in BMI) is associated with a slight (10 percent) increase in the risk of thyroid cancer.

HOW MIGHT OBESITY INCREASE THE RISK OF CANCER?

Several possible mechanisms have been suggested to explain how obesity might increase the risks of some cancers.

Obese people often have chronic low-level inflammation, which can, over time, cause deoxyribonucleic acid (DNA) damage that leads to cancer. Overweight and obese individuals are more likely than normal-weight individuals to have conditions or disorders that are linked to or that cause chronic local inflammation and that are risk factors for certain cancers. For example, chronic local inflammation induced by gastroesophageal reflux disease (GERD) or Barrett esophagus is a likely cause of esophageal adenocarcinoma. Obesity is a risk factor for gallstones, a condition characterized by chronic gallbladder inflammation, and a history of gallstones is a strong risk factor for gallbladder cancer. Chronic ulcerative colitis (a chronic inflammatory condition) and hepatitis (a disease of the liver causing inflammation) are risk factors for different types of liver cancer.

Fat tissue (also called "adipose tissue") produces excess amounts of estrogen, high levels of which have been associated with increased risks of breast, endometrial, ovarian, and some other cancers.

Obese people often have increased blood levels of insulin and insulin-like growth factor-1 (IGF-1). (This condition, known as "hyperinsulinemia" or "insulin resistance," precedes the development of type 2 diabetes.) High levels of insulin and IGF-1 may promote the development of colon, kidney, prostate, and endometrial cancers.

Fat cells produce adipokines, hormones that may stimulate or inhibit cell growth. For example, the level of an adipokine called "leptin," which seems to promote cell proliferation, in the blood increases with increasing body fat. And another adipokine, adiponectin – which is less abundant in obese people than in those of normal weight – may have antiproliferative effects.

Fat cells may also have direct and indirect effects on other cell growth regulators, including mammalian target of rapamycin (mTOR) and AMP-activated protein kinase.

Other possible mechanisms by which obesity could affect cancer risk include changes in the mechanical properties of the scaffolding that surrounds breast cells and altered immune responses, effects on the nuclear factor kappa beta system, and oxidative stress.

HOW MANY CANCER CASES MAY BE DUE TO OBESITY

A population-based study using BMI and cancer incidence data from the GLOBOCAN project estimated that, in 2012 in the United States, about 28,000 new cases of cancer in men (3.5 percent) and 72,000 in women (9.5 percent) were due to overweight or obesity. The percentage of cases attributed to overweight or obesity varied widely for different cancer types but was as high as 54 percent for gallbladder cancer in women and 44 percent for esophageal adenocarcinoma in men.

A 2016 study summarizing worldwide estimates of the fractions of different cancers attributable to overweight/obesity reported that, compared with other countries, the United States had the highest fractions attributable to overweight/obesity for colorectal cancer, pancreatic cancer, and postmenopausal breast cancer.

DOES AVOIDING WEIGHT GAIN OR LOSING WEIGHT DECREASE THE RISK OF CANCER?

Most of the data about whether avoiding weight gain or losing weight reduces cancer risk comes from cohort and case-control studies. As with observational studies of obesity and cancer risk, these studies can be difficult to interpret because people who lose weight or avoid weight gain may differ in other ways from people who do not.

Nevertheless, when the evidence from multiple observational studies is consistent, the association is more likely to be real. Many observational studies have provided consistent evidence that people who have lower weight gain during adulthood have lower risks of colon cancer, kidney cancer, and – for postmenopausal women – breast, endometrial, and ovarian cancers.

Fewer studies have examined possible associations between weight loss and cancer risk. Some of these have found decreased risks of breast, endometrial, colon, and prostate cancers among people who have lost weight. However, most of these studies were not able to evaluate whether the weight loss was intentional or unintentional (and possibly related to underlying health problems).

Stronger evidence for a relationship between weight loss and cancer risk comes from studies of people who have undergone bariatric surgery (surgery performed on the stomach or intestines to induce weight loss). Obese people who have bariatric surgery appear to have lower risks of obesity-related cancers than obese people who do not have bariatric surgery.

Nevertheless, the follow-up study of weight and breast cancer in the Women's Health Initiative (WHI) found that for women who were already overweight or obese at baseline, weight change (either gain or loss) was not associated with breast cancer risk during follow-up. However, for women who were of normal weight at baseline, gaining more than 5 percent of body weight was associated with increased breast cancer risk.

HOW DOES OBESITY AFFECT CANCER SURVIVORSHIP?

Most of the evidence about obesity in cancer survivors comes from people who were diagnosed with breast, prostate, or colorectal cancer. Research indicates that obesity may worsen several aspects of cancer survivorship, including quality of life, cancer recurrence, cancer progression, and prognosis (survival).

For example, obesity is associated with increased risks of treatment-related lymphedema in breast cancer survivors and incontinence in prostate cancer survivors treated with radical prostatectomy. In a large clinical trial of patients with stage II and stage III rectal cancer, those with a higher baseline BMI (particularly men) had an increased risk of local recurrence. Death from multiple myeloma is 50 percent more likely for people at the highest levels of obesity compared with people at normal weight.

Several randomized clinical trials in breast cancer survivors have reported weight-loss interventions that resulted in both weight loss and beneficial changes in biomarkers that have been linked to the association between obesity and prognosis. However, there is little evidence about whether weight loss improves cancer recurrence or prognosis. The National Cancer Institute (NCI)-sponsored Breast Cancer Weight Loss (BWEL) Study, a randomized phase III trial that is currently recruiting participants, will compare recurrence rate in women who are overweight and obese take part in a weight-loss program after breast cancer diagnosis with that in women who do not take part in the weight-loss program.

Chapter 36 | Childhood Obesity

Chapter Contents

Section 36.1 | **Childhood Obesity: Causes and Consequences**

This section contains text excerpted from the following sources: Text under the heading "Childhood Obesity: A Complex Health Issue" is excerpted from "Childhood Obesity Causes & Consequences," Centers for Disease Control and Prevention (CDC), March 19, 2021; Text under the heading "Prevalence of Childhood Obesity in the United States" is excerpted from "Childhood Obesity Facts," Centers for Disease Control and Prevention (CDC), April 5, 2021.

CHILDHOOD OBESITY: A COMPLEX HEALTH ISSUE

Childhood obesity is a complex health issue. It occurs when a child is well above the normal or healthy weight for her or his age and height. The causes of excess weight gain in young people are similar to those in adults, including behavior and genetics. Obesity is also influenced by a person's community as it can affect the ability to make healthy choices.

Behavior

Behaviors that influence excess weight gain include eating high-calorie, low-nutrient foods and beverages, medication use and sleep routines. Not getting enough physical activity and spending too much time on sedentary activities such as watching television or other screen devices can lead to weight gain.

In contrast, consuming healthy foods and being physically active can help children grow and maintain a healthy weight. Balancing energy or calories consumed from foods and beverages with the calories burned through activity plays a role in preventing excess weight gain. In addition, eating healthy foods and being physically active helps to prevent chronic diseases such as type 2 diabetes, some cancers, and heart disease.

Eat Well and Be Active!

A healthy diet follows the *2020-2025 Dietary Guidelines for Americans*. It emphasizes eating a variety of vegetables and fruits, whole grains, a variety of lean protein foods, and low-fat and fat-free dairy products. It also recommends limiting foods and beverages with added sugars, solid fats, or sodium.

The *Physical Activity Guidelines for Americans* recommends children aged 6–17 years do at least 60 minutes of moderate-to-vigorous physical activity every day. Children aged three through five years should be physically active throughout the day for growth and development.

Community Environment

It can be difficult to make healthy food choices and get enough physical activity in environments that do not support healthy habits. Places such as childcare centers, schools, or communities can affect diet and activity through the foods and drinks they offer and the opportunities for physical activity they provide. Other community factors include the affordability of healthy food options, peer and social supports, marketing and promotion, and policies that determine how a community is designed.

Consequences of Obesity

MORE IMMEDIATE HEALTH RISKS

Obesity during childhood can harm the body in a variety of ways. Children who have obesity are more likely to have:

- High blood pressure (HBP) and high cholesterol, which are risk factors for cardiovascular disease (CVD)
- Increased risk of impaired glucose tolerance, insulin resistance, and type 2 diabetes
- Breathing problems, such as asthma and sleep apnea
- Joint problems and musculoskeletal discomfort
- Fatty liver disease, gallstones, and gastroesophageal reflux (GERD) (i.e., heartburn)

Childhood obesity is also related to:

- Psychological problems, such as anxiety and depression
- Low self-esteem and lower self-reported quality of life (QOL)
- Social problems, such as bullying and stigma

FUTURE HEALTH RISKS

Children who have obesity are more likely to become adults with obesity. Adult obesity is associated with increased risk of several serious health conditions including heart disease, type 2 diabetes, and cancer.

If children have obesity, their obesity and disease risk factors in adulthood are likely to be more severe.

PREVALENCE OF CHILDHOOD OBESITY IN THE UNITED STATES

Childhood obesity is a serious problem in the United States, putting children and adolescents at risk for poor health. Obesity prevalence among children and adolescents is still too high.

For children and adolescents aged 2–19 years:

- The prevalence of obesity was 18.5 percent. About 13.7 million children and adolescents had obesity.
- Obesity prevalence was 13.9 percent among 2- to 5-year-olds, 18.4 percent among 6- to 11-year-olds, and 20.6 percent among 12- to 19-year-olds.
- Childhood obesity is more common among certain populations.
    - Hispanic (25.8 percent) and non-Hispanic Black children (22.0 percent) had higher obesity prevalence than non-Hispanic white children (14.1 percent).
    - Non-Hispanic Asian children (11.0 percent) had lower obesity prevalence than non-Hispanic Blacks and Hispanic children.

Section 36.2 | Body Mass Index as a Tool to Measure Childhood Overweight and Obesity

This section includes text excerpted from "Defining Childhood Obesity," Centers for Disease Control and Prevention (CDC), July 3, 2018.

BODY MASS INDEX FOR CHILDREN AND TEENS

Body mass index (BMI) is a measure used to determine childhood overweight and obesity. Overweight is defined as a BMI at or above the 85th percentile and below the 95th percentile for children and teens of the same age and sex. Obesity is defined as a BMI at or above the 95th percentile for children and teens of the same age and sex.

BMI is calculated by dividing a person's weight in kilograms by the square of height in meters. For children and teens, BMI is age- and sex-specific and is often referred to as "BMI-for-age." A child's weight status is determined using an age- and sex-specific percentile for BMI rather than the BMI categories used for adults. This is because children's body composition varies as they age and varies between boys and girls. Therefore, BMI levels among children and teens need to be expressed relative to other children of the same age and sex.

For example, a 10-year-old boy of average height (56 inches) who weighs 102 pounds would have a BMI of 22.9 kg/m. This would place the boy in the 95th percentile for BMI, and he would be considered obese. This means that the child's BMI is greater than the BMI of 95 percent of 10-year-old boys in the reference population.

The CDC Growth Charts are the most commonly used indicator to measure the size and growth patterns of children and teens in the United States.

The BMI does not measure body fat directly, but research has shown that BMI is correlated with more direct measures of body fat, such as skinfold thickness measurements, bioelectrical impedance, densitometry (underwater weighing), dual-energy x-ray absorptiometry (DXA) and other methods. BMI can be considered an alternative to direct measures of body fat. A trained healthcare

Table 36.1. BMI-for-Age

Weight Status Category	**Percentile Range**
Underweight	Less than the 5th percentile
Normal or Healthy Weight	5th percentile to less than the 85th percentile
Overweight	85th to less than the 95th percentile
Obese	95th percentile or greater

provider should perform appropriate health assessments in order to evaluate an individual's health status and risks.

Section 36.3 | Helping Children to Maintain a Healthy Weight

This section includes text excerpted from "Tips to Help Children Maintain a Healthy Weight," Centers for Disease Control and Prevention (CDC), January 8, 2021.

In the United States, the number of children with obesity has continued to rise over the past two decades. Obesity in childhood poses immediate and future health risks.

Parents, guardians, and teachers can help children maintain a healthy weight by helping them develop healthy eating habits and limiting calorie-rich temptations. You also want to help children be physically active, have reduced screen time, and get adequate sleep.

The goal for children who are overweight is to reduce the rate of weight gain while allowing normal growth and development. Children should not be placed on a weight reduction diet without the consultation of a healthcare provider.

DEVELOP HEALTHY EATING HABITS

To help children develop healthy eating habits:

- Provide plenty of vegetables, fruits, and whole-grain products.

- Include low-fat or nonfat milk or dairy products, including cheese and yogurt.
- Choose lean meats, poultry, fish, lentils, and beans for protein.
- Encourage your family to drink lots of water.
- Limit sugary drinks.
- Limit consumption of sugar and saturated fat.

Remember that small changes every day can lead to success!

LIMIT CALORIE-RICH TEMPTATIONS

Reducing the availability of high-fat and high-sugar or salty snacks can help your children develop healthy eating habits. Only allow your children to eat these foods rarely, so that they truly will be treats! Here are examples of easy-to-prepare, low-fat and low-sugar snacks that are 100 calories or less:

- One cup carrots, broccoli, or bell peppers with two tablespoons hummus
- A medium apple or banana
- One cup blueberries or grapes
- One-fourth cup of tuna wrapped in a lettuce leaf
- A few homemade oven-baked kale chips

HELP CHILDREN STAY ACTIVE

In addition to being fun for children, regular physical activity has many health benefits, including:

- Strengthening bones
- Decreasing blood pressure
- Reducing stress and anxiety
- Increasing self-esteem
- Helping with weight management

Children ages three through five years should be active throughout the day. Children and adolescents ages six through 17 years should be physically active at least 60 minutes each day. Include aerobic activity, which is anything that makes their hearts beat faster. Also include bone-strengthening activities such as running or jumping and muscle-strengthening activities such as climbing or push-ups.

Remember that children imitate adults. Start adding physical activity to your own routine and encourage your child to join you.

REDUCE SEDENTARY TIME

Although quiet time for reading and homework is fine, limit the time children watch television, play video games, or surf the web to no more than two hours per day. Additionally, the American Academy of Pediatrics (AAP) does not recommend television viewing for children aged two years or younger. Instead, encourage children to find fun activities to do with family members or on their own that simply involve more activity.

ENSURE ADEQUATE SLEEP

Too little sleep is associated with obesity, partly because inadequate sleep makes us eat more and be less physically active. Children need more sleep than adults, and the amount varies by age. See the recommended amounts of sleep and suggested habits to improve sleep (www.cdc.gov/sleep/features/getting-enough-sleep.html).

Chapter 37 | **Healthy Weight Loss**

Chapter Contents

Section 37.1 | **Healthy Weight Loss: An Overview**

This section contains text excerpted from the following sources: Text beginning with the heading "What Is Healthy Weight Loss?" is excerpted from "Losing Weight," Centers for Disease Control and Prevention (CDC), August 17, 2020.

WHAT IS HEALTHY WEIGHT LOSS?

It is natural for anyone trying to lose weight to want to lose it very quickly. But, people who lose weight gradually and steadily (about 1 to 2 pounds per week) are more successful at keeping weight off. Healthy weight loss is not just about a "diet" or "program." It is about an ongoing lifestyle that includes long-term changes in daily eating and exercise habits.

Once you have achieved a healthy weight, rely on healthy eating and physical activity to help you keep the weight off over the long term.

Losing weight is not easy, and it takes commitment. But, if you are ready to get started, we have got a step-by-step guide to help get you on the road to weight loss and better health.

EVEN MODEST WEIGHT LOSS CAN MEAN BIG BENEFITS

Even a modest weight loss of 5 to 10 percent of your total body weight is likely to produce health benefits, such as improvements in blood pressure, blood cholesterol, and blood sugars.

For example, if you weigh 200 pounds, a 5 percent weight loss equals 10 pounds, bringing your weight down to 190 pounds. While this weight may still be in the "overweight" or "obese" range, this modest weight loss can decrease your risk factors for chronic diseases related to obesity.

So even if the overall goal seems large, see it as a journey rather than just a final destination. You will learn new eating and physical activity habits that will help you live a healthier lifestyle. These habits may help you maintain your weight loss over time.

For example, the National Weight Control Registry (NWCR) noted that study participants who maintained a significant weight loss reported improvements in physical health as well as energy levels, physical mobility, general mood, and self-confidence.

Section 37.2 | Eating for a Healthy Weight

This section includes text excerpted from "Healthy Eating for a Healthy Weight," Centers for Disease Control and Prevention (CDC), April 19, 2021.

An eating plan that helps manage your weight includes a variety of healthy foods. Add an array of colors to your plate and think of it as eating the rainbow. Dark, leafy greens, oranges, and tomatoes – even fresh herbs – are loaded with vitamins, fiber, and minerals. Adding frozen peppers, broccoli, or onions to stews and omelets gives them a quick and convenient boost of color and nutrients.

According to the *Dietary Guidelines for Americans 2020–2025*, a healthy eating plan:

- Emphasizes fruits, vegetables, whole grains, and fat-free or low-fat milk and milk products
- Includes a variety of protein foods such as seafood, lean meats and poultry, eggs, legumes (beans and peas), soy products, nuts, and seeds
- Is low in saturated fats, *trans* fats, cholesterol, salt (sodium), and added sugars
- Stays within your daily calorie needs

The USDA's MyPlate Plan can help you identify what and how much to eat from the different food groups while staying within your recommended calorie allowance.

FRUITS

Fresh, frozen, or canned fruits are great choices. Try fruits beyond apples and bananas such as mango, pineapple or kiwi fruit. When fresh fruit is not in season, try a frozen, canned, or dried variety. Be aware that dried and canned fruit may contain added sugars or syrups. Choose canned varieties of fruit packed in water or in its own juice.

VEGETABLES

Add variety to grilled or steamed vegetables with an herb such as rosemary. You can also sauté (pan fry) vegetables in a nonstick pan with a small amount of cooking spray or try frozen or canned vegetables for a quick side dish – just microwave and serve. Look for canned vegetables without added salt, butter, or cream sauces. For variety, try a new vegetable each week.

CALCIUM-RICH FOODS

In addition to fat-free and low-fat milk, consider low-fat and fat-free yogurts without added sugars. These come in a variety of flavors and can be a great dessert substitute.

MEATS

If your favorite recipe calls for frying fish or breaded chicken, try healthier variations by baking or grilling. Maybe even try dry beans in place of meats. Ask friends and search the Internet and magazines for recipes with fewer calories? You might be surprised to find you have a new favorite dish!

COMFORT FOODS

Healthy eating is all about balance. You can enjoy your favorite foods, even if they are high in calories, fat, or added sugars. The key is eating them only once in a while and balancing them with healthier foods and more physical activity.

Some general tips for comfort foods:

- **Eat them less often.** If you normally eat these foods every day, cut back to once a week or once a month.
- **Eat smaller amounts.** If your favorite higher-calorie food is a chocolate bar, have a smaller size or only half a bar.
- **Try a lower-calorie version.** Use lower-calorie ingredients or prepare food differently. For example, if your macaroni and cheese recipe includes whole milk, butter, and full-fat cheese, try remaking it with nonfat milk, less butter, low-fat cheese, fresh spinach, and tomatoes. Just remember to not increase your portion size.

Section 37.3 | Improving Your Eating Habits

This section includes text excerpted from "Improving Your Eating Habits," Centers for Disease Control and Prevention (CDC), August 17, 2020.

When it comes to eating, we have strong habits. Some are good ("I always eat breakfast"), and some are not so good ("I always clean my plate"). Although many of our eating habits were established during childhood, it does not mean it is too late to change them.

Making sudden, radical changes to eating habits such as eating nothing but cabbage soup, can lead to short-term weight loss. However, such radical changes are neither healthy nor a good idea, and will not be successful in the long run. Permanently improving your eating habits requires a thoughtful approach in which you reflect, replace, and reinforce.

- Reflect on all of your specific eating habits, both bad and good; and, your common triggers for unhealthy eating.
- Replace your unhealthy eating habits with healthier ones.
- Reinforce your new, healthier eating habits.

REFLECT

- Create a list of your eating habits. Keep a food diary for a few days. Write down everything you eat and the time of day you eat it. This will help you uncover your habits. For example, you might discover that you always seek a sweet snack to get you through the mid-afternoon energy slump. It is good to note how you were feeling when you decided to eat, especially if you were eating when not hungry. Were you tired? Stressed out?
- Highlight the habits on your list that may be leading you to overeat. Common eating habits that can lead to weight gain are:
  - Eating too fast
  - Always cleaning your plate
  - Eating when not hungry

  - Eating while standing up (may lead to eating mindlessly or too quickly)
  - Always eating dessert
  - Skipping meals (or maybe just breakfast)
- Look at the unhealthy eating habits you have highlighted. Be sure you have identified all the triggers that cause you to engage in those habits. Identify a few you would like to work on improving first. Do not forget to pat yourself on the back for the things you are doing right. Maybe you usually eat fruit for dessert, or you drink low-fat or fat-free milk. These are good habits! Recognizing your successes will help encourage you to make more changes.
- Create a list of "cues" by reviewing your food diary to become more aware of when and where you are "triggered" to eat for reasons other than hunger. Note how you are typically feeling at those times. Often an environmental "cue," or a particular emotional state, is what encourages eating for nonhunger reasons.
- Common triggers for eating when not hungry are:
- Opening up the cabinet and seeing your favorite snack food
- Sitting at home watching television
- Before or after a stressful meeting or situation at work
- Coming home after work and having no idea what is for dinner
- Having someone offer you a dish they made "just for you!"
- Walking past a candy dish on the counter
- Sitting in the break room beside the vending machine
- Seeing a plate of doughnuts at the morning staff meeting.
- Swinging through your favorite drive-through every morning.
- Feeling bored or tired and thinking food might offer a pick-me-up.
- Circle the "cues" on your list that you face on a daily or weekly basis. While the Thanksgiving holiday may be a trigger to overeat, for now focus on cues you face more often. Eventually, you want a plan for as many eating cues as you can.

- Ask yourself these questions for each "cue" you have circled:
- Is there anything I can do to avoid the cue or situation? This option works best for cues that do not involve others. For example, could you choose a different route to work to avoid stopping at a fast-food restaurant on the way? Is there another place in the break room where you can sit so you are not next to the vending machine?
- For things I cannot avoid, can I do something differently that would be healthier? Obviously, you cannot avoid all situations that trigger your unhealthy eating habits, such as staff meetings at work. In these situations, evaluate your options. Could you suggest or bring healthier snacks or beverages? Could you offer to take notes to distract your attention? Could you sit farther away from the food so it will not be as easy to grab something? Could you plan ahead and eat a healthy snack before the meeting?

REPLACE

- Replace unhealthy habits with new, healthy ones. For example, in reflecting upon your eating habits, you may realize that you eat too fast when you eat alone. So, make a commitment to share a lunch each week with a colleague, or have a neighbor over for dinner one night a week. Another strategy is to put your fork down between bites. Also, minimize distractions, such as watching the news while you eat. Such distractions keep you from paying attention to how quickly and how much you are eating.
- Eat more slowly. If you eat too quickly, you may "clean your plate" instead of paying attention to whether your hunger is satisfied.
- Eat only when you are truly hungry instead of when you are tired, anxious, or feeling an emotion besides hunger. If you find yourself eating when you are experiencing an emotion besides hunger, such as boredom or anxiety, try to find a noneating activity to do instead. You may find a quick walk or phone call with a friend helps you feel better.

- Plan meals ahead of time to ensure that you eat a healthy well-balanced meal.

REINFORCE

Reinforce your new, healthy habits and be patient with yourself. Habits take time to develop. It does not happen overnight. When you do find yourself engaging in an unhealthy habit, stop as quickly as possible and ask yourself: Why do I do this? When did I start doing this? What changes do I need to make? Be careful not to berate yourself or think that one mistake "blows" a whole day's worth of healthy habits. You can do it! It just takes one day at a time!

Section 37.4 | **How to Cut Calories from Your Diet**

This section includes text excerpted from "Cutting Calories," Centers for Disease Control and Prevention (CDC), August 17, 2020.

GETTING STARTED WITH CALORIE CUTTING

Once you start looking, you can find ways to cut calories for your meals, snacks, and even beverages. Here are some examples to get you started.

Eat More, Weigh Less?

Eating fewer calories does not necessarily mean eating less food. To be able to cut calories without eating less and feeling hungry, you need to replace some higher-calorie foods with foods that are lower in calories and fill you up. In general, these foods contain a lot of water and are high in fiber.

Rethink Your Drink

Most people try to reduce their calorie intake by focusing on food, but another way to cut calories may be to change what you drink. You may find that you are consuming quite a few calories just in the beverages you have each day. Find out how you can make better drink choices to reduce your calorie intake.

How to Avoid Portion Size Pitfalls to Help Manage Your Weight

You may find that your portion sizes are leading you to eat more calories than you realize. Research shows that people unintentionally consume more calories when faced with larger portions. This can mean excessive calorie intake, especially when eating high-calorie foods.

How to Use Fruits and Vegetables to Help Manage Your Weight

Learn about fruits and vegetables and their role in your weight management plan. Tips to cut calories by substituting fruits and vegetables are included with meal-by-meal examples. You will also find snack ideas that are 100 calories or less. With these helpful tips, you will soon be on your way to adding more fruits and vegetables into your healthy eating plan.

Table 37.1. Ideas for Every Meal

Breakfast	**Substitution**	**Calories Reduced by**
Top your cereal with low-fat or fat-free milk instead of 2% or whole milk.	1 cup of fat-free milk instead of 1 cup of whole milk	63
Use a nonstick pan and cooking spray (rather than butter) to scramble or fry eggs.	1 spray of cooking spray instead of 1 pat of butter	34
Choose reduced-calorie margarine spread for toast rather than butter or stick margarine.	2 pats of reduced-calorie margarine instead of 2 pats of butter	36
Lunch	**Substitution**	**Calories Reduced by**
Add more vegetables such as cucumbers, lettuce, tomato, and onions to a sandwich instead of extra meat or cheese.	2 slices of tomatoes, ¼ cup of sliced cucumbers, and 2 slices of onions instead of an extra slice (3/4 ounce) of cheese and 2 slices (1 ounce) of ham	154

Table 37.1. Continued

Breakfast	**Substitution**	**Calories Reduced by**
Accompany a sandwich with salad or fruit instead of chips or French fries.	½ cup diced raw pineapple instead of 1-ounce bag of potato chips	118
Choose vegetable-based broth soups rather than cream- or meat-based soups.	1 cup of vegetable soup instead of 1 cup cream of chicken soup	45
When eating a salad, dip your fork into dressing instead of pouring lots of dressing on the salad.	½ tbsp. of regular ranch salad dressing instead of 2 TBSP of regular ranch dressing	109
When eating out, substitute a broth-based soup or a green lettuce salad for French fries or chips as a side dish.	A side salad with a packet of low-fat vinaigrette dressing instead of a medium order of French fries	270
Dinner	**Substitution**	**Calories Reduced by**
Have steamed or grilled vegetables rather than those sautéed in butter or oil. Try lemon juice and herbs to flavor the vegetables. You can also sauté with nonstick cooking spray.	½ cup steamed broccoli instead of ½ cup broccoli sautéed in 1/2 tbsp. of vegetable oil.	62
Modify recipes to reduce the amount of fat and calories. For example, when making lasagna, use part-skim ricotta cheese instead of whole-milk ricotta cheese. Substitute shredded vegetables, such as carrots, zucchini, and spinach for some of the ground meat in lasagna.	1 cup of part-skim ricotta cheese instead of 1 cup whole milk ricotta cheese	89
When eating out, have a cocktail or dessert instead of both during the same eating occasion.	Choosing one or the other saves you calories. A 12-ounce beer has about 153 calories. A slice of apple pie (1/6 of an 8" pie) has 277 calories.	153 if you have the apple pie without the drink 277 if you have a drink and no pie.

Table 37.1. Continued

Breakfast	Substitution	Calories Reduced by
When having pizza, choose vegetables as toppings and just a light sprinkling of cheese instead of fatty meats.	One slice of a cheese pizza instead of one slice of a meat and cheese pizza	60
Snacks	**Substitution**	**Calories Reduced by**
Choose air-popped popcorn instead of oil-popped popcorn and dry-roasted instead of oil-roasted nuts.	3 cups of air-popped popcorn instead of 3 cups of oil-popped popcorn	73
Avoid the vending machine by packing your own healthful snacks to bring to work. For example, consider vegetable sticks, fresh fruit, low fat or nonfat yogurt without added sugars, or a small handful of dry-roasted nuts.	An eight-ounce container of no sugar added nonfat yogurt instead of a package of 6 peanut butter crackers	82
Choose sparkling water instead of sweetened drinks or alcoholic beverages.	A bottle of carbonated water instead of a 12-ounce can of soda with sugar	136
Instead of cookies or other sweet snacks, have some fruit for a snack.	One large orange instead of 3 chocolate sandwich cookies	54

Section 37.5 | **Keeping It Off: Maintaining Weight Loss**

This section includes text excerpted from "Keeping It Off," Centers for Disease Control and Prevention (CDC), May 15, 2015. Reviewed May 2021.

If you have recently lost excess weight, congratulations! It is an accomplishment that will likely benefit your health now and in the future. Now that you have lost weight, let us talk about some ways to maintain that success. The following tips are some of the common characteristics among people who have successfully lost weight and maintained that loss over time.

WATCH YOUR DIET

- **Follow a healthy and realistic eating pattern.** You have embarked on a healthier lifestyle, now the challenge is maintaining the positive eating habits you have developed along the way. In studies of people who have lost weight and kept it off for at least a year, most continued to eat a diet lower in calories as compared to their preweight loss diet.
- **Keep your eating patterns consistent.** Follow a healthy eating pattern regardless of changes in your routine. Plan ahead for weekends, vacations, and special occasions. By making a plan, it is more likely you will have healthy foods on hand for when your routine changes.
- **Eat breakfast every day.** Eating breakfast is a common trait among people who have lost weight and kept it off. Eating a healthful breakfast may help you avoid getting "over-hungry" and then overeating later in the day.

BE ACTIVE

Get daily physical activity. People who have lost weight and kept it off typically engage in 60 to 90 minutes of moderate-intensity physical activity most days of the week while not exceeding calorie needs. This does not necessarily mean 60 to 90 minutes at one time. It might mean 20 to 30 minutes of physical activity three times a day. For example, a brisk walk in the morning, at lunchtime, and in the evening. Some people may need to talk to their healthcare provider before participating in this level of physical activity.

STAY ON COURSE

- Monitor your diet and activity. Keeping a food and physical activity journal can help you track your progress and spot trends. For example, you might notice that your weight creeps up during periods when you have a lot of business travel or when you have to work overtime. Recognizing this tendency can be a signal to try different behaviors, such as packing your own healthful food for

the plane and making time to use your hotel's exercise facility when you are traveling. Or if working overtime, maybe you can use your breaks for quick walks around the building.
- Monitor your weight. Check your weight regularly. When managing your weight loss, it is a good idea to keep track of your weight so you can plan accordingly and adjust your diet and exercise plan as necessary. If you have gained a few pounds, get back on track quickly.
- Get support from family, friends, and others. People who have successfully lost weight and kept it off often rely on support from others to help them stay on course and get over any "bumps." Sometimes having a friend or partner who is also losing weight or maintaining a weight loss can help you stay motivated.

Section 37.6 | **Why Weight Cycling Is Bad for Health**

Weight cycling is the process of losing weight for a short period and regaining it soon after. It is also called "yo-yo dieting" as the individual's weight fluctuates multiple times. It occurs as a result of extreme dieting that involves restrictive methods. During this process, the individual loses and gains almost the same amount of weight numerous times. It affects regular body functions and hormone regulation, which can lead to severe health disorders. Continued weight cycling may hamper the body's metabolism and make weight loss harder in the future. People involved in weight cycling are 40 percent more likely to suffer a heart attack or stroke. According to a 1998 study by the *Journal of Nutrition Reviews* and a 2009 study by the *International Journal of Exercise Science*, around 30 percent of women and 10 percent of men have experienced weight cycling, respectively.

Weight gain occurs when the energy from food intake in the form of calories is more than what is expended by any form of physical activity or body metabolism. Unchecked weight gain can lead to obesity and other associated health risks such as hypertension, diabetes, and cardiovascular ailments. Weight loss is the loss of body mass that results from physical exertion and nutritional changes. Weight loss from malnutrition can cause issues such as:

- Reduced immunity
- Decreased muscle strength
- Irregular periods in women
- Reduced thermoregulation (the innate ability of the human body to maintain an optimum core temperature)

It is crucial to maintain proper body weight through balanced nutrition and physical exercise to avoid obesity or malnutrition. Maintaining a healthy body weight can help avert life-threatening conditions in the future.

WEIGHT CYCLING AND HEALTH

The process of weight cycling affects the individual's mental and physical health. It leads to unsustainable weight loss/gain due to its strict diets and other inconsistencies, such as an unregulated exercise regime. Weight cycling is an erratic approach to weight loss as it does not follow a comprehensive plan. It causes stress and adapts the body to unhealthy routines leading to health problems such as:

- **Increased blood pressure.** Weight gain during weight cycling can cause an increase in blood pressure. It can also affect blood pressure levels negatively for an extended period.
- A heightened sense of frustration occurs due to erratic eating habits and extremely restrictive portion sizes. After experiencing a period of weight loss in weight cycling, sudden weight gain can cause frustration about an individual's health and life choices.
- **Higher risk of heart disease.** Weight cycling increases coronary heart disease risk, which is primarily caused

by the narrowing of arteries due to a buildup of plaque. Sudden weight gain has a higher potential to cause heart disease than being constantly overweight.

- Fatty liver caused by weight gain is one of the health risks of weight cycling as, during weight gain, the liver tends to store excess fat cells, which affect the metabolism of fat cells and sugar in the body. It can also lead to type 2 diabetes and, in severe cases, cirrhosis or chronic liver failure.
- **Muscle loss.** As a part of weight loss, the body loses muscle and fat but losing weight continuously can reduce the body's muscle mass. This reduced muscle mass can cause muscle weakness thereby leading to physical strain, reduced movement, and decreased strength. A considerable amount of protein intake is required to balance the body's high protein requirement during weight loss to avoid such conditions.
- Increased percentage of body fat is a common side effect of weight gain. Body fat stored in the belly area can cause reduced insulin levels leading to diabetic conditions.
- **Leptin imbalance.** The leptin hormone is decreased when the fat level in the body is reduced. This hormone provides a sensation of feeling full and thereby reducing intake. With weight loss, leptin decreases, leading to an increase in appetite, which can lead to unhealthy indulgences in food intake.

References

1. Scott. R, Jennifer. "Why Weight Cycling Is Bad for Your Health," Verywell Fit, January 7, 2020.
2. Thorpe, Matthew, MD, Ph.D. "10 Solid Reasons Why Yo-Yo Dieting Is Bad for You," Healthline, May 29, 2017.
3. Daller, John. A, MD. "Weight Cycling, Facts about Yo-Yo Dieting," OnHealth, WebMD, June 22, 2016.

Chapter 38 | Weight Loss and Nutrition Myths

Are you overwhelmed by daily decisions about what to eat, how much to eat, when to eat, and how much physical activity you need to be healthy? If so, do not be discouraged because you are not alone. With so many choices and decisions, it can be hard to know what to do and which information you can trust.

This chapter may help you make changes in your daily eating and physical activity habits so that you improve your well-being and reach or maintain a healthy weight.

FOOD MYTHS

Myth. To lose weight, you have to give up all your favorite foods.

Fact. You do not have to give up all your favorite foods when you are trying to lose weight. Small amounts of your favorite high-calorie foods may be part of your weight-loss plan. Just remember to keep track of the total calories you take in. To lose weight, you must burn more calories than you take in through food and beverages.

Tip. Limiting foods that are high in calories may help you lose weight.

Myth. Grain products such as bread, pasta, and rice are fattening. You should avoid them when trying to lose weight.

Fact. Grains themselves are not necessarily fattening – or unhealthy – although substituting whole grains for refined-grain products is healthier and may help you feel fuller. At least half of the grains you eat should be whole grains. Examples of whole

This chapter includes text excerpted from "Some Myths about Nutrition and Physical Activity," National Institute of Diabetes and Digestive and Kidney Diseases (NIDDK), April 2017. Reviewed May 2021.

grains include brown rice and whole-wheat bread, cereal, and pasta. Whole grains provide iron, fiber, and other important nutrients.

Tip. Try to replace refined or white bread with whole-wheat bread and refined pasta with whole-wheat pasta. Or add whole grains to mixed dishes, such as brown instead of white rice to stir fry.

Myth. Choosing foods that are gluten free will help you eat healthier.

Fact. Gluten-free foods are not healthier if you do not have celiac disease or are not sensitive to gluten. Gluten is a protein found in wheat, barley, and rye grains. A healthcare professional is likely to prescribe a gluten-free eating plan to treat people who have celiac disease or are sensitive to gluten. If you do not have these health problems but avoid gluten anyway, you may not get the vitamins, fiber, and minerals you need. A gluten-free diet is not a weight-loss diet and is not intended to help you lose weight.

Tip. Before you decide to avoid a whole food group, talk with your healthcare professional if you believe you have problems after you consume foods or drinks with wheat, barley, or rye.

Myth. You should avoid all fats if you are trying to be healthy or lose weight.

Fact. You do not have to avoid all fats if you are trying to improve your health or lose weight. Fat provides essential nutrients and should be an important part of a healthy eating plan. But because fats have more calories per gram than protein or carbohydrates, or "carbs," you need to limit fats to avoid extra calories. If you are trying to lose weight, consider eating small amounts of food with healthy fats, such as avocados, olives, or nuts. You also could replace whole-fat cheese or milk with lower-fat versions.

Tip. The *Dietary Guidelines for Americans 2015-2020* recommend consuming less than 10 percent of your daily calories from saturated fats. Try cutting back on solid-fat foods. Use olive oil instead of butter in cooking.

Myth. Dairy products are fattening and unhealthy.

Fact. Dairy products are an important food group because they have protein your body needs to build muscles and help organs work well, and calcium to strengthen bones. Most dairy products, such as milk and some yogurts, have added vitamin D to help your body use calcium, since many Americans do not get enough of these nutrients. Dairy products made from fat-free or low-fat milk have fewer calories than dairy products made from whole milk.

Tip. Adults should have three servings a day of fat-free or low-fat dairy products, including milk or milk products such as yogurt and cheese, or fortified soy beverages, as part of a healthy eating plan. If you cannot digest lactose, the sugar found in dairy products, choose fortified soy products, lactose-free or low lactose dairy products, or other foods and beverages with calcium and vitamin D:

- Calcium – soy-based beverages or tofu made with calcium sulfate, canned salmon, or dark leafy greens such as collards or kale
- Vitamin D – cereals or soy-based beverages

Myth. "Going vegetarian" will help you lose weight and be healthier.

Fact. Some research shows that a healthy vegetarian eating plan or one made up of foods that come mostly from plants, may be linked to lower levels of obesity, lower blood pressure, and a reduced risk of heart disease. But, going vegetarian will only lead to weight loss if you reduce the total number of calories you take in. Some vegetarians may make food choices that could lead to weight gain, such as eating a lot of food high in sugar, fats, and calories.

Eating small amounts of lean meats can also be part of a healthy plan to lose or maintain weight.

Tip. If you choose to follow a vegetarian eating plan, be sure you get enough of the nutrients your body needs to be healthy.

Chapter 39 | **Diet Pills and Supplements for Weight Loss Explained**

Chapter Contents

Section 39.1 | Dietary Supplements for Weight Loss

This section includes text excerpted from "Dietary Supplements for Weight Loss: Fact Sheet for Consumers," Office of Dietary Supplements (ODS), National Institutes of Health (NIH), March 22, 2021.

WHAT ARE WEIGHT-LOSS DIETARY SUPPLEMENTS AND WHAT DO THEY DO?

The proven ways to lose weight are eating healthful foods, cutting calories, and being physically active. But, making these lifestyle changes is not easy, so you might wonder if taking a dietary supplement that is promoted for weight loss might help.

This section describes what is known about the safety and effectiveness of many ingredients that are commonly used in weight-loss dietary supplements. Sellers of these supplements might claim that their products help you lose weight by blocking the absorption of fat or carbohydrates, curbing your appetite, or speeding up your metabolism. But, there is little scientific evidence that weight-loss supplements work. Many are expensive, some can interact or interfere with medications, and a few might be harmful.

If you are thinking about taking a dietary supplement to lose weight, talk with your healthcare provider. This is especially important if you have high blood pressure, diabetes, heart disease, liver disease, or other medical conditions.

WHAT ARE THE INGREDIENTS IN WEIGHT-LOSS DIETARY SUPPLEMENTS?

Weight-loss supplements contain many ingredients – such as herbs, fiber, and minerals – in different amounts and in many combinations. Sold in forms such as capsules, tablets, liquids, and powders, some products have dozens of ingredients.

Common ingredients in weight-loss supplements are described below in alphabetical order. You will learn what is known about whether each ingredient works and is safe. Figuring out whether these ingredients really help you lose weight safely is complicated, though. Most products contain more than one ingredient, and ingredients can work differently when they are mixed together.

You might be surprised to learn that makers of weight-loss supplements rarely carry out studies in people to find out whether their product works and is safe. And when studies are done, they usually involve only small numbers of people who take the supplement for just a few weeks or months. To know whether a weight-loss supplement can help people lose weight safely and keep it off, larger groups of people need to be studied for a longer time.

HOW ARE WEIGHT-LOSS DIETARY SUPPLEMENTS REGULATED?

The FDA is the federal agency that oversees dietary supplements in the United States. Unlike over-the-counter and prescription drugs – which must be approved by the FDA before they can be sold – dietary supplements do not require review or approval by the FDA before they are put on the market. Also, manufacturers do not have to provide evidence to the FDA that their products are safe or effective before selling these products.

When the FDA finds an unsafe dietary supplement, it can remove the supplement from the market or ask the supplement maker to recall it. The FDA and the Federal Trade Commission can also take enforcement action against companies that make false weight-loss claims about their supplements; add pharmaceutical drugs to their supplements; or claim that their supplements can diagnose, treat, cure, or prevent disease.

CAN WEIGHT-LOSS DIETARY SUPPLEMENTS BE HARMFUL?

Weight-loss supplements, like all dietary supplements, can have harmful side effects and might interact with prescription and over-the-counter medications. Many weight-loss supplements have ingredients that have not been tested in combination with one another, and their combined effects are unknown.

Tell your healthcare providers about any weight-loss supplements or other supplements you take. This information will help them work with you to prevent supplement-drug interactions, harmful side effects, and other risks.

Table 39.1. Common Ingredients in Weight-Loss Dietary Supplements

Ingredient	Does It Work?	Is It Safe?
African mango African mango seed extract is claimed to curb the formation of fat tissue.	African mango might help you lose a very small amount of weight.	African mango seems to be safe, but its safety has not been well studied. It can cause headache, sleeping problems, flatulence, and gas.
Beta-glucans Beta-glucans are soluble dietary fibers in bacteria, yeasts, fungi, oats, and barley. They might slow down the time it takes for food to travel through your digestive system, making you feel fuller.	Beta-glucans do not seem to have any effect on body weight.	Beta-glucans seem to be safe (at up to 10 grams [g] a day for 12 weeks). They can cause flatulence.
Bitter orange Bitter orange contains synephrine (a stimulant). It is claimed to burn calories, increase fat breakdown, and decrease appetite. Products with bitter orange usually also contain caffeine and other ingredients. Bitter orange is in some weight-loss dietary supplements that used to contain ephedra, another stimulant-containing herb that was banned from the U.S. market in 2004.	Bitter orange might slightly increase the number of calories you burn. It might also reduce your appetite a little, but whether it can help you lose weight is unknown.	Bitter orange might not be safe. Supplements with bitter orange can cause chest pain, anxiety, headache, muscle and bone pain, a faster heart rate, and higher blood pressure.

Table 39.1. Continued

Ingredient	Does It Work?	Is It Safe?
Caffeine Caffeine is a stimulant that can make you more alert, give you a boost of energy, burn calories, and increase fat breakdown. Often added to weight-loss dietary supplements, caffeine is found naturally in tea, guarana, kola (cola) nut, yerba mate, and other herbs. The labels of supplements that contain caffeine do not always list it, so you might not know if a supplement has caffeine.	Weight-loss dietary supplements with caffeine might help you lose a little weight or gain less weight over time. But, when you use caffeine regularly, you become tolerant of it. This tolerance might lessen any effect of caffeine on body weight over time.	Caffeine is safe for most adults at doses up to 400–500 milligrams (mg) a day. But, it can make you feel nervous, jittery, and shaky. It can also affect your sleep. At higher doses, it can cause nausea, vomiting, rapid heartbeat, and seizures. Combining caffeine with other stimulant ingredients can increase caffeine's effects.
Calcium Calcium is a mineral you need for healthy bones, muscles, nerves, blood vessels, and many of your body's functions. It is claimed to burn fat and decrease fat absorption.	Calcium – either from food or in weight-loss dietary supplements probably does not help you lose weight or prevent weight gain.	Calcium is safe at the recommended amounts of 1,000 to 1,200 mg a day for adults. Too much calcium (more than 2,000–2,500 mg a day) can cause constipation and decrease your body's absorption of iron and zinc. Also, too much calcium from supplements (but not foods) might increase your risk of kidney stones.

Table 39.1. Continued

Ingredient	Does It Work?	Is It Safe?
Capsaicin Capsaicin comes from chili peppers and makes them taste hot. It is claimed to help burn fat and calories and to help you feel full and eat less.	Capsaicin has not been studied enough to know if it will help you lose weight.	Capsaicin is safe (at up to 33 mg a day for 4 weeks or 4 mg a day for 12 weeks), but it can cause stomach pain, burning sensations, nausea, and bloating.
Carnitine Your body makes carnitine, and it is also found in meat, fish, poultry, milk, and dairy products. In your cells, it helps break down fats.	Carnitine supplements might help you lose a small amount of weight.	Carnitine supplements seem to be safe (at up to 2 g a day for 1 year or 4 g a day for 56 days). They can cause nausea, vomiting, diarrhea, abdominal cramps, and a fishy body odor.
Chitosan Chitosan comes from the shells of crabs, shrimp, and lobsters. It is claimed to bind fat in the digestive tract so that your body cannot absorb it.	Chitosan binds only a tiny amount of fat, not enough to help you lose much weight.	Chitosan seems to be safe (at up to 15 g a day for 6 months). But, it can cause flatulence, bloating, mild nausea, constipation, indigestion, and heartburn. If you are allergic to shellfish, you could have an allergic reaction to chitosan.

Table 39.1. Continued

Ingredient	Does It Work?	Is It Safe?
Chromium Chromium is a mineral that you need to regulate your blood sugar levels. It is claimed to increase muscle mass and fat loss and decrease appetite and food intake.	Chromium might help you lose a very small amount of weight and body fat.	Chromium in food and supplements is safe at recommended amounts, which range from 20 to 45 micrograms a day for adults. In larger amounts, chromium can cause watery stools, headache, weakness, nausea, vomiting, constipation, dizziness, and hives.
Coleus forskohlii *Coleus forskohlii* is a plant that grows in India, Thailand, and other subtropical areas. Forskolin, made from the plant's roots, is claimed to help you lose weight by decreasing your appetite and increasing the breakdown of fat in your body.	Forskolin has not been studied much. But, so far, it does not seem to have any effect on body weight or appetite.	Forskolin seems to be safe (at 500 mg a day for 12 weeks), but it has not been well studied. It can cause frequent bowel movements and loose stools.
Conjugated linoleic acid (CLA) CLA is a fat found mainly in dairy products and beef. It is claimed to reduce your body fat.	CLA may help you lose a very small amount of weight and body fat.	CLA seems to be safe (at up to 6 g a day for 1 year). It can cause an upset stomach, constipation, diarrhea, loose stools, and indigestion.
Fucoxanthin Fucoxanthin comes from brown seaweed and other algae. It is claimed to help with weight loss by burning calories and decreasing fat.	Fucoxanthin has not been studied enough to know if it will help you lose weight. Only one study in people included fucoxanthin (the other studies were in animals).	Fucoxanthin seems to be safe (at 2.4 mg a day for 16 weeks), but it has not been studied enough to know for sure.

Table 39.1. Continued

Ingredient	Does It Work?	Is It Safe?
Garcinia cambogia *Garcinia cambogia* is a tree that grows throughout Asia, Africa, and the Polynesian islands. Hydroxycitric acid in the fruit is claimed to decrease the number of new fat cells your body makes, suppress your appetite and thus reduce the amount of food you eat, and limit the amount of weight you gain.	*Garcinia cambogia* has little to no effect on weight loss.	*Garcinia cambogia* seems to be fairly safe. But, it can cause headache, nausea, and symptoms in the upper respiratory tract, stomach, and intestines.
Glucomannan Glucomannan is a soluble dietary fiber from the root of the konjac plant. It is claimed to absorb water in the gut to help you feel full.	Glucomannan has little to no effect on weight loss. But, it might help lower total cholesterol, LDL ("bad") cholesterol, triglycerides, and blood sugar levels.	Most forms of glucomannan seem to be safe (at up to 15.1 g a day for several weeks in a powder or capsule form). It can cause loose stools, flatulence, diarrhea, constipation, and abdominal discomfort.
Green coffee bean extract Green coffee beans are unroasted coffee beans. Green coffee bean extract is claimed to decrease fat accumulation and help convert blood sugar into energy that your cells can use.	Green coffee bean extract might help you lose a small amount of weight.	Green coffee bean extract seems to be safe (at up to 200 mg a day for 12 weeks). It might cause headache and urinary tract infections. Green coffee beans contain the stimulant caffeine, which can cause problems at high doses or when it is combined with other stimulants (see the section on Caffeine).

Table 39.1. Continued

Ingredient	Does It Work?	Is It Safe?
Green tea and green tea extract Green tea (also called "*Camellia sinensis*") is a common beverage all over the world. Green tea and green tea extract in some weight-loss supplements are claimed to reduce body weight by increasing the calories your body burns, breaking down fat cells, and decreasing fat absorption and the amount of new fat your body makes.	Green tea might help you lose a small amount of weight.	Drinking green tea is safe, but taking green tea extract might not be. Green tea extract can cause constipation, abdominal discomfort, nausea, and increased blood pressure. In some people, it has been linked to liver damage.
Guar gum Guar gum is a soluble dietary fiber in some dietary supplements and food products. It is claimed to make you feel full, lower your appetite, and decrease the amount of food you eat.	Guar gum probably does not help you lose weight.	Guar gum seems to be safe (at up to 30 g a day for 6 months) when it is taken with enough fluid. But, it can cause abdominal pain, flatulence, diarrhea, nausea, and cramps.
Hoodia Hoodia is a plant from southern Africa, where it is used as an appetite suppressant.	There has not been much research on hoodia, but it probably will not help you eat less or lose weight. Analyses showed that some "hoodia" supplements sold in the past contained very little hoodia or none at all. It is not known whether this is true of hoodia supplements sold today.	Hoodia might not be safe. It can cause rapid heart rate, increased blood pressure, headache, dizziness, nausea, and vomiting.
Probiotics Probiotics are microorganisms in foods, such as some yogurts, and some dietary supplements that help maintain or restore beneficial bacteria in your digestive tract.	It is unclear whether probiotic supplements have any effect on weight or body fat.	Probiotics are safe in healthy people but may cause gas or other gastrointestinal problems.

Table 39.1. Continued

Ingredient	Does It Work?	Is It Safe?
Pyruvate Pyruvate is naturally present in your body. Pyruvate in weight-loss supplements is claimed to increase fat breakdown, reduce body weight and body fat, and improve exercise performance.	Pyruvate in supplements might help you lose a small amount of weight.	Pyruvate seems to be safe (at up to 30 g a day for 6 weeks). It can cause diarrhea, gas, bloating, and rumbling noises in the intestines due to gas.
Raspberry ketone Raspberry ketone, found in red raspberries, is claimed to be a "fat burner."	Raspberry ketone has only been studied as a weight-loss aid in combination with other ingredients and not alone. Its effects on body weight are unknown.	Raspberry ketone has not been studied enough to tell if it is safe.
Vitamin D Your body needs vitamin D for good health and strong bones. People who are obese tend to have lower levels of vitamin D, but there is no known reason why taking vitamin D would help people lose weight.	Vitamin D does not help you lose weight.	Vitamin D from foods and dietary supplements is safe at the recommended amounts of 600?800 IU a day for adults. Too much vitamin D (more than 4,000 IU a day) can be toxic and cause nausea, vomiting, poor appetite, constipation, weakness, and irregular heartbeat.
White kidney bean/bean pod White kidney bean or bean pod (also called "*Phaseolus vulgaris*") is a legume grown around the world. An extract of this bean is claimed to block the absorption of carbohydrates and suppress your appetite.	*Phaseolus vulgaris* extract might help you lose a small amount of weight and body fat.	*Phaseolus vulgaris* seems to be safe (at up to 3,000 mg a day for 12 weeks). But, it might cause headaches, soft stools, flatulence, and constipation.

Table 39.1. Continued

Ingredient	Does It Work?	Is It Safe?
Yohimbe Yohimbe is a West African tree. Yohimbe, which contains a compound called "yohimbine," is an ingredient found in some dietary supplements claiming to increase weight loss, improve libido, increase muscle mass, or treat male sexual dysfunction.	Yohimbe does not help you lose weight.	Yohimbe might not be safe (especially at yohimbine doses of 20 mg or higher). Use it only with guidance from your healthcare provider because the side effects can be severe. Yohimbe can cause headaches, high blood pressure, anxiety, agitation, rapid heartbeat, heart attack, heart failure, and death.

Fraudulent and Adulterated Products

Be very cautious when you see weight-loss supplements with tempting claims, such as "magic diet pill," "melt away fat," and "lose weight without diet or exercise." If the claim sounds too good to be true, it probably is. These products might not help you lose weight – and they could be dangerous.

Weight-loss products marketed as dietary supplements are sometimes adulterated with prescription drugs or controlled substances. These ingredients will not be listed on the product label, and they could harm you.

Interactions with Medications

Like most dietary supplements, some weight-loss supplements can interact or interfere with other medicines or supplements you take. If you take dietary supplements and medications on a regular basis, be sure to talk about this with your healthcare provider.

CHOOSING A SENSIBLE APPROACH TO WEIGHT LOSS

Weight-loss supplements can be expensive, and they might not work. The best way to lose weight and keep it off is to follow a healthy eating pattern, reduce calories, and exercise regularly under the guidance of your healthcare provider.

As a bonus, lifestyle changes that help you lose weight might also improve your mood and energy level and lower your risk of heart disease, diabetes, and some types of cancer.

Section 39.2 | Beware of Miracle Weight-Loss Products

This section contains text excerpted from the following sources: Text beginning with the heading "Tainted Products" is excerpted from "Beware of Products Promising Miracle Weight Loss," U.S. Food and Drug Administration (FDA), January 5, 2015. Reviewed May 2021; Text beginning with the heading "The Truth behind Weight Loss Ads" is excerpted from "The Truth behind Weight Loss Ads," Federal Trade Commission (FTC), August 2019.

TAINTED PRODUCTS

For example, the FDA has found weight-loss products tainted with the prescription drug ingredient sibutramine. This ingredient was in an FDA-approved drug called "Meridia," which was removed from the market in October 2010 because it caused heart problems and strokes.

"We have also found weight-loss products marketed as supplements that contain dangerous concoctions of hidden ingredients including active ingredients contained in approved seizure medications, blood pressure medications, and antidepressants," says Jason Humbert, a senior regulatory manager at the FDA. Most recently, the FDA has found a number of products marketed as dietary supplements containing fluoxetine, the active ingredient found in Prozac, a prescription drug marketed for the treatment of depression and other conditions. Another product contained triamterene, a powerful diuretic sometimes known as "water pills" that can have serious side effects and should only be used under the supervision of a healthcare professional.

Many of these tainted products are imported, sold online, and heavily promoted on social media sites. Some can also be found on store shelves.

And if you are about to take what you think of as "natural" dietary supplements, such as bee pollen or Garcinia cambogia, you should be aware that the FDA has found some of these products also contain hidden active ingredients contained in prescription drugs.

"The only natural way to lose weight is to burn more calories than you take in," says James P. Smith, M.D. That means a combination of healthful eating and physical activity.

DIETARY SUPPLEMENTS ARE NOT FDA-APPROVED

Under the Federal Food, Drug, and Cosmetics Act (as amended by the Dietary Supplement Health and Education Act of 1994), dietary supplement firms do not need the FDA approval prior to marketing their products. It is the company's responsibility to make sure its products are safe and that any claims made about such products are true.

But, just because you see a supplement product on a store shelf does not mean it is safe, Humbert says. The FDA has received numerous reports of harm associated with the use of weight-loss products, including increased blood pressure, heart palpitations (a pounding or racing heart), stroke, seizure, and death. When safety issues are suspected, the FDA must investigate and, when warranted, take steps to have these products removed from the market.

The FDA has issued over 30 public notifications and recalled seven tainted weight-loss products in 2014. The agency also has issued warning letters, seized products, and criminally prosecuted people responsible for marketing these illegal diet products. In addition, the FDA maintains an online list of tainted weight-loss products.

To help people with long-term weight management, the FDA has approved prescription drugs such as Belviq, Qysmia, and Contrave, but these products are intended for people at least 18 years of age who:

- Have a body mass index (BMI, a standard measure of body fat) of 30 or greater (considered obese); or
- Have a BMI of 27 or greater (considered overweight) and have at least one other weight-related health condition.

Moreover, if you are going to embark on any type of weight control campaign, you should talk to your healthcare professional about it first, Smith says.

KNOW THE WARNING SIGNS

Look for potential warning signs of tainted products, such as:

- Promises of a quick fix, for example, "lose 10 pounds in one week"

- Use of the words “guaranteed” or “scientific breakthrough”
- Products marketed in a foreign language
- Products marketed through mass e-mails
- Products marketed as herbal alternatives to an FDA-approved drug or as having effects similar to prescription drugs

ADVICE FROM THE FDA

Generally, if you are using or considering using any product marketed as a dietary supplement, the FDA suggests that you:

- Check with your healthcare professional or a registered dietitian about any nutrients you may need in addition to your regular diet.
- Ask yourself if it sounds too good to be true.
- Be cautious if the claims for the product seem exaggerated or unrealistic.
- Watch out for extreme claims such as “quick and effective” or “totally safe.”
- Be skeptical about anecdotal information from personal “testimonials” about incredible benefits or results from using a product.

THE TRUTH BEHIND WEIGHT LOSS ADS

Would not it be nice if you could lose weight simply by taking a pill, wearing a patch, or rubbing in a cream? Unfortunately, claims that you can lose weight without changing your habits just are not true, and some of these products could even hurt your health. So do not be hooked by ads that woo you with wild promises – or by glowing product reviews and “news articles” that are often fake. All you will lose is money. Doctors, dieticians, and other experts agree: The best way to lose weight is to eat less and exercise more.

FALSE PROMISES IN ADS

Dishonest advertisers will say just about anything to get you to buy their weight-loss products.

Here are some of the (false) promises from weight-loss ads:

- Lose weight without dieting or exercising. (You will not)
- You do not have to watch what you eat to lose weight. (You do)
- If you use this product, you will lose weight permanently. (Wrong)
- To lose weight, all you have to do is take this pill. (Not true)
- You can lose 30 pounds in 30 days. (Nope)
- This product works for everyone. (It does not)
- Lose weight with this patch or cream. (You cannot)

Here is the truth:

- Any promise of miraculous weight loss is simply untrue.
- There is no magic way to lose weight without a sensible diet and regular exercise.
- No product will let you eat all the food you want and still lose weight.
- Permanent weight loss requires permanent lifestyle changes, so do not trust any product that promises once-and-for-all results.
- FDA-approved fat-absorption blockers or appetite suppressants will not result in weight loss on their own; those products are to be taken with a low-calorie, low-fat diet and regular exercise.
- Products promising lightning-fast weight loss are always a scam. Worse, they can ruin your health.
- Even if a product could help some people lose weight in some situations, there is no one-size-fits-all product guaranteed to work for everyone. Everyone's habits and health concerns are unique.

- Nothing you wear or apply to your skin will cause you to lose weight.

FALSE STORIES ONLINE

Dishonest advertisers place false stories online through fake news websites, blogs, banner ads, and social media to sell bogus weight-loss products. This is what they do:

Post false "news" stories. They create so-called news reports online about how an ingredient (such as garcinia cambogia) found in a diet pill is supposedly effective for weight loss.

- Use logos of legitimate news outlets. They place the stolen logos of real news organizations, or they use names and web addresses that look like those of well-known news outlets and websites.
- Feature phony investigations. They say these false stories are "investigations" into the effectiveness of a product, and even add public photos of known reporters to make you think the report is real.
- Pay for positive online reviews. Sometimes they write glowing online reviews themselves or pay others to do so. Sometimes they just cut and paste positive comments from other fake sites.
- Use stock or altered photos. Very often they use images showing a dramatic weight loss, but these images are just stock or altered photographs.

OTHER THINGS TO CONSIDER

"Free" trial offers are often not free at all. Many people who have signed up for "free" trials have wound up paying a lot of money and have been billed for recurring shipments they did not want.

The FDA has found tainted weight-loss products. In recent years, the FDA has discovered hundreds of dietary supplements containing potentially harmful drugs or other chemicals not listed on the product label. Many of these products are for weight loss and bodybuilding.

Using an electronic muscle stimulator alone will not work. You might have seen ads for electronic muscle stimulators claiming they will tone, firm, and strengthen abdominal muscles, help you lose weight, or get rock-hard abs. But, according to the FDA, while these devices may temporarily strengthen, tone, or firm a muscle, they have not been shown to help you lose weight … or get those "six-pack" abs.

Chapter 40 | Popular Fad Diets

The many popular diets and diet plans on the market today can be confusing and overwhelming for consumers to navigate. People who want to lose weight are bombarded with advertisements for various diets all claiming to provide the secret to rapid weight loss with little or no effort. Some of these diets eliminate or restrict various foods, while others focus on including only certain foods. A diet can be considered a fad if it promises to deliver drastic weight loss in a short amount of time, without exercise, and if it is based on an unbalanced approach to nutrition. Many popular fad diets can be organized by type: high protein, low carbohydrate, fasting, food-specific, liquid only, and so on.

HIGH-PROTEIN DIETS

High-protein diets promote an eating plan based largely on foods containing protein, usually meat, eggs, cheese, and other dairy products. The theory behind high-protein diets is that the body must work harder to digest protein, and in doing so, more calories are burned. Studies have found that diets high in protein can cause certain health problems, as the body works to process excess protein. High-protein diets can cause rapid initial weight loss as the body eliminates water while processing extra protein. Typically, any weight lost on a high-protein diet will be regained.

LOW-CARBOHYDRATE DIETS

The main premise of low-carbohydrate diets is the severe restriction of calories from carbohydrates (sugar). Most low-carbohydrate diets suggest replacing foods high in carbohydrates with foods high in protein. In this way, low-carbohydrate diets are similar to high-protein diets. A low-carbohydrate diet is often high in fat. A high-fat diet causes a condition known as "ketosis," which can act as an appetite suppressant. The theory of low-carbohydrate diets is that the suppressed appetite will result in the dieter consuming fewer calories overall. Studies of low-carbohydrate diets have shown that dieters are at risk for health problems including kidney malfunction and heart disease. Many people who follow a low-carbohydrate diet report feeling sluggish and tired, and typically any weight that is lost will be regained.

DETOXIFYING DIETS

Detoxifying diets are often high-fiber diets, and sometimes include increased consumption of fats and oils. The theory of this type of detoxification is that the fiber helps the dieter to feel full, therefore consuming fewer calories throughout the day. It is also believed that a high-fiber diet will cleanse the digestive system through the elimination of more solid waste. Side effects of a high-fiber detoxifying diet often include gastrointestinal distress, bloating, cramps, and dehydration. Studies have shown no permanent weight loss from this type of detoxifying diet.

FASTING DIETS

Fasting diets require dieters to consume nothing but clear liquids for a short period of time, typically one to five days. This is believed to help rid the body of toxins. Fasting can result in temporary weight loss due to consuming far fewer calories than normal, though the weight generally returns once the fast is ended. Fasting produces a host of side effects, including dizziness, lethargy, and feeling weak or tired.

FOOD-SPECIFIC DIETS

Food-specific diets recommend consumption of a single type of food, such as grapefruit, cabbage, or protein shakes. These diets are based on the theory that certain foods have special properties that promote weight loss. Food-specific diets do not provide the range of vitamins, minerals, and other nutrients needed to support bodily functions. If maintained over an extended period of time, the side effects of food-specific diets can be serious.

POPULAR DIET PLANS

The Atkins Diet

The Atkins Diet is a low-carbohydrate, high-protein diet created by Dr. Robert Atkins, an American cardiologist. The main premise of the Atkins Diet is that eating too many carbohydrates causes obesity and other health problems. A diet that is low in carbohydrates produces metabolic activity that results in less hunger and also in weight loss. The Atkins Diet is structured in four phases: induction; weight loss; premaintenance; lifetime maintenance. Dieters move through the four phases at their own pace. Early phases of the Atkins Diet allow consumption of seafood, poultry, meat, eggs, cheese, salad vegetables, oils, butter, and cream. Later phases allow consumption of food, such as nuts, fruits, wine, beans, whole grains, and other vegetables. The Atkins Diet recommends avoidance of certain food, such as fruit, bread, most grains, starchy vegetables, and dairy products other than cheese, cream, and butter. The Atkins Diet may help people feel full longer and may result in weight loss as long as the diet in continued. Side effects may result from consuming low amounts of fiber and certain vitamins and minerals, while consuming larger amounts of saturated fat, cholesterol, and red meat.

The Zone Diet

The Zone Diet was created by Dr. Barry Spears and is based on the genetic evolution of humans. The main premise of the Zone Diet is that humans should maintain a diet similar to that of our ancient hunter-gatherer ancestors. The Zone Diet focuses on lean protein, natural carbohydrates (fruit) and natural fiber (vegetables) while avoiding or eliminating processed carbohydrates, such as grains and products made from grains. The Zone Diet recommends a food plan that is made up of 40 percent natural carbohydrates. 30 percent fat, and 30 percent protein. The emphasis is on food choices, not amount of calories. This percentage should apply to every meal and snack that is eaten. Close evaluation of the Zone Diet has revealed that at its core, the Zone Diet is a very low-calorie eating plan that is lacking in certain nutrients, vitamins, and minerals.

Weight Watchers

Weight Watchers was founded by Jean Nidetch in 1963. The Weight Watchers program focuses on weight loss through diet, exercise, and the use of support networks. Members are given the option of joining a group or following the program online. In either case, educational materials and support are available to assist members. The Weight Watchers support network is considered a critical aspect of the program, as it is believed that dieters need constant positive reinforcement in order to achieve and maintain long-term weight loss. The Weight Watchers program is structured in two phases: weight loss and maintenance. During weight loss, dieters work to lose weight slowly, with the goal of one to two pounds per week. Once the goal weight has been attained, dieters move into the maintenance phase, during which they gradually adjust their food intake until they are neither losing nor gaining weight. In general, Weight Watchers is viewed as providing a healthy approach to dieting.

Ornish Lifestyle Medicine

The Ornish Lifestyle Medicine program was created by Dr. Dean Ornish. The main premise of the program is that foods are neither good nor bad, but some are healthier than others. The Ornish diet focuses on fruits, vegetables, whole grains, legumes, soy products, nonfat dairy, natural egg whites, and fats that contain omega-3 fatty acids. The Ornish diet is plant-based; meat, poultry, and fish are excluded. Portion control is recommended, but caloric intake is not restricted unless a person is trying to lose weight. The program recommends small, frequent meals spread out throughout the day to support constant energy and avoid hunger. The consumption of caffeine is discouraged though allowed in small amounts. The Ornish program recommends exercise and low-dose multivitamin supplements. In general, the Ornish program is viewed as a healthy diet.

DIET SAFETY

Fad diets may produce initial weight loss results, but the potential for undesirable side effects should not be ignored. The human body needs simple carbohydrates (glucose) for energy and brain function. Low-carbohydrate and high-protein diets are not nutritionally balanced enough to meet the needs of children and some adults, particularly women who are pregnant, plan to become pregnant, or are nursing a baby. If maintained for an extended period of time, high-protein, low-carbohydrate diets can result in health problems, such as heart disease, kidney problems, and certain cancers.

Weight loss is achieved by eating fewer calories than are consumed by physical activity. Because most fad diets require people to consume very few calories, these diets can result in weight loss. However, because most fad diets are not nutritionally balanced and cannot be maintained for long periods of time, people usually find that any weight lost is regained once they stop following the diet and return to their old eating habits. The most effective weight-loss strategies are those that include a healthy, balanced diet combined with exercise.

References

1. "Diet Fads vs. Diet Truths," January 2004.
2. Nordqvist, Christian. "The Eight Most Popular Diets Today," *Medical News Today*, October 1, 2015.
3. "Nutrition Fact Sheet," Alaska Department of State Health Services, Nutrition Services Section, 2005.

Part 7 | The Role of Nutrition in People with Other Medical Concerns

Chapter 41 | **Nutrition and Diabetes**

Chapter Contents

Section 41.1 | **How to Count Carbs When You Eat Out**

This section includes text excerpted from "Eat Well," Centers for Disease Control and Prevention (CDC), September 19, 2019.

Managing blood sugar is the key to living well with diabetes, and eating well is the key to managing blood sugar. But, what does it mean to eat well? Simply put, eat healthy foods in the right amounts at the right times so your blood sugar stays in your target range as much as possible.

Work with your dietitian or diabetes educator to create a healthy eating plan, and check out the resources in this section for tips, strategies, and ideas to make it easier to eat well.

DIABETES MEAL PLANNING

A meal plan is your guide for when, what, and how much to eat to get the nutrition you need while keeping your blood sugar levels in your target range. A good meal plan will consider your goals, tastes, and lifestyle, as well as any medicines you are taking.

A good meal plan will also:

- Include more nonstarchy vegetables, such as broccoli, spinach, and green beans.
- Include fewer added sugars and refined grains, such as white bread, rice, and pasta with less than 2 grams of fiber per serving.
- Focus on whole foods instead of highly processed foods as much as possible.

Carbohydrates in the food you eat raise your blood sugar levels. How fast carbs raise your blood sugar depends on what the food is and what you eat with it. For example, drinking fruit juice raises blood sugar faster than eating whole fruit. Eating carbs with foods that have protein, fat, or fiber slows down how quickly your blood sugar rises.

You will want to plan for regular, balanced meals to avoid high or low blood sugar levels. Eating about the same amount of carbs at each meal can be helpful. Counting carbs and using the plate method are two common tools that can make planning meals easier too.

Counting Carbs

Keeping track of how many carbs you eat and setting a limit for each meal can help keep your blood sugar levels in your target range. Work with your doctor or a registered dietitian to find out how many carbs you can eat each day and at each meal, and then refer to this list of common foods that contain carbs and serving sizes.

The Plate Method

It is easy to eat more food than you need without realizing it. The plate method is a simple, visual way to make sure you get enough nonstarchy vegetables and lean protein while limiting the amount of higher-carb foods you eat that have the highest impact on your blood sugar.

Start with a 9-inch dinner plate (about the length of a business envelope):

- Fill half with nonstarchy vegetables, such as salad, green beans, broccoli, cauliflower, cabbage, and carrots.
- Fill one quarter with a lean protein, such as chicken, turkey, beans, tofu, or eggs.
- Fill one quarter with carb foods. Foods that are higher in carbs include grains, starchy vegetables (such as potatoes and peas), rice, pasta, beans, fruit, and yogurt. A cup of milk also counts as a carb food.

Then choose water or a low-calorie drink, such as unsweetened iced tea to go with your meal.

About Portion Size

Portion size and serving size are not always the same. A portion is the amount of food you choose to eat at one time, while a serving is a specific amount of food, such as one slice of bread or 8 ounces (1 cup) of milk.

These days, portions at restaurants are quite a bit larger than they were several years ago. One entrée can equal 3 or 4 servings! Studies show that people tend to eat more when they are served more food, so getting portions under control is really important for managing weight and blood sugar.

If you are eating out, have half of your meal wrapped up to go so you can enjoy it later. At home, measure out snacks; do not eat straight from the bag or box. At dinnertime, reduce the temptation to go back for seconds by keeping the serving bowls out of reach.

EATING OUT

Three in five Americans say they eat dinner out at least once a week, and as you have probably noticed, restaurant portions have gotten a lot bigger. Unless you have a plan in place, that can be a recipe for regular overeating.

While you cannot directly control the way the food is prepared or the calories in each dish, you can plan ahead, ask questions, and order food that both tastes good and is good for you. With practice, it will get easier to separate the healthier choices from the not so healthy and to keep portions under control. Some tips:

Plan Ahead

- Decide what you are going to order before you go so you do not feel rushed or tempted by less healthy choices.
- If your meal will be later than normal, have a snack that contains fiber and protein – a small handful of nuts is a great choice – before you go out to avoid getting too hungry. Then cut back by that amount when you eat your meal.

Start Smart

- Drink a big glass of water as soon as you sit down. It has been shown to help you eat less.
- Skip the chips and salsa or bread that comes to your table before you order. Better yet, ask your server to remove them.

Order Wisely

- Choose baked, steamed, grilled, or broiled instead of fried, breaded, crispy, or creamy to reduce fat and calories.
- Ask for veggies instead of fries or other high-calorie side dishes.
- Avoid items that seem healthy but are not, such as salads loaded with dressing, cheese, croutons, and bacon.
- Avoid added sugar – do not order dishes that have BBQ, glazed, sticky, honey, or teriyaki in their name.
- Order sauces, salad dressing, and spreads on the side and use sparingly. Try dipping your fork in the dressing before taking each bite to enjoy the flavor for fewer calories.

Share and Savor

- Share your main dish or eat half and wrap up the rest for later.
- Enjoy the occasional sweet treat (minus the guilt) by cutting back on carbs during your meal, and get a dessert to share with the table. You will not miss out – the first few bites are usually the tastiest.

CARB COUNTING

Counting carbohydrates, or carbs – keeping track of the carbs in all your meals, snacks, and drinks – can help you match your activity level and medicines to the food you eat. Many people with diabetes count carbs to make managing blood sugar easier, which can also help them:

- Stay healthy longer
- Feel better and improve their quality of life (QOL)
- Prevent or delay diabetes complications, such as kidney disease, eye disease, heart disease, and stroke

If you take mealtime insulin, you will count carbs to match your insulin dose to the amount of carbs in your foods and drinks. You may also take additional insulin if your blood sugar is higher than your target when eating.

What Are the Different Types of Carbs?

There are 3 types of carbs:

1. Sugars, such as the natural sugar in fruit and milk or the added sugar in soda and many other packaged foods
2. Starches, including wheat, oats, and other grains; starchy vegetables, such as corn and potatoes; and dried beans, lentils, and peas
3. Fiber, the part of plant foods that are not digested but helps you stay healthy

Sugars and starches raise your blood sugar, but fiber does not.

How Are Carbs Measured?

Carbs are measured in grams. On packaged foods, you can find total carb grams on the Nutrition Facts label. You can also check this list (www.cdc.gov/diabetes/managing/eat-well/diabetes-and-carbs/carbohydrate-choice-lists.html) or use a carb-counting app to find grams of carbs in foods and drinks.

For diabetes meal planning, 1 carb serving is about 15 grams of carbs. This is not always the same as what you think of as a serving of food. For example, most people would count a small baked potato as 1 serving. However, at about 30 grams of carbs, it counts as 2 carb servings.

How Many Carbs Should You Eat?

There is no "one size fits all" answer – everyone is different because everyone's body is different. The amount you can eat and stay in your target blood sugar range depends on your age, weight, activity level, and other factors.

On average, people with diabetes should aim to get about half of their calories from carbs. That means if you normally eat about 1,800 calories a day to maintain a healthy weight, about 800 to 900 calories can come from carbs. At 4 calories per gram, that is 200–225 carb grams a day. Try to eat about the same amount of carbs at each meal to keep your blood sugar levels steady throughout the day (not necessary if you use an insulin pump or give yourself multiple daily injections – you will take a fast-acting or short-acting insulin at mealtimes to match the amount of carbs you eat).

This sample menu has about 1,800 calories and 200 grams of carbs:

- Breakfast
  - ½ cup rolled oats (28g)
  - 1 cup low-fat milk (13g)
  - 2/3 medium banana (20g)
  - ¼ cup chopped walnuts (4g)
  - Total carbs: 65 grams
- Lunch
  - 2 slices whole-wheat bread (24g)
  - 4 oz. low-sodium turkey meat (1g)
  - 1 slice low-fat Swiss cheese (1g)
  - ½ large tomato (3g)
  - 1 tbs. yellow mustard (1g)
  - ¼ cup shredded lettuce (0g)
  - 8 baby carrots (7g)
  - 6 oz. plain fat-free Greek yogurt (7g)
  - ¾ cup blueberries (15g)
  - Total carbs: 59 grams
- Dinner
  - 6 ounces baked chicken breast (0g)
  - 1 cup brown rice (45g)
  - 1 cup steamed broccoli (12g)
  - 2 tbs. margarine (0g)
  - Total carbs: 57 grams
- Snack
  - 1 low-fat string cheese stick (1g)
  - 2 tangerines (18g)
  - Total carbs: 19 grams

How Can You Find Out More about Carb Counting?

Talk with your dietitian about the right amount of carbs for you, and be sure to update your meal plan if your needs change (e.g., if you get more active, you may increase how many carbs you eat).

Ask about tasty, healthy recipes that can help you stay on top of your carb intake – which will make it easier to manage your blood sugar levels, too.

DIABETES AND KIDNEY DISEASE: WHAT TO EAT?

One meal plan for diabetes, another for chronic kidney disease (CKD). Find out how you can eat well for both.

If you have diabetes and CKD, you are definitely not alone – about 1 in 3 American adults with diabetes also has CKD. The right diet helps your body function at its best, but figuring out what to eat can be a major challenge. What is good for you on one meal plan may not be good on the other.

Your first step: Meet with a registered dietitian who is trained in both diabetes and CKD nutrition. Together you will create a diet plan to keep blood sugar levels steady and reduce how much waste and fluid your kidneys have to handle.

Medicare and many private insurance plans may pay for your appointment. Ask if your policy covers medical nutrition therapy (MNT). MNT includes a nutrition plan designed just for you, which the dietitian will help you learn to follow.

Diabetes and CKD diets share a lot of the same foods, but there are some important differences.

Diabetes Diet

A healthy diabetes diet looks pretty much like a healthy diet for anyone: lots of fruits, veggies, healthy fats, and lean protein; less salt, sugar, and foods high in refined carbs (cookies, crackers, and soda, just to name a few). Your individual carb goal is based on your age, activity level, and any medicines you take. Following your meal plan will help keep your blood sugar levels in your target range, which will also prevent more damage to your kidneys.

Kidney Diet

With a CKD diet, you will avoid or limit certain foods to protect your kidneys, and you will include other foods to give you energy and keep you nourished. Your specific diet will depend on whether you are in early-stage or late-stage CKD or if you are on dialysis.

FOODS TO LIMIT

Eat less salt/sodium. That is a good move for diabetes and really important for CKD. Over time, your kidneys lose the ability to control your sodium-water balance. Less sodium in your diet will help lower blood pressure and decrease fluid buildup in your body, which is common in kidney disease.

Focus on fresh, homemade food and eat only small amounts of restaurant food and packaged food, which usually have lots of sodium. Look for low sodium (5 percent or less) on food labels.

In a week or two, you will get used to less salt in your food, especially if you dial up the flavor with herbs, spices, mustard, and flavored vinegars. But, do not use salt substitutes unless your doctor or dietitian says you can. Many are very high in potassium, which you may need to limit.

Depending on your stage of kidney disease, you may also need to reduce the potassium, phosphorus, and protein in your diet. Many foods that are part of a typical healthy diet may not be right for a CKD diet.

Phosphorus is a mineral that keeps your bones strong and other parts of your body healthy. Your kidneys cannot remove extra phosphorus from your blood very well. Too much weakens bones and can damage your blood vessels, eyes, and heart. Meat, dairy, beans, nuts, whole-grain bread, and dark-colored sodas are high in phosphorus. Phosphorus is also added to lots of packaged foods.

The right level of potassium keeps your nerves and muscles working well. With CKD, too much potassium can build up in your blood and cause serious heart problems. Oranges, potatoes, tomatoes, whole-grain bread, and many other foods are high in potassium. Apples, carrots, and white bread are lower in potassium. Your doctor may prescribe a potassium binder, a medicine that helps your body get rid of extra potassium.

Eat the right amount of protein. More protein than you need makes your kidneys work harder and may make CKD worse. But, too little is not healthy either. Both animal and plant foods have protein. Your dietitian can help you figure out the right combination and amount of protein to eat.

Diabetes and Chronic Kidney Disease Foods

Below are just a few examples of foods a person with both diabetes and CKD can eat. Your dietitian can give you lots more suggestions and help you find recipes for tasty meals:

- Fruits such as berries, grapes, cherries, apples, plums
- Veggies such as cauliflower, onions, eggplant, turnips
- Proteins such as lean meats (poultry, fish), eggs, unsalted seafood
- Carbs such as white bread, bagels, sandwich buns, unsalted crackers, pasta
- Drinks such as water, clear diet sodas, unsweetened tea

Here is one way your CKD diet and diabetes diet can work together: If you drink orange juice to treat low blood sugar, switch to kidney-friendly apple or grape juice. You will get the same blood-sugar boost with a lot less potassium.

Late-Stage Chronic Kidney Disease

Your nutrition needs will change with late-stage CKD. If you are on dialysis, you may need to eat more, especially more protein. Your appetite can change because food tastes different.

Dialysis filters your blood like kidneys do, but it does not work as well as healthy kidneys. Fluid can build up in your body between treatments. You may need to limit how much fluid you drink, and watch for swelling around your eyes or in your legs, arms, or belly.

Your blood sugar levels can actually get better with late-stage CKD, possibly because of changes in how your body uses insulin. But, when you are on dialysis, your blood sugar can increase because the fluid used to filter your blood is high in glucose (sugar). Your need for insulin and other diabetes medicines will be hard to predict, so your doctor will monitor you closely.

See Your Dietitian

Chronic kidney disease and diabetes both change over time, and so will your diet. Be sure to check in with your dietitian as recommended. You will get the support and confidence you need to manage your meals, solve any problems, and be your healthiest.

Section 41.2 | Nutrition Tips to Prevent Type 2 Diabetes

This section includes text excerpted from "Choose More than 50 Ways to Prevent Type 2 Diabetes," National Institute of Diabetes and Digestive and Kidney Diseases (NIDDK), September 2014. Reviewed May 2021.

REDUCE PORTION SIZES

Portion size is the amount of food you eat, such as 1 cup of fruit or 6 ounces of meat. If you are trying to eat smaller portions, eat a half of a bagel instead of a whole bagel or have a 3-ounce hamburger instead of a 6-ounce hamburger. Three ounces is about the size of your fist or a deck of cards.

Put Less on Your Plate

- Drink a large glass of water 10 minutes before your meal so you feel less hungry.
- Keep meat, chicken, turkey, and fish portions to about 3 ounces.
- Share one dessert.

Eat a Small Meal

- Use teaspoons, salad forks, or child-size forks, spoons, and knives to help you take smaller bites and eat less.
- Make less food look like more by serving your meal on a salad or breakfast plate.
- Eat slowly. It takes 20 minutes for your stomach to send a signal to your brain that you are full.
- Listen to music while you eat instead of watching TV (people tend to eat more while watching TV).

HOW MUCH SHOULD YOU EAT?

Try filling your plate like this:

- 1/4 protein
- 1/4 grains
- 1/2 vegetables and fruit
- Dairy (low-fat or skim milk)

MAKE HEALTHY FOOD CHOICES

Find ways to make healthy food choices. This can help you manage your weight and lower your chances of getting type 2 diabetes.

Choose to eat more vegetables, fruits, and whole grains. Cut back on high-fat foods, such as whole milk, cheeses, and fried foods. This will help you reduce the amount of fat and calories you take in each day.

Snack on a Veggie

- Buy a mix of vegetables when you go food shopping.
- Choose veggie toppings, such as spinach, broccoli, and peppers for your pizza.
- Try eating foods from other countries. Many of these dishes have more vegetables, whole grains, and beans.
- Buy frozen and low-salt (sodium) canned vegetables. They may cost less and keep longer than fresh ones.
- Serve your favorite vegetable and a salad with low-fat macaroni and cheese.

Cook with Care

- Stir fry, broil, or bake with nonstick spray or low-salt broth. Cook with less oil and butter.
- Try not to snack while cooking or cleaning the kitchen.
- Cook with smaller amounts of cured meats (smoked turkey and turkey bacon). They are high in salt.

Cook in Style

- Cook with a mix of spices instead of salt.

- Try different recipes for baking or broiling meat, chicken, and fish.
- Choose foods with little or no added sugar to reduce calories.
- Choose brown rice instead of white rice.

Eat Healthy on the Go

- Have a big vegetable salad with low-calorie salad dressing when eating out. Share your main dish with a friend or have the other half wrapped to go.
- Make healthy choices at fast-food restaurants. Try grilled chicken (with skin removed) instead of a cheeseburger.
- Skip the fries and chips and choose a salad.
- Order a fruit salad instead of ice cream or cake.

Chapter 42 | **Nutrition and Heart Disease**

Chapter Contents

Section 42.1 | Eating for a Healthy Heart

This section includes text excerpted from "Heart-Healthy Eating," Office on Women's Health (OWH), U.S. Department of Health and Human Services (HHS), January 3, 2019.

Heart-healthy eating is an important way to lower your risk of heart disease and stroke. Heart disease is the number one cause of death for American women. Stroke is the number three cause of death. To get the most benefit for your heart, you should choose more fruits, vegetables, and foods with whole grains and healthy protein. You also should eat less food with added sugar, calories, and unhealthy fats.

WHY IS HEART-HEALTHY EATING IMPORTANT?

Heart-healthy eating, along with regular exercise or physical activity, can lower your risk of heart disease and stroke.

WHAT FOODS SHOULD YOU EAT TO HELP LOWER YOUR RISK FOR HEART DISEASE AND STROKE?

You should choose these foods most of the time:

- **Fruits and vegetables.** At least half of your plate should be fruits and vegetables.
- **Whole grains.** At least half of your grains should be whole grains. Whole grains include:
    - Whole wheat
    - Whole oats
    - Oatmeal
    - Whole-grain corn
    - Brown rice
    - Wild rice
    - Whole rye
    - Whole-grain barley
    - Buckwheat
    - Bulgur
    - Millet
    - Sorghum

- **Fat-free or low-fat dairy products.** These include milk, calcium-fortified soy drinks (soy milk), cheese, yogurt, and other milk products.
- Seafood, skinless poultry, lean meats, beans, eggs, and unsalted nuts.

WHAT FOODS SHOULD YOU LIMIT TO LOWER YOUR RISK OF HEART DISEASE AND STROKE?

You should limit:

- **Saturated fats.** This type of fat is usually found in pizza, ice cream, fried chicken, many cakes and cookies, bacon, and hamburgers. Check the Nutrition Facts label for saturated fat. Less than 10 percent of your daily calories should be from saturated fats.
- ***Trans* fats.** These are found mainly in commercially prepared baked goods, snack foods, fried foods, and margarine. The U.S. Food and Drug Administration (FDA) is taking action to remove artificial *trans* fats from our food supply because of their risk to heart health. Check the Nutrition Facts label and choose foods with no *trans* fats as much as possible.
- **Cholesterol**. This is found in foods made from animals, such as bacon, whole milk, cheese made from whole milk, ice cream, full-fat frozen yogurt, and eggs. Fruits and vegetables do not contain cholesterol. Eggs are a major source of dietary cholesterol for Americans, but studies show that eating one egg a day does not increase the risk for heart disease in healthy people. You should eat less than 300 milligrams of cholesterol per day. Check the Nutrition Facts label for cholesterol. Foods with 20 percent or more of the "Daily Value" of cholesterol are high in cholesterol.
- **Sodium**. This is found in salt, but most of the sodium we eat does not come from salt that we add while cooking or at the table. Most of our sodium comes from breads and rolls, cold cuts, pizza, hot dogs, cheese, pasta dishes, and condiments (such as ketchup

and mustard). Limit your daily sodium to less than 2,300 milligrams (equal to a teaspoon), unless your doctor says something else. Check the Nutrition Facts label for sodium. Foods with 20 percent or more of the "Daily Value" of sodium are high in sodium.

- **Added sugars**. Foods such as fruit and dairy products naturally contain sugar. But, you should limit foods that contain added sugars. These include sodas, sports drinks, cake, candy, and ice cream. Check the Nutrition Facts label for added sugars and limit how much food you eat with added sugars. Look for these other names for sugar in the list of ingredients:
  - Corn syrup
  - Corn sweetener
  - Fructose
  - Glucose
  - Sucrose
  - Dextrose
  - Lactose
  - Maltose
  - Honey
  - Molasses
  - Raw sugar
  - Invert sugar
  - Syrup
  - Caramel
  - Fruit juice concentrates

HOW CAN YOU TELL WHAT IS IN THE FOODS YOU EAT?

Most packaged foods have a Nutrition Facts label. This label has information about how many calories, saturated fat, *trans* fat, cholesterol, sodium, and added sugars are in each serving. It also lists the amounts of certain vitamins and minerals.

For food that does not have a Nutrition Facts label, such as fresh salmon or a raw apple, you can check the FDA's Nutrition Facts (www.fda.gov/food/food-labeling-nutrition/nutrition-information-raw-fruits-vegetables-and-fish) posters. The posters show whether a food is high or low in cholesterol, saturated fat, or sodium.

HOW MANY CALORIES SHOULD YOU EAT?

The number of calories you should eat each day depends on your age, sex, body size, physical activity, and other factors.

For instance, a woman between 31 and 50 years old who is of normal weight and is moderately active (gets 30 minutes of exercise on most days of the week) should eat and drink about 2,000 calories each day to maintain her weight. To find your personalized daily calorie limit, use the MyPlate Plan tool (www.myplate.gov/myplate-plan).

WHAT TOOLS CAN HELP YOU CHOOSE FOODS THAT ARE GOOD FOR YOUR HEART?

Get a personalized food plan for your age, sex, height, weight, and physical activity level. This easy-to-use online calculator is based on the most recent *Dietary Guidelines for Americans*.

- Get your personalized MyPlate Plan (www.choosemyplate.gov/MyPlatePlan) now.

The following eating plans were developed by independent research scientists at the National Heart, Lung, and Blood Institute (NHLBI) at the National Institutes of Health (NIH):

- Dietary Approaches to Stop Hypertension (DASH) eating plan. The DASH diet helps lower your blood pressure and is regularly rated the best overall diet by the *U.S. News and World Report*. It can also be used to help prevent heart disease.
- Therapeutic Lifestyle Changes (TLC) diet (www.nhlbi.nih.gov/files/docs/public/heart/chol_tlc.pdf). The TLC diet helps lower your cholesterol and is often in the top five diets rated by *U.S. News and World Report*.

To be top rated, a diet must be easy to follow, nutritious, and safe and effective for weight loss. Top rated diets must also help prevent diabetes and heart disease.

HOW DOES SODIUM IN FOOD AFFECT YOUR HEART?

Eating foods high in sodium may cause high blood pressure, also called "hypertension." Hypertension is a risk factor for heart disease and stroke. You should limit the amount of sodium you eat each day to less than 2,300 milligrams (about one teaspoon of salt), including the sodium found in packaged foods that you cannot see. You should limit your sodium intake to less than 1,500 milligrams (about two-thirds of a teaspoon of salt) if you:

- Have high blood pressure (HBP)
- Are African American
- Are 51 years or older
- Have diabetes
- Have chronic kidney disease (CKD)

You can lower the amount of sodium you eat each day by:

- **Eating fewer processed foods.** Most of the salt we eat comes from processed foods rather than salt we add to foods we cook.
- **Checking the sodium content on the Nutrition Facts label.** The sodium content in similar foods can vary a lot. For instance, the sodium content in regular tomato soup may be 700 milligrams (about a third of a teaspoon) per cup in one brand and 1,100 milligrams (about a half a teaspoon) per cup in another brand.
- **Seasoning your food with herbs and spices instead of salt.** Look for salt-free seasoning combinations in your grocery store.

HOW DOES POTASSIUM IN FOOD AFFECT YOUR HEART?

Potassium lessens the harmful effects of sodium on blood pressure. Try to eat or drink at least 4,700 milligrams of potassium a day. Good sources of potassium include:

- Bananas (442 milligrams for a medium banana)
- Milk, nonfat and low fat (up to 370 milligrams per cup)
- Orange juice (496 milligrams per 8-ounce glass of 100 percent orange juice)

- Plain yogurt, nonfat or low fat (up to 579 milligrams per 8-ounce carton)
- Prunes and prune juice (707 milligrams per 8-ounce glass)
- Spinach (up to 419 milligrams per half cup)
- Sweet potatoes (542 milligrams for a medium-sized sweet potato)
- Tomatoes and tomato products (664 milligrams for one-half cup of tomato paste; 405 milligrams for one-half cup of tomato sauce)
- White potatoes (738 milligrams per small potato)

HOW DOES CHOLESTEROL IN FOOD AFFECT YOUR HEART?

Cholesterol is a waxy, fat-like substance made by your body. It also is found in foods made from animals, such as meat and dairy. Fruits and vegetables do not contain cholesterol. There are two types of cholesterol: HDL, or "good cholesterol," and LDL, or "bad cholesterol." Higher levels of total cholesterol and LDL or "bad" cholesterol raise your risk for heart disease. Almost half of American women have high or borderline high cholesterol.

You can lower your cholesterol and LDL or "bad" cholesterol by:

- **Limiting foods that are high in saturated fats, *trans* fats, and cholesterol.** Find a list of these foods in the "What foods should you limit to lower the risk of heart disease and stroke?"
- **Limiting cholesterol.** Try to eat or drink less than 300 milligrams of cholesterol each day. For comparison, a fast-food double-patty plain cheeseburger has about 100 milligrams of cholesterol.

IS EATING SEAFOOD GOOD FOR YOUR HEART?

Yes. Seafood contains a type of fat called "omega-3 fatty acids." Research suggests that eating about eight ounces of seafood with omega-3 fatty acids per week can lower your risk of dying from heart disease.

Seafood that naturally contain more oil and are better sources of omega-3 fatty acids include:

- Salmon
- Trout
- Mackerel
- Anchovies
- Sardines

Lean fish (such as cod, haddock, and catfish) have less omega-3 fatty acids.

IS DRINKING ALCOHOL GOOD FOR YOUR HEART?

Maybe. Some research shows a link between moderate drinking and a lower risk of heart disease and stroke. For women, moderate drinking is up to one drink per day. For men, it is up to two drinks per day. One drink is:

- One glass of wine (five ounces)
- One can of beer (12 ounces)
- One shot of 80-proof hard liquor (1.5 ounces)

The reasons behind the possible benefit of moderate drinking on heart disease are not clear. But, we also know that moderate drinking is linked to breast cancer, violence, and injuries. So, if you do not already drink, you should not start because of possible health benefits.

You should also not drink alcohol if:

- You are pregnant or may be pregnant. There is no amount of alcohol that is known to be safe during pregnancy.
- You have another health condition that makes alcohol harmful
- You are taking a medicine that is affected by alcohol

WHO CAN HELP YOU WORK OUT AN EATING PLAN THAT IS BEST FOR YOU?

You may want to talk with a registered dietitian. A dietitian is a nutrition expert who can give you advice about what foods to eat and how much of each type. Ask your doctor to recommend a dietitian. You can also contact the Academy of Nutrition and Dietetics (www.eatright.org).

HOW CAN YOU GET FREE OR LOW-COST NUTRITION COUNSELING?

If you are at risk of heart disease or another chronic disease that is affected by what you eat, most insurance plans cover nutrition counseling at no cost to you.

If you have insurance, check with your insurance provider before you visit a health professional for diet counseling to find out what types of services are covered.

- If you have Medicare, find out how Medicare covers nutrition counseling (www.medicare.gov/coverage/nutrition-therapy-services).
- If you have Medicaid, the benefits covered are different in each state, but certain benefits must be covered by every Medicaid program.

Section 42.2 | How to Lower Cholesterol with Diet

This section includes text excerpted from "How to Lower Cholesterol with Diet," MedlinePlus, National Institutes of Health (NIH), February 27, 2019.

WHAT IS CHOLESTEROL?

Your body needs some cholesterol to work properly. But, if you have too much in your blood, it can stick to the walls of your arteries and narrow or even block them. This puts you at risk for coronary artery disease and other heart diseases.

Cholesterol travels through the blood on proteins called "lipoproteins." One type, LDL, is sometimes called the "bad" cholesterol. A high LDL level leads to a buildup of cholesterol in your arteries. Another type, HDL, is sometimes called the "good" cholesterol. It carries cholesterol from other parts of your body back to your liver. Then your liver removes the cholesterol from your body.

Table 42.1. Calories Intake

Calories per Day	Total Fat	Saturated Fat
1,500	42–58 grams	10 grams
2,000	56–78 grams	13 grams
2,500	69–97 grams	17 grams

WHAT ARE THE TREATMENTS FOR HIGH CHOLESTEROL?

The treatments for high cholesterol are heart-healthy lifestyle changes and medicines. The lifestyle changes include healthy eating, weight management, and regular physical activity.

HOW CAN YOU LOWER CHOLESTEROL WITH DIET?

Heart-healthy lifestyle changes include a diet to lower your cholesterol. The DASH eating plan is one example. Another is the Therapeutic Lifestyle Changes diet, which recommends that you:

Choose healthier fats. You should limit both total fat and saturated fat. No more than 25 to 35 percent of your daily calories should come from dietary fats, and less than seven percent of your daily calories should come from saturated fat. Depending upon how many calories you eat per day, here are the maximum amounts of fats that you should eat:

Saturated fat is a bad fat because it raises your LDL (bad cholesterol) level more than anything else in your diet. It is found in some meats, dairy products, chocolate, baked goods, and deep-fried and processed foods.

Trans fat is another bad fat; it can raise your LDL and lower you HDL (good cholesterol). *Trans* fat is mostly in foods made with hydrogenated oils and fats, such as stick margarine, crackers, and French fries.

Instead of these bad fats, try healthier fats, such as lean meat, nuts, and unsaturated oils such as canola, olive, and safflower oils.

Limit foods with cholesterol. If you are trying to lower your cholesterol, you should have less than 200 mg a day of cholesterol.

Cholesterol is in foods of animal origin, such as liver and other organ meats, egg yolks, shrimp, and whole-milk dairy products.

Eat plenty of soluble fiber. Foods high in soluble fiber help prevent your digestive tract from absorbing cholesterol. These foods include:

- Whole-grain cereals, such as oatmeal and oat bran
- Fruits such as apples, bananas, oranges, pears, and prunes
- Legumes such as kidney beans, lentils, chick peas, black-eyed peas, and lima beans

Eat lots of fruits and vegetables. A diet rich in fruits and vegetables can increase important cholesterol-lowering compounds in your diet. These compounds, called "plant stanols" or "sterols," work like soluble fiber.

Eat fish that are high in omega-3 fatty acids. These acids will not lower your LDL level, but they may help raise your HDL level. They may also protect your heart from blood clots and inflammation and reduce your risk of heart attack. Fish that are a good source of omega-3 fatty acids include salmon, tuna (canned or fresh), and mackerel. Try to eat these fish two times a week.

Limit salt. You should try to limit the amount of sodium (salt) that you eat to no more than 2,300 milligrams (about one teaspoon of salt) a day. That includes all the sodium you eat, whether it was added in cooking or at the table, or already present in food products. Limiting salt will not lower your cholesterol, but it can lower your risk of heart diseases by helping to lower your blood pressure. You can reduce your sodium by instead choosing low-salt and "no added salt" foods and seasonings at the table or while cooking.

Limit alcohol. Alcohol adds extra calories, which can lead to weight gain. Being overweight can raise your LDL level and lower your HDL level. Too much alcohol can also increase your risk of heart diseases because it can raise your blood pressure and triglyceride level. One drink is a glass of wine, beer, or a small amount of hard liquor, and the recommendation is that:

- Men should have no more than two drinks containing alcohol a day.
- Women should have no more than one drink containing alcohol a day.

Section 42.3 | Lowering Your Blood Pressure with the DASH Eating Plan

This section includes text excerpted from "Your Guide to Lowering Your Blood Pressure with DASH," National Heart, Lung, and Blood Institute (NHLBI), August 2015. Reviewed May 2021.

What you eat affects your chances of developing high blood pressure (HBP or hypertension). Research shows that HBP can be prevented – and lowered – by following the Dietary Approaches to Stop Hypertension (DASH) eating plan, which includes eating less sodium.

High blood pressure is blood pressure higher than 140/90 mmHg*, and prehypertension is blood pressure between 120/80 and 139/89 mmHg. High blood pressure is dangerous because it makes your heart work too hard, hardens the walls of your arteries, and can cause the brain to hemorrhage or the kidneys to function poorly or not at all. If not controlled, HBP can lead to heart and kidney disease, stroke, and blindness.

But, HBP can be prevented – and lowered – if you take these steps:

- Follow a healthy eating plan, such as DASH, that includes foods lower in sodium.
- Maintain a healthy weight.
- Be moderately physically active for at least two hours and 30 minutes per week.
- If you drink alcoholic beverages, do so in moderation.

If you already have HBP and your doctor has prescribed medicine, take your medicine, as directed, and follow these steps.

THE DASH EATING PLAN

The DASH eating plan is rich in fruits, vegetables, fat-free or low-fat milk and milk products, whole grains, fish, poultry, beans, seeds, and nuts. It also contains less sodium; sweets, added sugars, and beverages containing sugar; fats; and red meats than the typical American diet. This heart-healthy way of eating is also lower in saturated fat, trans fat, and cholesterol and rich in nutrients that are associated with lowering blood pressure – mainly potassium, magnesium, calcium, protein, and fiber.

HOW DO YOU MAKE THE DASH?

The DASH eating plan requires no special foods and has no hard-to-follow recipes. It simply calls for a certain number of daily servings from various food groups.

The number of servings depends on the number of calories you are allowed each day. Your calorie level depends on your age and, especially, how active you are. Think of this as an energy balance system – if you want to maintain your current weight, you should take in only as many calories as you burn by being physically active. If you need to lose weight, eat fewer calories than you burn or increase your activity level to burn more calories than you eat.

What is your physical activity level? Are you mostly:

- Sedentary? You do only light physical activity that is part of your typical day-to-day routine.
- Moderately active? You do physical activity equal to walking about one to three miles a day at three to four miles per hour, plus light physical activity.
- Active? You do physical activity equal to walking more than three miles per day at three to four miles per hour, plus light physical activity.

Now that you know how many calories you are allowed each day. This shows roughly the number of servings from each food group that you can eat each day.

Next, compare DASH with your current eating pattern. This should help you decide what changes you need to make in your food choices – and in the sizes of the portions you eat.

Increase or decrease the serving sizes for your own calorie level. This chart also shows the two levels of sodium, 2,300 and 1,500 milligrams (mg), that DASH allows each day. Because fruits and vegetables are naturally lower in sodium than many other foods, DASH makes it easier to eat less sodium. Try it at the 2,300 mg level (about one teaspoon of table salt). Then, talk to your doctor about gradually lowering it to 1,500 mg a day. Keep in mind:

The less sodium you eat, the more you may be able to lower your blood pressure.

Choose and prepare foods with less sodium and salt, and do not bring the salt shaker to the table. Be creative – try herbs, spices, lemon, lime, vinegar, wine, and salt-free seasoning blends in cooking and at the table. And, because most of the sodium that we eat comes from processed foods, be sure to read food labels to check the amount of sodium in different food products. Aim for foods that contain five percent or less of the Daily Value of sodium. Foods with 20 percent or more Daily Value of sodium are considered high. These include baked goods, certain cereals, soy sauce, and some antacids – the range is wide.

DASH TIPS FOR GRADUAL CHANGE

Make these changes over a couple of days or weeks to give yourself a chance to adjust and make them part of your daily routine:

- Add a serving of vegetables at lunch one day and dinner the next, and add fruit at one meal or as a snack.
- Increase your use of fat-free and low-fat milk products to three servings a day.
- Limit lean meats to six ounces a day – three ounces a meal, which is about the size of a deck of cards. If you usually eat large portions of meats, cut them back over a couple of days – by half or a third at each meal.
- Include two or more vegetarian-style, or meatless, meals each week.

MAKE THE DASH FOR LIFE

DASH can help you prevent and control HBP. It also can help you lose weight, if you need to. It meets your nutritional needs and has other health benefits for your heart. So get started today, and make the DASH for a healthy life.

Chapter 43 | **Food Allergies and Intolerances**

Chapter Contents

Section 43.1 | **About Food Allergies**

This section contains text excerpted from the following sources: Text in this section begins with excerpts from "Food Allergy," MedlinePlus, National Institutes of Health (NIH), March 9, 2021; Text beginning with the heading "Major Food Allergens" is excerpted from "Food Allergies," U.S. Food and Drug Administration (FDA), April 26, 2021.

Food allergy is an abnormal response to a food triggered by your body's immune system.

In adults, the foods that most often trigger allergic reactions include fish, shellfish, peanuts, and tree nuts, such as walnuts. Problem foods for children can include eggs, milk, peanuts, tree nuts, soy, and wheat.

The allergic reaction may be mild. In rare cases it can cause a severe reaction called "anaphylaxis." Symptoms of food allergy include:

- Itching or swelling in your mouth
- Vomiting, diarrhea, or abdominal cramps and pain
- Hives or eczema
- Tightening of the throat and trouble breathing
- Drop in blood pressure

Your healthcare provider may use a detailed history, elimination diet, and skin and blood tests to diagnose a food allergy.

When you have food allergies, you must be prepared to treat an accidental exposure. Wear a medical alert bracelet or necklace, and carry an auto-injector device containing epinephrine (adrenaline).

You can only prevent the symptoms of food allergy by avoiding the food. After you and your healthcare provider have identified the foods to which you are sensitive, you must remove them from your diet.

MAJOR FOOD ALLERGENS

Congress passed the Food Allergen Labeling and Consumer Protection Act of 2004 (FALCPA). This law identified the following eight foods as major food allergens:

- Milk
- Eggs

- Fish
- Shellfish
- Tree nuts
- Peanuts
- Wheat
- Soybeans

At the time of the law's passage, the eight major allergens accounted for 90 percent of food allergies and serious allergic reactions in the United States. The FALCPA requires that foods or ingredients that contain a "major food allergen" be specifically labeled with the name of the allergen source. Congress passed this law to make it easier for consumers who are allergic to foods and their caregivers to identify and avoid foods that contain major food allergens. The U.S. Food and Drug Administration (FDA) enforces the provisions of this law in most packaged food products. This includes dietary supplements but does not include meat, poultry, and egg products (which are regulated by the U.S. Department of Agriculture (USDA)); alcoholic beverages subject to Alcohol and Tobacco Tax and Trade Bureau labeling regulations; raw agricultural commodities; drugs; cosmetics; and most foods sold at retail or food service establishments that are not prepackaged with a label.

FOOD LABELS AND ALLERGENS

People with food allergies should read labels and avoid the foods they are allergic to. The law requires that food labels identify the food source of all major food allergens used to make the food. This requirement is met if the common or usual name of an ingredient already identifies that allergen's food source name (e.g., buttermilk). Otherwise, the allergen's food source must be declared at least once on the food label in one of two ways.

The name of the food source of a major food allergen must appear:

In parentheses following the name of the ingredient.

Examples: "lecithin (soy)," "flour (wheat)," and "whey (milk)" (OR)

Immediately after or next to the list of ingredients in a "contains" statement.

Example: "Contains wheat, milk, and soy."

The FALCPA's labeling requirements extend to retail and food-service establishments that package, label, and offer products for human consumption. However, the FALCPA's labeling requirements do not apply to foods that are placed in a wrapper or container (such as paper or a box for a sandwich) following a customer's order at the point of purchase.

Consumers may also see advisory statements, such as "may contain [allergen]" or "produced in a facility that also uses [allergen]." These are used to address "cross-contact," which can occur when multiple foods with different allergen profiles are produced in the same facility using shared equipment or on the same production line, as the result of ineffective cleaning, or from the generation of dust or aerosols containing an allergen.

The FDA guidance for the food industry states that advisory statements should not be used as a substitute for adhering to current good manufacturing practices and must be truthful and not misleading.

WHAT TO DO IF SYMPTOMS OF AN ALLERGIC REACTION OCCUR?

Symptoms of food allergies typically appear from within a few minutes to a few hours after a person has eaten the food to which she or he is allergic. A severe, life-threatening allergic reaction is called "anaphylaxis."

Symptoms of allergic reactions can include:

- Hives
- Flushed skin or rash
- Tingling or itchy sensation in the mouth
- Face, tongue, or lip swelling
- Vomiting and/or diarrhea
- Abdominal cramps
- Coughing or wheezing
- Dizziness and/or lightheadedness
- Swelling of the throat and vocal cords
- Difficulty breathing
- Loss of consciousness

People with a known food allergy who begin experiencing any of these symptoms should stop eating the food immediately, evaluate the need to use emergency medication (such as epinephrine) and seek medical attention. Some of these symptoms are not always due to a food allergen. So, it is important to seek proper care and diagnosis from a healthcare provider to determine if the symptoms or reaction experienced was due to a food allergen.

Section 43.2 | Reading Food Labels for Allergen Content

This section includes text excerpted from "Have Food Allergies? Read the Label," U.S. Food and Drug Administration (FDA), January 29, 2021.

Food labels can help consumers with food allergies avoid foods or ingredients that they or their families are allergic to.

This is because a federal law, the Food Allergen Labeling and Consumer Protection Act (FALCPA) of 2004, requires that the labels of most packaged foods marketed in the U.S. disclose – in simple-to-understand terms – when they are made with a "major food allergen."

Eight foods, and ingredients containing their proteins, are defined as major food allergens. These foods account for the large majority of severe food allergic reactions:

- Milk
- Egg
- Fish, such as bass, flounder, or cod
- Crustacean shellfish, such as crab, lobster, or shrimp
- Tree nuts, such as almonds, pecans, or walnuts
- Wheat
- Peanuts
- Soybeans

The law requires that food labels identify the food source of all major food allergens used to make the food. This requirement is met if the common or usual name of an ingredient already identifies that allergen's food source name (e.g., buttermilk). Otherwise, the allergen's food source must be declared at least once on the food label in one of two ways.

The name of the food source of a major allergen must appear:

In parentheses following the name of the ingredient.

Examples: "lecithin (soy)," "flour (wheat)," and "whey (milk)"

-OR-

Immediately after or next to the list of ingredients in a "contains" statement.

Example: "Contains wheat, milk, and soy."

"So first look for a 'Contains' statement and if your allergen is listed, put the product back on the shelf," says Carol D'Lima, food technologist with the Office of Nutrition and Food Labeling at the U.S. Food and Drug Administration (FDA). "If there is no 'Contains' statement, it is very important to read the entire ingredient list to see if your allergen is present. If you see its name even once, it is back to the shelf for that food too."

There are many different ingredients that contain the same major food allergen, but sometimes the ingredients' names do not indicate their specific food sources. For example, casein, sodium caseinate, and whey are all milk proteins. Although the same allergen can be present in multiple ingredients, its "food source name" (e.g., milk) must appear in the ingredient list just once to comply with labeling requirements.

Sesame is not a major food allergen under the FALCPA of 2004, but the FDA recently issued a draft guidance document to encourage manufacturers to clearly declare sesame in the ingredient list. In most cases, sesame does have to appear in the ingredient statement; an exception is when sesame is part of a flavoring or spice or if a term is used for a food, such as tahini, or contains, sesame. In those cases, it may be declared as simply "spice" or "flavor" on the label, so consumers may not know sesame is present.

"CONTAINS" AND "MAY CONTAIN" HAVE DIFFERENT MEANINGS

If a "Contains" statement appears on a food label, it must include the food source names of all major food allergens used as ingredients. For example, if "whey," "egg yolks," and a "natural flavor" that contained peanut proteins are listed as ingredients, the "Contains" statement must identify the words "milk," "egg," and "peanuts." Some manufacturers voluntarily include a separate advisory statement, such as "may contain" or "produced in a facility," on their labels when there is a chance that a food allergen could be present. A manufacturer might use the same equipment to make different products. Even after cleaning this equipment, a small amount of an allergen (such as peanuts) that was used to make one product (such as cookies) may become part of another product (such as crackers). In this case, the cracker label might state "may contain peanuts." Be aware that the "may contain" statement is voluntary, says D'Lima. "Not all manufacturers use it."

WHEN IN DOUBT, LEAVE IT OUT

Manufacturers can change their products' ingredients at any time, so D'Lima says it is a good idea to check the ingredient list every time you buy the product – even if you have eaten it before and did not have an allergic reaction.

"If you are unsure about whether a food contains any ingredient to which you are sensitive, do not buy the product, or check with the manufacturer first to ask what it contains," says D'Lima. "We all want convenience, but it is not worth playing Russian roulette with your life or that of someone under your care."

Section 43.3 | Lactose Intolerance

This section includes text excerpted from "Lactose Intolerance," National Diabetes Information Clearinghouse (NDIC), National Institute of Diabetes and Digestive and Kidney Diseases (NIDDK), February 2018.

ABOUT LACTOSE INTOLERANCE

What Is Lactose Intolerance?

Lactose intolerance is a condition in which you have digestive symptom, such as bloating, diarrhea, and gas – after you consume foods or drinks that contain lactose. Lactose is a sugar that is naturally found in milk and milk products, such as cheese or ice cream.

In lactose intolerance, digestive symptoms are caused by lactose malabsorption. Lactose malabsorption is a condition in which your small intestine cannot digest, or break down, all the lactose you eat or drink.

Not everyone with lactose malabsorption has digestive symptoms after they consume lactose. Only people who have symptoms are lactose intolerant.

Most people with lactose intolerance can consume some amount of lactose without having symptoms. Different people can tolerate different amounts of lactose before having symptoms.

Lactose intolerance is different from a milk allergy. A milk allergy is an immune system disorder.

How Common Is Lactose Malabsorption?

While most infants can digest lactose, many people begin to develop lactose malabsorption – a reduced ability to digest lactose – after infancy. Experts estimate that about 68 percent of the world's population has lactose malabsorption.

Lactose malabsorption is more common in some parts of the world than in others. In Africa and Asia, most people have lactose malabsorption. In some regions, such as northern Europe, many people carry a gene that allows them to digest lactose after infancy, and lactose malabsorption is less common. In the United States, about 36 percent of people have lactose malabsorption.

While lactose malabsorption causes lactose intolerance, not all people with lactose malabsorption have lactose intolerance.

Who Is More Likely to Have Lactose Intolerance?

You are more likely to have lactose intolerance if you are from, or your family is from, a part of the world where lactose malabsorption is more common. In the United States, the following ethnic and racial groups are more likely to have lactose malabsorption:

- African Americans
- American Indians

- Asian Americans
- Hispanics/Latinos

Because these ethnic and racial groups are more likely to have lactose malabsorption, they are also more likely to have the symptoms of lactose intolerance.

Lactose intolerance is least common among people who are from, or whose families are from, Europe.

What Are the Complications of Lactose Intolerance?

Lactose intolerance may affect your health if it keeps you from getting enough nutrients, such as calcium and vitamin D. Milk and milk products, which contain lactose, are some of the main sources of calcium, vitamin D, and other nutrients.

You need calcium throughout your life to grow and have healthy bones. If you do not get enough calcium, your bones may become weak and more likely to break. This condition is called "osteoporosis." If you have lactose intolerance, you can change your diet to make sure you get enough calcium while also managing your symptoms.

SYMPTOMS AND CAUSES

What Are the Symptoms of Lactose Intolerance?

If you have lactose intolerance, you may have symptoms within a few hours after you have milk or milk products, or other foods that contain lactose. Your symptoms may include:

- Bloating
- Diarrhea
- Gas
- Nausea
- Pain in your abdomen
- Stomach "growling" or rumbling sounds
- Vomiting

Your symptoms may be mild or severe, depending on how much lactose you have.

What Causes Lactose Intolerance?

Lactose intolerance is caused by lactose malabsorption. If you have lactose malabsorption, your small intestine makes low levels of lactase – the enzyme that breaks down lactose – and cannot digest all the lactose you eat or drink.

The undigested lactose passes into your colon. Bacteria in your colon break down the lactose and create fluid and gas. In some people, this extra fluid and gas causes lactose intolerance symptoms.

In some cases, your genes are the reason for lactose intolerance. Genes play a role in the following conditions, and these conditions can lead to low levels of lactase in your small intestine and lactose malabsorption:

- **Lactase nonpersistence.** In people with lactase nonpersistence, the small intestine makes less lactase after infancy. Lactase levels get lower with age. Symptoms of lactose intolerance may not begin until later childhood, the teen years, or early adulthood. Lactase nonpersistence, also called "primary lactase deficiency," is the most common cause of low lactase levels.
- **Congenital lactase deficiency.** In this rare condition, the small intestine makes little or no lactase, starting at birth.

Not all causes of lactose intolerance are genetic. The following can also lead to lactose intolerance:

- **Injury to the small intestine.** Infections, diseases, or other conditions that injure your small intestine, such as Crohn disease or celiac disease, may cause it to make less lactase. Treatments, such as medicines, surgery, or radiation therapy for other conditions may also injure your small intestine. Lactose intolerance caused by injury to the small intestine is called "secondary lactose intolerance." If the cause of the injury is treated, you may be able to tolerate lactose again.
- **Premature birth.** In premature babies, or babies born too soon, the small intestine may not make enough

lactase for a short time after birth. The small intestine usually makes more lactase as the baby gets older.

What Is the Difference between Lactose Intolerance and Milk Allergies?

Lactose intolerance and milk allergies are different conditions with different causes. Lactose intolerance is caused by problems digesting lactose, the natural sugar in milk. In contrast, milk allergies are caused by your immune system's response to one or more proteins in milk and milk products.

A milk allergy most often appears in the first year of life, while lactose intolerance typically appears later. Lactose intolerance can cause uncomfortable symptoms, while a serious allergic reaction to milk can be life-threatening.

DIAGNOSIS OF LACTOSE INTOLERANCE

How Do Doctors Diagnose Lactose Intolerance?

To diagnose lactose intolerance, your doctor will ask about your symptoms, family and medical history, and eating habits.

Your doctor may perform a physical exam and tests to help diagnose lactose intolerance or to check for other health problems. Other conditions, such as irritable bowel syndrome, celiac disease, inflammatory bowel disease, or small bowel bacterial overgrowth can cause symptoms similar to those of lactose intolerance.

Your doctor may ask you to stop eating and drinking milk and milk products for a period of time to see if your symptoms go away. If your symptoms do not go away, your doctor may order additional tests.

PHYSICAL EXAM

During a physical exam, your doctor may:

- Check for bloating in your abdomen
- Use a stethoscope to listen to sounds within your abdomen
- Tap on your abdomen to check for tenderness or pain

What Tests Do Doctors Use to Diagnose Lactose Intolerance?

Your doctor may order a hydrogen breath test to see how well your small intestine digests lactose.

HYDROGEN BREATH TEST

Doctors use this test to diagnose lactose malabsorption and lactose intolerance. Normally, a small amount of hydrogen, a type of gas, is found in your breath. If you have lactose malabsorption, undigested lactose causes you to have high levels of hydrogen in your breath. For this test, you will drink a liquid that contains a known amount of lactose. Every 30 minutes over a few hours, you will breathe into a balloon-type container that measures the amount of hydrogen in your breath. During this time, a healthcare professional will ask about your symptoms. If both your breath hydrogen levels rise and your symptoms get worse during the test, your doctor may diagnose lactose intolerance.

TREATMENT FOR LACTOSE INTOLERANCE

How Can You Manage Your Lactose Intolerance Symptoms?

In most cases, you can manage the symptoms of lactose intolerance by changing your diet to limit or avoid foods and drinks that contain lactose, such as milk and milk products.

Some people may only need to limit the amount of lactose they eat or drink, while others may need to avoid lactose altogether. Using lactase products can help some people manage their symptoms.

LACTASE PRODUCTS

Lactase products are tablets or drops that contain lactase, the enzyme that breaks down lactose. You can take lactase tablets before you eat or drink milk products. You can also add lactase drops to milk before you drink it. The lactase breaks down the lactose in foods and drinks, lowering your chances of having lactose intolerance symptoms.

Check with your doctor before using lactase products. Some people, such as young children and pregnant and breastfeeding women, may not be able to use them.

How Do Doctors Treat Lactose Intolerance?

Treatments depend on the cause of lactose intolerance. If your lactose intolerance is caused by lactase nonpersistence or congenital lactase deficiency, no treatments can increase the amount of lactase your small intestine makes. Your doctor can help you change your diet to manage your symptoms.

If your lactose intolerance is caused by an injury to your small intestine, your doctor may be able to treat the cause of the injury. You may be able to tolerate lactose after treatment.

While some premature babies are lactose intolerant, the condition usually improves without treatment as the baby gets older.

EATING, DIET, AND NUTRITION

How Should You Change Your Diet If You Have Lactose Intolerance?

Talk with your doctor or a dietitian about changing your diet to manage lactose intolerance symptoms while making sure you get enough nutrients. If your child has lactose intolerance, help your child follow the dietary plan recommended by a doctor or dietitian. To manage your symptoms, you may need to reduce the amount of lactose you eat or drink. Most people with lactose intolerance can have some lactose without getting symptoms.

FOODS THAT CONTAIN LACTOSE

You may not need to completely avoid foods and beverages that contain lactose, such as milk or milk products. If you avoid all milk and milk products, you may get less calcium and vitamin D than you need.

People with lactose intolerance can handle different amounts of lactose. Research suggests that many people could have 12 grams of lactose – the amount in about one cup of milk – without symptoms or with only mild symptoms.

You may be able to tolerate milk and milk products if you:

- Drink small amounts of milk at a time and have it with meals
- Add milk and milk products to your diet a little at a time and see how you feel

- Try eating yogurt and hard cheeses, such as cheddar or Swiss, which are lower in lactose than other milk products
- Use lactase products to help digest the lactose in milk and milk products

LACTOSE-FREE AND LACTOSE-REDUCED MILK AND MILK PRODUCTS

Using lactose-free and lactose-reduced milk and milk products may help you lower the amount of lactose in your diet. These products are available in many grocery stores and are just as healthy for you as regular milk and milk products.

CALCIUM AND VITAMIN D

If you are lactose intolerant, make sure you get enough calcium and vitamin D each day. Milk and milk products are the most common sources of calcium.

Many foods that do not contain lactose are also sources of calcium. Examples include:

- Fish with soft bones, such as canned salmon or sardines
- Broccoli and leafy green vegetables
- Oranges
- Almonds, Brazil nuts, and dried beans
- Tofu
- Products with labels that show they have added calcium, such as some cereals, fruit juices, and soy milk

Vitamin D helps your body absorb and use calcium. Be sure to eat foods that contain vitamin D, such as eggs and certain kinds of fish, such as salmon. Some ready-to-eat cereals and orange juice have added vitamin D. Some milk and milk products also have added vitamin D. If you can drink small amounts of milk or milk products without symptoms, choose products that have added vitamin D. Also, being outside in the sunlight helps your body make vitamin D.

Talk with your doctor or dietitian about whether you are getting the nutrients you need. For safety reasons, also talk with your doctor before using dietary supplements or any other complementary or alternative medicines (CAMs) or practices. Also, talk with your doctor about sun exposure and sun safety.

WHAT FOODS AND DRINKS CONTAIN LACTOSE

Lactose is in all milk and milk products and may be found in other foods and drinks.

Milk and milk products may be added to boxed, canned, frozen, packaged, and prepared foods. If you have symptoms after consuming a small amount of lactose, you should be aware of the many products that may contain lactose, such as:

- Bread and other baked goods, such as pancakes, biscuits, cookies, and cakes
- Processed foods, including breakfast cereals, instant potatoes, soups, margarine, salad dressings, and flavored chips and other snack foods
- Processed meats, such as bacon, sausage, hot dogs, and lunch meats
- Milk-based meal replacement liquids and powders, smoothies, and protein powders and bars
- Nondairy liquid and powdered coffee creamers, and nondairy whipped toppings

You can check the ingredient list on packaged foods to see if the product contains lactose. The following words mean that the product contains lactose:

- Milk
- Lactose
- Whey
- Curds
- Milk by-products
- Dry milk solids
- Nonfat dry milk powder

A small amount of lactose may be found in some prescription and over-the-counter (OTC) medicines. Talk with your doctor about the amount of lactose in medicines you take, especially if you typically cannot tolerate even small amounts of lactose.

Section 43.4 | Eating Disorders

This section includes text excerpted from "Eating Disorders," MentalHealth.gov, U.S. Department of Health and Human Services (HHS), March 21, 2019.

Eating disorders involve extreme emotions, attitudes, and behaviors involving weight and food.

ANOREXIA NERVOSA

Anorexia nervosa is an eating disorder that makes people lose more weight than is considered healthy for their age and height. Persons with this disorder may have an intense fear of weight gain, even when they are underweight. They may diet or exercise too much, or use other methods to lose weight.

Causes of Anorexia Nervosa

The exact causes of anorexia nervosa are not known. Many factors probably are involved. Genes and hormones may play a role. Social attitudes that promote very thin body types may also be involved. Family conflicts are no longer thought to contribute to this or other eating disorders.

Risk factors for anorexia include:

- Being more worried about, or paying more attention to, weight and shape
- Having an anxiety disorder as a child
- Having a negative self-image
- Having eating problems during infancy or early childhood
- Having certain social or cultural ideas about health and beauty
- Trying to be perfect or overly focused on rules

Anorexia usually begins during the teen years or young adulthood. It is more common in females, but may also be seen in males. The disorder is seen mainly in white women who are high academic achievers and who have a goal-oriented family or personality.

Symptoms of Anorexia Nervosa

To be diagnosed with anorexia, a person must:

- Have an intense fear of gaining weight or becoming fat, even when she or he is underweight
- Refuse to keep weight at what is considered normal for her or his age and height (15 percent or more below the normal weight)
- Have a body image that is very distorted, be very focused on body weight or shape, and refuse to admit the seriousness of weight loss
- Have not had a period for three or more cycles (in women)

People with anorexia may severely limit the amount of food they eat, or eat and then make themselves throw up. Other behaviors include:

- Cutting food into small pieces or moving them around the plate instead of eating
- Exercising all the time, even when the weather is bad, they are hurt, or their schedule is busy
- Going to the bathroom right after meals
- Refusing to eat around other people
- Using pills to make themselves urinate (water pills or diuretics), have a bowel movement (enemas and laxatives), or decrease their appetite (diet pills)

Other symptoms of anorexia may include:

- Blotchy or yellow skin that is dry and covered with fine hair
- Confused or slow thinking, along with poor memory or judgement
- Depression
- Dry mouth
- Extreme sensitivity to cold (wearing several layers of clothing to stay warm)
- Loss of bone strength
- Wasting away of muscle and loss of body fat

BINGE EATING

Binge eating is when a person eats a much larger amount of food in a shorter period of time than she or he normally would. During binge eating, the person also feels a loss of control.

Considerations

A binge eater often:

- Eats 5,000–15,000 calories in one sitting
- Often snacks, in addition to eating three meals a day
- Overeats throughout the day

Binge eating by itself usually leads to becoming overweight.

Binge eating may occur on its own or with another eating disorder, such as bulimia. People with bulimia typically eat large amounts of high-calorie foods, usually in secret. After this binge eating they often force themselves to vomit or take laxatives.

Causes of Binge Eating

The cause of binge eating is unknown. However, binge eating often begins during or after strict dieting.

BULIMIA

Bulimia is an illness in which a person binges on food or has regular episodes of overeating and feels a loss of control. The person then uses different methods – such as vomiting or abusing laxatives – to prevent weight gain.

Many (but not all) people with bulimia also have anorexia nervosa.

Causes of Bulimia

Many more women than men have bulimia. The disorder is most common in adolescent girls and young women. The affected person is usually aware that her eating pattern is abnormal and may feel fear or guilt with the binge-purge episodes.

The exact cause of bulimia is unknown. Genetic, psychological, trauma, family, society, or cultural factors may play a role. Bulimia is likely due to more than one factor.

Symptoms of Bulimia

In bulimia, eating binges may occur as often as several times a day for many months.

People with bulimia often eat large amounts of high-calorie foods, usually in secret. People can feel a lack of control over their eating during these episodes.

Binges lead to self-disgust, which causes purging to prevent weight gain. Purging may include:

- Forcing yourself to vomit
- Excessive exercise
- Using laxatives, enemas, or diuretics (water pills)

Purging often brings a sense of relief.

People with bulimia are often at a normal weight, but they may see themselves as being overweight. Because the person's weight is often normal, other people may not notice this eating disorder.

Symptoms that other people can see include:

- Compulsive exercise
- Suddenly eating large amounts of food or buying large amounts of food that disappear right away
- Regularly going to the bathroom right after meals
- Throwing away packages of laxatives, diet pills, emetics (drugs that cause vomiting), or diuretics

Chapter 44 | Celiac Disease and a Gluten-Free Diet

WHAT IS CELIAC DISEASE?

Celiac disease is a chronic digestive and immune disorder that damages the small intestine. The disease is triggered by eating foods containing gluten. Gluten is a protein found naturally in wheat, barley, and rye, and is common in foods, such as bread, pasta, cookies, and cakes. Many products contain gluten, such as prepackaged foods, lip balms and lipsticks, toothpaste, vitamin and nutrient supplements, and, rarely, medicines.

Celiac disease can be serious. The disease can cause long-lasting digestive problems and keep your body from getting all the nutrients it needs, and it can also affect the body outside the small intestine.

Celiac disease is different from gluten sensitivity or wheat intolerance. If you have gluten sensitivity, you may have symptoms like those of celiac diseases, such as abdominal pain and tiredness. Unlike celiac disease, gluten sensitivity does not damage the small intestine.

Celiac disease is also different from a wheat allergy, a type of food allergy. In both cases, your body's immune system reacts to wheat. However, some symptoms of wheat allergies, such as having itchy eyes or a hard time breathing, are different from celiac disease. Wheat allergies also do not cause long-term damage to the small intestine.

This chapter includes text excerpted from "Celiac Disease," National Institute of Diabetes and Digestive and Kidney Diseases (NIDDK), November 15, 2014. Reviewed May 2021.

HOW DO DOCTORS TREAT CELIAC DISEASE?

Gluten-Free Diet

Doctors treat celiac disease by helping people to follow a gluten-free diet. Gluten is a protein found naturally in certain grains, including wheat, barley, and rye. Gluten is also added to many other foods and products. In people who have celiac disease, consuming gluten triggers an abnormal immune system reaction that damages the small intestine.

Symptoms greatly improve for most people with celiac disease who stick to a gluten-free diet. For most people, following a gluten-free diet will heal damage in the small intestine and prevent more damage. Many people see symptoms improve within days to weeks of starting the diet.

Your doctor will explain the gluten-free diet and may refer you to a registered dietitian who specializes in treating people who have celiac disease. The dietitian will teach you how to avoid gluten while following a healthy diet and recommend substitutes for foods that contain gluten. She/he will help you to:

- Check food and product labels for gluten
- Design everyday meal plans
- Make healthy choices about foods and drinks

Avoiding Medicines and Other Products That May Contain Gluten

In addition to prescribing a gluten-free diet, your doctor will want you to avoid all hidden sources of gluten. If you have celiac disease, ask a pharmacist about ingredients in:

- Herbal and nutritional supplements
- Prescription and over-the-counter (OTC) medicines
- Vitamin and mineral supplements

Medicines are rare sources of gluten. Even if gluten is present in a medicine, it is likely to be in such small quantities that it would not cause any symptoms.

Other products can be hidden sources of gluten. You may take in small amounts of gluten if you consume these products, use them around your mouth, or transfer them from your hands to your mouth by accident. Products that may contain gluten include:

- Children's modeling dough, such as Play-Doh
- Cosmetics
- Lipstick, lip gloss, and lip balm
- Skin and hair products
- Toothpaste and mouthwash
- Communion wafers

Reading product labels can sometimes help you avoid gluten. Some companies label their products as being gluten free. In the United States, products labeled gluten free must have less than 20 parts per million of gluten, which should not be a problem for the vast majority of people. If a label does not tell you what is in a product, ask the company that makes the product for an ingredients list. You cannot assume that the product is gluten free.

Treatments for Symptoms or Complications

A gluten-free diet will treat or prevent many of the symptoms and complications of celiac disease. Some symptoms may take longer to get better than others, and some symptoms may need additional help.

Dermatitis herpetiformis may not go away until a person has been following a gluten-free diet for six months to two years. In some cases, doctors may prescribe medicine, such as dapsone, to help treat dermatitis herpetiformis until the rash is under control with a gluten-free diet alone.

In untreated celiac disease, damage to the small intestine can lead to malabsorption and malnutrition. When you are diagnosed with celiac disease, your doctor may test you for low levels of certain vitamins and minerals and may recommend or prescribe supplements if you need them. For safety reasons, talk with your doctor before using dietary supplements, such as vitamins, or any complementary or alternative medicines or medical practices.

When you are diagnosed with celiac disease, your doctor may recommend additional testing if you are at risk for certain complications. For example, doctors may order a bone mineral density test to check for osteoporosis.

HOW WILL YOU NEED TO CHANGE YOUR DIET IF YOU HAVE CELIAC DISEASE?

If you have celiac disease, you will need to remove foods and drinks that contain gluten from your diet. Following a gluten-free diet can relieve celiac disease symptoms and heal damage to the small intestine. People with celiac disease need to follow a gluten-free diet for life to prevent symptoms and intestinal damage from coming back. Your doctor or a registered dietitian can guide you on what to eat and drink to maintain a balanced diet.

If you or your child has been diagnosed with celiac disease, you may find support groups helpful as you learn about and adjust to a gluten-free lifestyle. Your doctor or a registered dietitian may be able to recommend support groups and other reliable sources of information.

WHAT FOODS AND DRINKS CONTAIN GLUTEN

Gluten occurs naturally in certain grains, including:

- Wheat and types of wheat, such as durum, emmer, and semolina
- Barley, which may be found in malt, malt extract, malt vinegar, and brewer's yeast
- Rye
- Triticale, a cross between wheat and rye

Gluten is found in foods that contain ingredients made from these grains, including baked goods, baking mixes, bread, cereals, and pasta. Drinks, such as beer, lagers, ale, flavored liquors, and malt beverages may also contain gluten.

Many food ingredients and additives, such as colorings, flavorings, starches, and thickeners are made from grains that contain gluten. These ingredients are added to many processed foods, including foods that are boxed, canned, frozen, packaged, or prepared. Therefore, gluten may be found in a variety of foods, including candy, condiments, hot dogs and sausages, ice cream, salad dressing, and soups.

Cross-Contact

Cross-contact occurs when foods or products that contain gluten come into contact with gluten-free foods. Cross-contact can spread gluten to gluten-free foods, making the gluten-free foods unsafe for people with celiac disease to consume. Cross-contact can occur at any time, including when foods are grown, processed, stored, prepared, or served.

HOW CAN YOU IDENTIFY AND AVOID FOODS AND DRINKS THAT CONTAIN GLUTEN?

A registered dietitian can help you learn to identify and avoid foods and drinks that contain gluten when you shop, prepare foods at home or eat out.

For example, when you shop and eat at home:

- Carefully read food labels to check for grains that contain gluten, such as wheat, barley, rye, and ingredients or additives made from those grains.
- Check for gluten-free food labeling.
- Do not eat foods if you are not sure whether they contain gluten. If possible, contact the company that makes the food or visit the company's website for more information.
- Store and prepare your gluten-free foods separately from other family members' foods that contain gluten to prevent cross-contact.

When you eat out at restaurants or social gatherings:

- Before you go out to eat, search online for restaurants that offer a gluten-free menu.
- Review restaurant menus online or call ahead to make sure a restaurant can accommodate you safely.
- At the restaurant, let the server know that you have celiac disease. Ask about food ingredients, how food is

prepared, and whether a gluten-free menu is available. Ask to talk with the chef if you would like more details about the menu.
- When attending social gatherings, let the host know you have celiac disease and find out if gluten-free foods will be available. If not, or if you are unsure, bring gluten-free foods that are safe for you to eat.

WHAT SHOULD YOU EAT IF YOU HAVE CELIAC DISEASE?

If you have celiac disease, you will need to follow a gluten-free diet. Your doctor and a registered dietitian can help you plan a healthy, balanced diet to make sure that you get the nutrients you need.

Gluten-Free Foods

Many foods, such as meat, fish, fruits, vegetables, rice, and potatoes, without additives or some seasonings, are naturally gluten free. Flour made from gluten-free foods, such as potatoes, rice, corn, soy, nuts, cassava, amaranth, quinoa, buckwheat, or beans is safe to eat.

You can also buy packaged gluten-free foods, such as gluten-free types of baked goods, bread, and pasta. These foods are available from many grocery stores, restaurants, and at specialty food companies. Packaged gluten-free foods tend to cost more than the same foods that have gluten, and restaurants may charge more for gluten-free types of foods.

Talk with your doctor or a registered dietitian about whether you should include oats in your diet and how much. Research suggests that most people with celiac disease can safely eat moderate amounts of oats. If you do eat oats, make sure they are gluten free. Cross-contact between oats and grains that contain gluten is common and can make oats unsafe for people with celiac disease.

Gluten-Free Labeling

The U.S. Food and Drug Administration (FDA) requires that foods labeled "gluten free" meet specific standards. One requirement is that foods with the terms "gluten free," "no gluten," "free of gluten," or "without gluten" on the label must contain less than 20 parts per million of gluten. This amount of gluten is too small to cause problems in most people with celiac disease.

The FDA rule does not apply to foods regulated by the U.S. Department of Agriculture (USDA), including meat, poultry, and some egg products. The rule also does not apply to most alcoholic beverages, which are regulated by the U.S. Department of the Treasury (USDT).

SHOULD YOU START A GLUTEN-FREE DIET BEFORE YOU TALK WITH YOUR DOCTOR?

No. If you think you might have celiac disease, you should talk with your doctor about testing to diagnose celiac disease before you begin a gluten-free diet. If you avoid gluten before you have tested, the test results may not be accurate.

Also, if you start avoiding gluten without advice from a doctor or a registered dietitian, your diet may not provide enough of the nutrients you need, such as fiber, iron, and calcium. Some packaged gluten-free foods may be higher in fat and sugar than the same foods that contain gluten. If you are diagnosed with celiac disease, your doctor and dietitian can help you plan a healthy gluten-free diet.

If you do not have celiac disease or another health problem related to gluten, your doctor may not recommend a gluten-free diet. In recent years, more people without celiac disease have begun avoiding gluten, believing that a gluten-free diet is healthier or could help them lose weight. However, researchers have found no evidence that a gluten-free diet promotes better health or weight loss for the general population.

Chapter 45 | **Cancer and Nutrition**

Chapter Contents

Section 45.1 | **Nutrition in Cancer Care**

This section includes text excerpted from "Eating Hints: Before, during, and after Cancer Treatment," National Cancer Institute (NCI), January 15, 2018.

PEOPLE WITH CANCER HAVE DIFFERENT DIET NEEDS

People with cancer often need to follow diets that are different from what you think of as healthy. For most people, a healthy diet includes:

- Lots of fruits, vegetables, and whole-grain bread and cereals
- Modest amounts of meat and milk products
- Small amounts of fat, sugar, alcohol, and salt

When you have cancer, though, you need to eat to keep up your strength to deal with the side effects of treatment. When you are healthy, eating enough food is often not a problem. But, when you are dealing with cancer and treatment, this can be a real challenge.

When you have cancer, you may need extra protein and calories. At times, your diet may need to include extra milk, cheese, and eggs. If you have trouble chewing and swallowing, you may need to add sauces and gravies. Sometimes, you may need to eat low-fiber foods instead of those with high fiber. A dietitian can help you with any diet changes you may need to make.

SIDE EFFECTS FROM CANCER TREATMENT CAN LEAD TO EATING PROBLEMS

Cancer treatments are designed to kill cancer cells. But, these treatments can also damage healthy cells. Damage to healthy cells can cause side effects that lead to eating problems. Common eating problems during cancer treatment include:

- Appetite loss
- Changes in sense of taste or smell
- Constipation
- Diarrhea
- Dry mouth
- Lactose intolerance

- Nausea
- Sore mouth
- Sore throat and trouble swallowing
- Vomiting
- Weight gain
- Weight loss

Some people have appetite loss or nausea because they are stressed about cancer and treatment. But, once people know what to expect, they often feel better.

TALK WITH YOUR DOCTOR, NURSE, OR DIETITIAN

Talk with your doctor or nurse if you are not sure what to eat during cancer treatment. Ask her or him to refer you to a dietitian. A dietitian is the best person to talk with about your diet. She or he can help choose foods and drinks that are best for you during treatment and after.

Make a list of questions for your meeting with the dietitian. Ask about your favorite foods and recipes and if you can eat them during cancer treatment. You might want to find out how other patients manage their eating problems. You can also bring this book and ask the dietitian to mark sections that are right for you.

If you are already on a special diet for diabetes, kidney or heart disease, or other health problems, it is even more important to speak with a doctor and dietitian. Your doctor and dietitian can advise you about how to follow your special diet while coping with eating problems caused by cancer treatment.

WAYS TO GET THE MOST FROM FOODS AND DRINKS

During treatment, you may have good days and bad days when it comes to food. Here are some ways to manage:

- Eat plenty of protein and calories when you can. This helps you keep up your strength and helps rebuild tissues harmed by cancer treatment.
- Eat when you have the biggest appetite. For many people, this is in the morning. You might want to eat

a bigger meal early in the day and drink liquid meal replacements later on.

- It is okay if you feel like you cannot eat a lot of different foods. Eat the foods that sound good until you are able to eat more, even if it is the same thing again and again. You might also drink liquid meal replacements for extra nutrition.
- Do not worry if you cannot eat at all some days. Spend this time finding other ways to feel better and start eating when you can. Tell your doctor if you cannot eat for more than two days.
- Drink plenty of liquids. It is even more important to get plenty to drink on days when you cannot eat. Drinking a lot helps your body get the liquid it needs. Most adults should drink 8 to 12 cups of liquid a day. You may find this easier to do if you keep a water bottle nearby.

TAKING SPECIAL CARE WITH FOOD TO AVOID INFECTIONS

Some cancer treatments can make you prone to infections. When this happens, you need to take special care in the way you handle and prepare food. Be careful to:

- Keep hot foods hot and cold foods cold.
- Put leftovers in the refrigerator as soon as you have finished eating.
- Scrub all raw fruits and vegetables with a brush and water before you eat them.
- Soak berries and other foods that are not easily scrubbed in water, then rinse.
- Scrub fruits and vegetables that have rough surfaces and peels, such as melons, oranges, and avocados, with a brush and water before you cut or peel them.
- Soak frozen fruits and vegetables in water and rinse if you are not going to cook them (for a smoothie, for instance). If cooking, you do not need to wash frozen fruits and vegetables.

- Wash your hands, knives, and countertops before and after you prepare food. This step is most important when preparing raw meat, chicken, turkey, and fish.
- Wash your hands each time you touch raw meat, chicken, turkey, or fish. Use one cutting board for meat and another one for fruits and vegetables.
- Thaw meat, chicken, turkey, and fish in the refrigerator or defrost them in the microwave. Cook meat, chicken, turkey, and eggs thoroughly. Eggs should be hard, not runny. Meats should not have any pink inside. To be sure meat, chicken, turkey, and fish is safe, use a meat thermometer and cook to the safe temperature.
- Make sure your juices and milk products are pasteurized.
- Eat nuts that are shelled and roasted.

Do Not

- Eat raw fish or shellfish, such as sushi and uncooked oysters
- Eat raw nuts
- Use foods, condiments, or drinks that are past their freshness date
- Buy food from bulk bins
- Eat at buffets, salad bars, or self-service restaurants
- Eat foods that show signs of mold, including moldy cheeses, such as bleu cheese and Roquefort
- Eat any perishable foods that have been sitting at room temperature longer than two hours
- Eat leftovers that have been in the refrigerator longer than three days
- Leave meat, chicken, turkey, or fish sitting out to thaw

Section 45.2 | **Antioxidants and Cancer Prevention**

This section includes text excerpted from "Antioxidants and Cancer Prevention," National Cancer Institute (NCI), February 6, 2017. Reviewed May 2021.

WHAT ARE FREE RADICALS, AND DO THEY PLAY A ROLE IN CANCER DEVELOPMENT?

Free radicals are highly reactive chemicals that have the potential to harm cells. They are created when an atom or a molecule (a chemical that has two or more atoms) either gains or loses an electron (a small negatively charged particle found in atoms). Free radicals are formed naturally in the body and play an important role in many normal cellular processes. At high concentrations, however, free radicals can be hazardous to the body and damage all major components of cells, including DNA, proteins, and cell membranes. The damage to cells caused by free radicals, especially the damage to DNA, may play a role in the development of cancer and other health conditions.

Abnormally high concentrations of free radicals in the body can be caused by exposure to ionizing radiation and other environmental toxins. When ionizing radiation hits an atom or a molecule in a cell, an electron may be lost, leading to the formation of a free radical. The production of abnormally high levels of free radicals is the mechanism by which ionizing radiation kills cells. Moreover, some environmental toxins, such as cigarette smoke, some metals, and high-oxygen atmospheres, may contain large amounts of free radicals or stimulate the body's cells to produce more free radicals.

Free radicals that contain the element oxygen are the most common type of free radicals produced in living tissue. Another name for them is "reactive oxygen species," (ROS).

WHAT ARE ANTIOXIDANTS?

Antioxidants are chemicals that interact with and neutralize free radicals, thus preventing them from causing damage. Antioxidants are also known as "free radical scavengers."

The body makes some of the antioxidants that it uses to neutralize free radicals. These antioxidants are called "endogenous antioxidants." However, the body relies on external (exogenous) sources, primarily the diet, to obtain the rest of the antioxidants it needs. These exogenous antioxidants are commonly called "dietary antioxidants." Fruits, vegetables, and grains are rich sources of dietary antioxidants. Some dietary antioxidants are also available as dietary supplements.

Examples of dietary antioxidants include beta-carotene, lycopene, and vitamins A, C, and E (alpha-tocopherol). The mineral element selenium is often thought to be a dietary antioxidant, but the antioxidant effects of selenium are most likely due to the antioxidant activity of proteins that have this element as an essential component (i.e., selenium-containing proteins), and not to selenium itself.

CAN ANTIOXIDANT SUPPLEMENTS HELP PREVENT CANCER?

In laboratory and animal studies, the presence of increased levels of exogenous antioxidants has been shown to prevent the types of free radical damage that have been associated with cancer development. Therefore, researchers have investigated whether taking dietary antioxidant supplements can help lower the risk of developing or dying from cancer in humans.

Many observational studies, including case-control studies and cohort studies, have been conducted to investigate whether the use of dietary antioxidant supplements is associated with reduced risks of cancer in humans. Overall, these studies have yielded mixed results. Because observational studies cannot adequately control for biases that might influence study outcomes, the results of any individual observational study must be viewed with caution.

Randomized controlled clinical trials, however, lack most of the biases that limit the reliability of observational studies. Therefore, randomized trials are considered to provide the strongest and most reliable evidence of the benefit and/or harm of a health-related intervention. To date, nine randomized controlled trials of dietary antioxidant supplements for cancer prevention have been conducted worldwide. Many of the trials were sponsored by the National Cancer Institute.

SHOULD PEOPLE ALREADY DIAGNOSED WITH CANCER TAKE ANTIOXIDANT SUPPLEMENTS?

Several randomized controlled trials, some including only small numbers of patients, have investigated whether taking antioxidant supplements during cancer treatment alters the effectiveness or reduces the toxicity of specific therapies. Although these trials had mixed results, some found that people who took antioxidant supplements during cancer therapy had worse outcomes, especially if they were smokers.

In some preclinical studies, antioxidants have been found to promote tumor growth and metastasis in tumor-bearing mice and to increase the ability of circulating tumor cells to metastasize. Until more is known about the effects of antioxidant supplements in cancer patients, these supplements should be used with caution. Cancer patients should inform their doctors about their use of any dietary supplement.

Chapter 46 | Nutrition and Oral Health

Tooth development begins in the fetus as early as six weeks of age when the basic material that makes up teeth starts to form. The impact of nutrition on oral health and dental development begins in the womb, with the mother's nutritional status and eating patterns playing a vital role in the process. Studies have shown that adequate nutrition is a key factor in defining the health of teeth and periodontal tissues and in maintaining salivary secretions at their optimum. Early nutritional imbalances can lead to developmental malformations of the dentition, while malnutrition can result in enamel hypoplasia (thin tooth enamel), poor periodontal health, increased risk of oral infectious disease, and the early onset of dental erosion.

IMPORTANCE OF BALANCED DIET

Nutrition plays a vital role in boosting the body's immune system and preventing infections and inflammations. Malnutrition – deficiencies of essential nutrients, such as vitamins and minerals – can have a negative impact on general health and result in cavities and gum disease. Gum disease may start as gingivitis, an inflammation of the gums usually caused by a bacterial infection which, if unchecked, may progress to periodontal disease, a condition that affects the supporting tissues of the teeth.

SOME IMPORTANT MICRONUTRIENTS

Studies show that nutrition and oral health are interrelated. Poor nutrition can cause oral and dental problems and, conversely, problems with oral health can trigger nutritional deficiencies. Food habits and eating patterns greatly impact the decay resistance of teeth in children and teens, and a well-balanced diet is an important factor in maintaining periodontal health in the adults and elderly.

A number of micronutrients (vitamins and minerals) are critical to the maintenance of healthy teeth and gums. These include:

Vitamin D (Calciferol)

Vitamin D plays a vital role in maintaining musculoskeletal health by aiding in calcium absorption. Its direct effect on bone metabolism makes it an essential nutrient in preventing tooth loss and maintaining periodontal health. Vitamin D is also involved in certain immunoregulatory pathways and reduces the risk of periodontitis or inflammation of periodontal tissues. Dietary sources of vitamin D include fish liver oils, fatty fish, mushrooms, egg yolks, liver, and fortified foods, such as breakfast cereals, milk, and orange juice. The vitamin is also synthesized in the skin by the action of ultraviolet radiation of the sun on certain sterols (substances in many plants that help lower cholesterol).

Vitamin C (Ascorbic Acid)

Vitamin C is essential for maintaining the integrity of the connective tissue and dentine, the hard material that makes up much of a tooth. It is also necessary for the proper functioning of the immune system. The deficiency of vitamin C can lead to scurvy, a disease characterized by gingivitis (spongy, bleeding gums). Rich sources of vitamin C include citrus fruits, such as oranges, limes, grapefruit, green leafy vegetables, tomatoes, and berries.

CHOOSING A HEALTHY DIET

- Fruits and vegetables are especially important in maintaining good oral health. Salads are ideal, as chewing raw vegetables stimulates the secretion of saliva, which helps to wash acid and food remnants from the mouth.

- Nuts are also good. Their low-carbohydrate content reduces the risk of cavities. In addition to providing such benefits as minerals and vitamins, they also serve as rich sources of proteins that are important for maintaining overall health.
- Dairy products, such as milk, cheese, and yogurt, are excellent sources of proteins, as well as calcium, a mineral that is critical for the development and maintenance of healthy teeth and periodontal tissue.
- Lean meat, eggs, legumes, and green leafy vegetables, such as collards and spinach, are also rich sources of calcium and can help to build strong teeth and maintain good oral health.

FLUORIDATED WATER AND ORAL HEALTH

Drinking fluoridated water is highly beneficial for maintaining healthy teeth. Fluoride helps prevent tooth decay, and water washes away food debris in the mouth. The presence of food particles encourages the growth of bacteria that break down the sugars in food to release acids. These acids wear away the mineralized oral tissues, including enamel (the hard protective covering of the teeth), cementum (the exterior surface of the roots), and dentine. Water not only removes food residue in the mouth but also dilutes the acid produced by cavity-causing bacteria. Drinking water also prevents dehydration and xerostomia (dry mouth, or insufficient saliva). Saliva is an important factor in maintaining the integrity of oral structures. It helps lubricate, chew, and digest food; kill microorganisms in food; dilute sugars; and buffer acid in the mouth. Saliva also helps remineralize tooth enamel with calcium and phosphorous. Insufficient salivary secretions can increase the risk of gingivitis, dental cavities, and oral thrush, a fungal infection of the mouth.

FOODS TO AVOID FOR BETTER ORAL HEALTH

The connection between sugar and cavities has been studied for a long time, and it has been established that fermentable carbohydrates and sugars play a major role in the development of dental cavities. These cariogenic (cavity-causing) foods are acted upon by bacteria in the mouth, such as *streptococci* and *lactobacilli*, and are converted to acids. The acids demineralize teeth by dissolving calcium and phosphorus and causing tooth erosion. Normally, the demineralization of teeth is offset by remineralization with saliva, which is saturated with calcium and phosphorus. But, if the acidic environment in the mouth persists, it interferes with the remineralization process, leading to tooth decay.

Although cariogenic foods include a variety of sugars, such as glucose, lactose, fructose, and maltose – either naturally occurring or added to food – sucrose (table sugar) is by far the most cariogenic of all. Avoiding high-sugar food, such as candies, confectionery, and sugar-sweetened drinks, is undoubtedly the most important prophylactic measure in controlling tooth decay and maintaining good oral health. While acids resulting from bacterial fermentation of sugars in the mouth are major causes of cavities, dietary acids can also, to some extent, contribute to decay by lowering pH below critical levels. Thus, foods and drinks with lower pH can cause tooth erosion. Vinegar-containing foods, as well as acids, naturally occurring in fruit or added to candies and sports drinks, can promote cavities and should be consumed in smaller amounts or eliminated from the diet entirely.

References

1. Touger-Decker, Riva; Cor van Loveren. "Sugars and Dental Caries," *American Journal of Clinical Nutrition* (AJCN), October 2003.
2. "The Best and Worst Foods for Your Teeth," Health Encyclopedia, University of Rochester Medical Center (URMC), 2016.

Part 8 | Additional Help and Information

Chapter 47 | Glossary of Nutrition and Diet Terms

added sugars: Sugars and syrups that are added to foods during processing or preparation. Added sugars do not include naturally occurring sugars such as lactose in milk or fructose in fruits.

adequate intake (AI): A recommended average daily nutrient intake level based on observed or experimentally determined approximations or estimates of mean nutrient intake by a group (or groups) of apparently healthy people.

alcoholism: A disease characterized by a dependency on alcohol. Excessive alcohol use can have a negative impact on bone health.

anorexia nervosa: An eating disorder characterized by an irrational fear of weight gain. Individuals with anorexia nervosa can experience nutritional and hormonal problems that negatively impact bone health.

arthritis: A general term for conditions that cause inflammation (swelling) of the joints and surrounding tissues. Some forms of arthritis may occur simultaneously with osteoporosis and Paget disease.

balance: The ability to maintain your body's stability while moving or standing still. Along with flexibility and strength, improving balance can significantly reduce the risk of falling.

blood cholesterol: Cholesterol that travels in the serum of the blood as distinct particles containing both lipids and proteins (lipoproteins). Also referred to as "serum cholesterol."

body mass index (BMI): A measure of weight in kilograms (kg) relative to height in meters squared (m^2). BMI is considered a reasonably reliable indicator of total body fat, which is related to the risk of disease and death.

This glossary contains terms excerpted from documents produced by several sources deemed reliable.

bone mineral density (BMD) testing: A test that measures bone strength and fracture risk.

breast cancer: A disease in which abnormal tumor cells develop in the breast. Women who have had breast cancer may be at increased risk for osteoporosis and fracture because of possible reduced levels of estrogen, chemotherapy or surgery, or early menopause.

calcium: A mineral that is an essential nutrient for bone health. It is also needed for the heart, muscles and nerves to function properly and for blood to clot.

calorie: A unit commonly used to measure energy content of foods and beverages as well as energy use (expenditure) by the body. A kilocalorie is equal to the amount of energy (heat) required to raise the temperature of 1 kilogram of water 1 °C.

carbohydrates: One of the macronutrients and a source of energy. They include sugars, starches, and fiber.

cardiovascular disease (CVD): Heart disease as well as diseases of the blood vessel system (arteries, capillaries, veins) that can lead to heart attack, chest pain (angina), or stroke.

celiac disease: An inherited intestinal disorder in which the body cannot tolerate gluten, which is found in foods made with wheat, rye, and barley. Bone loss is a complication of untreated celiac disease.

collagen: A family of fibrous proteins that are components of osteogenesis imperfecta is caused by a genetic defect that affects the body's production of collagen.

constipation: A decrease in frequency of stools or bowel movements with hardening of the stool.

DASH eating plan: The DASH (Dietary Approaches to Stop Hypertension) was designed to increase intake of foods expected to lower blood pressure while being heart healthy and meeting Institute of Medicine's (IOM) nutrient recommendations.

diabetes: A disease in which the body does not produce or properly use insulin. Insulin is a hormone that is needed to convert sugar, starches, and other food into energy.

dietary cholesterol: Cholesterol found in foods of animal origin, including meat, seafood, poultry, eggs, and dairy products.

dietary fiber: Nondigestible carbohydrates and lignin that are intrinsic and intact in plants.

eating behaviors: Individual behaviors that affect food and beverage choices and intake patterns, such as what, where, when, why, and how much people eat.

eating pattern (also called "dietary pattern"): The combination of foods and beverages that constitute an individual's complete dietary intake over time.

energy drink: A beverage that contains caffeine as an ingredient, along with other ingredients, such as taurine, herbal supplements, vitamins, and added sugars.

enrichment: The addition of specific nutrients (i.e., iron, thiamin, riboflavin, and niacin) to refined grain products in order to replace losses of the nutrients that occur during processing.

essential nutrient: A vitamin, mineral, fatty acid, or amino acid required for normal body functioning that either cannot be synthesized by the body at all, or cannot be synthesized in amounts adequate for good health, and thus must be obtained from a dietary source.

fats: One of the macronutrients and a source of energy.

fiber: Total fiber is the sum of dietary fiber and functional fiber. Dietary fiber consists of nondigestible carbohydrates and lignin that are intrinsic and intact in plants (i.e., the fiber naturally occurring in foods). Functional fiber consists of isolated, nondigestible carbohydrates that have beneficial physiological effects in humans.

flexibility: The range of motion of a muscle or group of muscles. Along with balance and strength, improving flexibility can significantly reduce the risk of falling.

food categories: A method of grouping similar foods in their as consumed forms, for descriptive purposes. The USDA's Agricultural Research Service (ARS) has created 150 mutually exclusive food categories to account for each food or beverage item reported in What We Eat in America (WWEIA), the food intake survey component of the National Health and Nutrition Examination Survey.

food groups: A method of grouping similar foods for descriptive and guidance purposes. Food groups in the USDA Food Patterns are defined as vegetables, fruits, grains, dairy, and protein foods. Some of these groups are divided into subgroups.

foodborne disease: Caused by consuming contaminated foods or beverages. Many different disease-causing microbes, or pathogens, can contaminate foods, so there are many different foodborne infections.

fortification: As defined by the U.S. Food and Drug Administration (FDA), the deliberate addition of one or more essential nutrients to a food, whether or not it is normally contained in the food.

gynecologist: A doctor who diagnoses and treats conditions of the female reproductive system and associated disorders.

high-intensity sweeteners: Ingredients commonly used as sugar substitutes or sugar alternatives to sweeten and enhance the flavor of foods and beverages. People may choose these sweeteners in place of sugar for a number of reasons, including that they contribute few or no calories to the diet.

hydrogenation: A chemical reaction that adds hydrogen atoms to an unsaturated fat, thus saturating it and making it solid at room temperature.

hypertension: A condition, also known as "high blood pressure," in which blood pressure remains elevated over time. Hypertension makes the heart work too hard, and the high force of the blood flow can harm arteries and organs, such as the heart, kidneys, brain, and eyes.

inflammatory bowel disease (IBD): Diseases, including ulcerative colitis and Crohn disease, that cause swelling in the intestine and/or digestive track, which may result in diarrhea, abdominal pain, fever, and weight loss.

lactose intolerance: Inability to digest lactose, the natural sugar found in milk and other dairy products. Individuals with lactose intolerance who avoid dairy products may be at increased risk for osteoporosis.

lean meat: Any meat or poultry that contains less than 10 g of fat, 4.5 g or less of saturated fats, and less than 95 mg of cholesterol per 100 g and per labeled serving size, based on the USDA definitions for food label use.

low-density lipoprotein (LDL-cholesterol): Blood cholesterol often called "bad" cholesterol; carries cholesterol to arteries and tissues. A high LDL-cholesterol level in the blood leads to a buildup of cholesterol in arteries.

menopause: The cessation of menstruation in women. Bone health in women often deteriorates after menopause due to a decrease in the female hormone estrogen.

micronutrient: An essential nutrient, as a trace mineral or vitamin, that is required by an organism in minute amounts.

mixed dishes: Savory food items eaten as a single entity that include foods from more than one food group. These foods often are mixtures of grains, protein foods, vegetables, and/or dairy.

nutrient density: Nutrient-dense foods are those that provide substantial amounts of vitamins and minerals and relatively fewer calories.

osteoporosis: Literally means "porous bone." This disease is characterized by too little bone formation, excessive bone loss, or a combination of both, leading to bone fragility and an increased risk of fractures of the hip, spine, and wrist.

pathogen: Any microorganism that can cause or is capable of causing disease.

peak bone mass: The amount of bone tissue in the skeleton. Bone tissue can keep growing until around age 30. At that point, bones have reached their maximum strength and density, known as "peak bone mass."

physical activity: Any bodily movement produced by the contraction of skeletal muscle that increases energy expenditure above a basal level; generally refers to the subset of physical activity that enhances health.

portion size: The amount of a food served or consumed in one eating occasion. A portion is not a standardized amount, and the amount considered to be a portion is subjective and varies.

poultry: All forms of chicken, turkey, duck, geese, guineas, and game birds (e.g., quail, pheasant).

processed meat: All meat or poultry products preserved by smoking, curing, salting, and/or the addition of chemical preservatives.

protein: One of the macronutrients; a major functional and structural component of every animal cell. Proteins are composed of amino acids, nine of which are indispensable (essential), meaning they cannot be synthesized by humans and therefore must be obtained from the diet.

refined grains: Grains and grain products with the bran and germ removed; any grain product that is not a whole-grain product.

rheumatoid arthritis (RA): An inflammatory disease that causes pain, swelling, stiffness, and loss of function in the joints.

seafood: Marine animals that live in the sea and in freshwater lakes and rivers.

serving size: A standardized amount of a food, such as a cup or an ounce, used in providing information about a food within a food group, such as in dietary guidance.

simple carbohydrates: Sugars composed of a single sugar molecule (monosaccharide) or two joined sugar molecules (a disaccharide), such as glucose, fructose, lactose, and sucrose.

solid fats: Fats that are usually not liquid at room temperature. Solid fats are found in animal foods, except for seafood, and can be made from vegetable oils through hydrogenation.

starches: Many glucose units linked together into long chains. Examples of foods containing starch include vegetables (e.g., potatoes, carrots), grains (e.g., brown rice, oats, wheat, barley, corn), and legumes, beans and peas (e.g., kidney beans, garbanzo beans, lentils, split peas).

sugar-sweetened beverages: Liquids that are sweetened with various forms of added sugars. These beverages include, but are not limited to, soda (regular, not sugar-free), fruitades, sports drinks, energy drinks, sweetened waters, and coffee and tea beverages with added sugars.

sugars: Composed of one unit (a monosaccharide, such as glucose or fructose) or two joined units (a disaccharide, such as lactose or sucrose).

***trans* fatty acids:** Unsaturated fatty acids that are structurally different from the unsaturated fatty acids that occur naturally in plant foods.

variety: A diverse assortment of foods and beverages across and within all food groups and subgroups selected to fulfill the recommended amounts without exceeding the limits for calories and other dietary components.

vitamin A: A family of fat-soluble compounds that play an important role in vision, bone growth, reproduction, cell division, and cell differentiation. Too much vitamin A (in the form of retinol) has been linked to bone loss and an increase in the risk of hip fracture.

vitamin D: A nutrient that the body needs to absorb calcium.

whole fruits: All fresh, frozen, canned, and dried fruit but not fruit juice.

whole grains: Grains and grain products made from the entire grain seed, usually called the "kernel," which consists of the bran, germ, and endosperm. If the kernel has been cracked, crushed, or flaked, it must retain the same relative proportions of bran, germ, and endosperm as the original grain in order to be called whole grain. Many, but not all, whole grains are also sources of dietary fiber.

Chapter 48 | Nutrition Support Organizations and Programs

GOVERNMENT ORGANIZATIONS

Administration on Aging (AOA)

Washington, DC 20201
Phone: 202-619-0724
Fax: 202-357-3555
Website: www.acl.gov
E-mail: aoainfo@aoa.gov

Centers for Disease Control and Prevention (CDC)

1600 Clifton Rd.
Atlanta, GA 30329-4027
Toll-Free: 800-CDC-INFO (800-232-4636)
Phone: 404-639-3311
Toll-Free TTY: 888-232-6348
Website: www.cdc.gov
E-mail: cdcinfo@cdc.gov

Eunice Kennedy Shriver National Institute of Child Health and Human Development (NICHD)

P.O. Box 3006
Rockville, MD 20847
Toll-Free: 800-370-2943
Toll-Free TTY: 888-320-6942
Toll-Free Fax 866-760-5947
Website: www.nichd.nih.gov
E-mail: NICHDInformation ResourceCenter@mail.nih.gov

Food and Nutrition Information Center (FNIC)

10301 Baltimore Ave.
Beltsville, MD 20705-2351
Phone: 301-504-5414
Website: www.nal.usda.gov/fnic
E-mail: FNIC@ars.usda.gov

Resources in this chapter were compiled from several sources deemed reliable; all contact information was verified and updated in May 2021.

Food Safety and Inspection Service (FSIS)
1400 Independence Awe., S.W. Rm. 2932-S
Washington, DC 20250-3700
Toll-Free: 877-744-2968
Website: www.fsis.usda.gov
E-mail: fsis@usda.gov

MedlinePlus
8600 Rockville Pike
Bethesda, MD 20894
Toll-Free: 888-FIND-NLM (888-346-3656)
Phone: 301-594-5983
Website: www.medlineplus.gov

MyPlate, U.S. Department of Agriculture (USDA)
1320 Braddock Pl.
Alexandria, VA 22314
https://www.myplate.gov/contact-us
E-mail: usdaprivacy@usda.gov

National Cancer Institute (NCI)
9609 Medical Center Dr.
BG 9609, MSC 9760
Bethesda, MD 20892-9760
Toll-Free: 800-4-CANCER (800-422-6237)
Website: www.cancer.gov
E-mail: NCIinfo@nih.gov

National Center for Complementary and Integrative Health (NCCIH)
9000 Rockville Pike
Bethesda, MD 20892
Toll-Free: 888-644-6226
Toll-Free TTY: 866-464-3615
Website: www.nccih.nih.gov
E-mail: info@nccih.nih.gov

National Heart, Lung, and Blood Institute (NHLBI)
31 Center Dr., Bldg. 31
Bethesda, MD 20892
Toll-Free: 877-NHLBI4U (877-645-2448)
Website: www.nhlbi.nih.gov
E-mail: nhlbiinfo@nhlbi.nih.gov

National Institute of Diabetes and Digestive and Kidney Diseases (NIDDK)
9000 Rockville Pike
Bethesda, MD 20892
Toll-Free: 800-860-8747
Phone: 301-496-4000
TTY: 301-402-9612
Toll-Free TTY: 866-569-1162
Website: www.niddk.nih.gov
E-mail: healthinfo@niddk.nih.gov

National Institute on Aging (NIA)
31 Center Dr., MSC 2292
Bldg. 31, Rm. 5C27
Bethesda, MD 20892
Toll-Free: 800-222-2225
Toll-Free TTY: 800-222-4225
Website: www.nia.nih.gov
E-mail: niaic@nia.nih.gov

National Institutes of Health (NIH)
9000 Rockville Pike
Bethesda, MD 20892
Phone: 301-496-4000
TTY: 301-402-9612
Website: www.nih.gov

NIH News in Health
Bldg. 31, Rm. 5B52
Bethesda, MD 20892-2094
Phone: 301-451-8224
Website: newsinhealth.nih.gov
E-mail: nihnewsinhealth@od.nih.gov

Office of Dietary Supplements (ODS)
6100 Executive Blvd.
Rm. 3B01, MSC 7517
Bethesda, MD 20892-7517
Toll-Free: 888-723-3366
Phone: 301-435-2920
Fax: 301-480-1845
Website: ods.od.nih.gov
E-mail: ods@nih.gov

President's Council on Sports, Fitness & Nutrition (PCSFN)
1101 Wootton Pkwy., Ste. 420
Rockville, MD 20852
Website: www.health.gov

U.S. Department of Agriculture (USDA)
1400 Independence Ave., S.W.
Washington, DC 20250
Phone: 202-720-2791
Website: www.usda.gov

U.S. Department of Health and Human Services (HHS)
200 Independence Ave., S.W.
Washington, DC 20201
Toll-Free: 877-696-6775
Website: www.hhs.gov

U.S. Department of Veterans Affairs (VA)
810 Vermont Ave., N.W.
Washington, DC 20420
Toll-Free: 800-273-8255
Website: www.veteranshealthlibrary.va.gov

U.S. Food and Drug Administration (FDA)
10903 New Hampshire Ave.
Silver Spring, MD 20993-0002
Toll-Free: 888-INFO-FDA (888-463-6332)
Website: www.fda.gov

U.S. National Library of Medicine (NLM)
8600 Rockville Pike
Bethesda, MD 20894
Toll-Free: 888-FIND-NLM (888-346-3656)
Phone: 301-594-5983
Website: www.nlm.nih.gov

PRIVATE ORGANIZATIONS

Academy of Nutrition and Dietetics
120 S. Riverside Plaza, Ste. 2190
Chicago, IL 60606-6995
Toll-Free: 800-877-1600
Phone: 312-899-0040
Website: www.eatrightpro.org
E-mail: accounting@eatright.org

American Academy of Pediatrics (AAP)
345 Park Blvd.
Itasca, IL 60143
Toll-Free: 800-433-9016
Fax: 847-434-8000
Website: www.aap.org
E-mail: mcc@aap.org

American College of Sports Medicine (ACSM)
401 West Michigan St.
Indianapolis, IN 46202-3233
Phone: 317-637-9200
Fax: 317-634-7817
Website: www.acsm.org

American Council on Exercise (ACE)
4851 Paramount Dr.
San Diego, CA 92123
Toll-Free: 888-825-3636
Phone: 858-576-6500
Fax: 858-576-6564
Website: www.acefitness.org
E-mail: support@acefitness.org

American Diabetes Association (ADA)
2451 Crystal Dr., Ste. 900
Arlington, VA 22202
Toll-Free: 800-DIABETES (800-342-2383)
Website: www.diabetes.org
E-mail: privacy@diabetes.org

American Heart Association (AHA)
7272 Greenville Ave.
Dallas, TX 75231
Toll-Free: 800-AHA-USA1 (800-242-8721)
Website: www.heart.org

American Institute for Cancer Research
1560 Wilson Blvd., Ste. 1000
Arlington, VA 22209
Toll-Free: 800-843-8114
Fax: 202-328-7226
Website: www.aicr.org
E-mail: aicrweb@aicr.org

American Public Health Association (APHA)
800 I St., N.W.
Washington, DC 20001
Toll-Free: 888-320-APHA (888-320-2742)
Phone: 202-777-2742
TTY: 202-777-2500
Fax: 202-777-2534
Website: www.apha.org
E-mail: comments@apha.org

American Society for Metabolic and Bariatric Surgery (ASMBS)
14407 S.W. 2nd Pl., Ste. F-3
Newberry, FL 32669
Phone: 352-331-4900
Website: asmbs.org
E-mail: info@asmbs.org

Association of Diabetes Care & Education Specialists (ADCES)
125 S. Wacker Dr., Ste. 600
Chicago, IL 60606
Toll-Free: 800-338-3633
Website: www.diabeteseducator.org

Asthma and Allergy Foundation of America (AAFA)
1235 S. Clark St., Ste. 305
Arlington, VA 22202
Toll-Free: 800-7-ASTHMA (800-727-8462)
Website: www.aafa.org
E-mail: info@aafa.org

Celiac Disease Foundation
20350 Ventura Blvd., Ste. 240
Woodland Hills, CA 91364
Phone: 818-716-1513
Website: www.celiac.org

Center for Science in the Public Interest (CSPI)
1220 L St., N.W., Ste. 300
Washington, DC 20005
Toll-Free: 866-293-CSPI (866-293-2774)
Website: www.cspinet.org
E-mail: cspi@cspinet.org

Cleveland Clinic
9500 Euclid Ave.
Cleveland, OH 44195
Toll-Free: 800-223-2273
TTY: 216-444-0261
Website: my.clevelandclinic.org

Food Allergy Research & Education (FARE)
7901 Jones Branch Dr., Ste. 240
Toll-Free: 800-929-4040
Phone: 703-691-3179
Fax: 703-691-2713
Website: www.foodallergy.org
E-mail: contactfare@foodallergy.org

Institute of Food Technologists (IFT)
525 West Van Buren, Ste. 1000
Chicago, IL 60607
Toll-Free: 800-IFT-FOOD (800-438-3663)
Fax: 312-782-8348
Website: www.ift.org
E-mail: info@ift.org

International Food Information Council (IFIC)
900 19th St., N.W.
Washington, DC 20006
Website: ific.org
E-mail: info@ific.org

International Foundation for Gastrointestinal Disorders (IFFGD)
3015 Dunes West Blvd., Ste. 512
Mount Pleasant, SC 29466
Phone: 414-964-1799
Website: www.iffgd.org
E-mail: iffgd@iffgd.org

National Association of Anorexia Nervosa and Associated Disorders (ANAD)
701 N. Fairfax St.
Alexandria, VA 22314
Toll-Free: 800-892-2757
Phone: 703-836-7112
Website: www.anad.org
E-mail: hello@anad.org

National Eating Disorders Association (NEDA)
1500 Bdwy., Ste. 1101
New York, NY 10036
Toll-Free: 800-931-2237
Phone: 212-575-6200
Website: www.nationaleatingdisorders.org
E-mail: info@nationaleatingdisorders.org

The Obesity Society (TOS)
1110 Bonifant St., Ste. 500
Silver Spring, MD 20910
Phone: 301-563-6526
Website: www.obesity.org
E-mail: contact@obesity.org

INDEX

INDEX

Page numbers followed by 'n' indicate a footnote. Page numbers in *italics* indicate a table or illustration.

A

C

D

E

F

G

H

I

M

N

O

Q

R

S

V

W

X

Y

Z